VERNACULAR BO

Vernacular Bodies

The Politics of Reproduction in
Early Modern England

MARY E. FISSELL

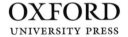

OXFORD
UNIVERSITY PRESS

OXFORD

UNIVERSITY PRESS

Great Clarendon Street, Oxford OX2 6DP

Oxford University Press is a department of the University of Oxford.
It furthers the University's objective of excellence in research, scholarship,
and education by publishing worldwide in

Oxford New York

Auckland Cape Town Dar es Salaam Hong Kong Karachi
Kuala Lumpur Madrid Melbourne Mexico City Nairobi
New Delhi Shanghai Taipei Toronto

With offices in

Argentina Austria Brazil Chile Czech Republic France Greece
Guatemala Hungary Italy Japan Poland Portugal Singapore
South Korea Switzerland Thailand Turkey Ukraine Vietnam

Oxford is a registered trade mark of Oxford University Press
in the UK and in certain other countries

Published in the United States
by Oxford University Press Inc., New York

British Library Cataloguing in Publication Data

Data available

Library of Congress Cataloging in Publication Data

Data available

Typeset by SNP Best-set Typesetter Ltd., Hong Kong
Printed in Great Britain
on acid-free paper by
Biddles Ltd.
King's Lynn, Norfolk

ISBN 0-19-926998-2   978-0-19-926988-4
ISBN 0-19-920270-2 (Pbk.)   978-0-19-920270-6 (Pbk.)

1 3 5 7 9 10 8 6 4 2

In Memoriam Maggy Brown, 1965–1998

Acknowledgements

This book has had a very long gestation, and a lot of midwives. It is a great pleasure to thank the many individuals and institutions who have helped me along the way. First, I am very grateful to those organizations that funded the research and writing—ideas are easy to find, but the time to work them through much harder. I am grateful to the Folger Shakespeare Library for a fellowship funded by the National Endowment for the Humanities, and to the National Library of Medicine Publication Grant (NIH 1 G13 LM07054-01); most of the book was written with their help, and in their reading rooms. I have been fortunate in having had much aid from libraries and librarians, including Stephen Greenberg and his colleagues at the National Library of Medicine, Georgianna Ziegler, Betsy Walsh, and all the others at the Folger, Christine Ruggere and Linda Bright in my own department at Johns Hopkins, the Eisenhower Express on the Homewood campus, those at the Wellcome Institute, the John Rylands Library, and the many librarians at the British Library who were unfailingly helpful and courteous even when working with staff shortages. Many thanks to the journal *Representations* for letting me include part of an article I published first with them, 'The Politics of Reproduction in the English Reformation', *Representations* (2004). For the images, institutions are credited in individual captions, but I would like thank the people who helped me get those pictures: Aude Fitzsimons at Magdalene College, Cambridge, Susan Harris at the Bodleian, Michael Woods and Beryl Blair at the British Library, Clare Brown at Lambeth Palace Library, Michael Scot at the Folger Library, and Susan Pugh at the National Monuments Record Centre. Thank you all.

Many colleagues and friends read chapters of the various incarnations of this book, and mere mention of their names here cannot come close to expressing my gratitude to them: Kathleen Crowther-Heyck, Amy Erickson, Lori-Ann Ferrell, Monica Green, Ann Hughes, Diarmaid MacCulloch, Harry Marks, John Marshall, and Helen Weinstein. Colleagues at Harvard, Penn, Stanford, Wisconsin, Yale, and York have helped me to refine my thoughts when I presented papers to them, as did my colleagues in the Folger seminar on eighteenth-century women. Several super-heroes read the entire manuscript, and their enthusiasm and trenchant comments have been invaluable: many, many thanks to Susan Amussen, Laura Gowing, Mary Henninger-Voss, Pamela Long, Charles Rosenberg, and an anonymous referee for the Press.

At my own institution, I am especially grateful to my colleagues Harry Marks and Dan Todes; we've soldiered in the junior-faculty trenches together and their support for me and the project, especially in the long years when I could never get it funded, have been much appreciated. John Marshall has offered me his wisdom and many a needed reality check about the history of early modern England. My graduate students—the late Maggy Brown, Kathleen Crowther-Heyck, Sue Ferry, Melissa Grafe, Alexa Green, Shoshanna Green, Massimo Petrozzi, and Nissa Strottman—have done far more than just tolerate an absent-minded professor; their questions and interests have helped me far more than they can know. Several colleagues and old friends have lived with this project for almost as long as I have. Peter D'Angio took me to the movies and thereby inadvertently sparked my curiosity about the Reformation, a curiosity that pushed the book back a hundred years and entailed me asking him many technical questions. Helen Weinstein read most of the first draft of the book whilst roasting aubergines; the aubergines were a lot better than that draft. Mary Henninger-Voss has read just about everything I have written for the past several years, and her careful ear has improved my writing immensely. Susan Abrams has been a constant source of encouragement. Laura Gowing and I found ourselves writing parallel books, and her help and enthusiasm have been wonderful—I should be so lucky as to write the next one in tandem also. It has been a privilege and a pleasure to work with Louisa Lapworth, Ruth Parr, and Kay Rogers at Oxford University Press, and with Bonnie Blackburn as copy-editor. Carisa Greenfield and Sharon Halm took care of my young son Sam in such a thoughtful way that I was free to wander back to the 1640s while he was with them. And Sam, of course, made me want to re-emerge from early modern texts at the end of the day.

The book is dedicated to the memory of Maggy Brown, a bright star of a historian who died much too young. It saddens me that I cannot hand Maggy her own copy of this book when she had to hear about it so often in the process. I'm sadder still that she won't be handing me hers.

M.E.F.

Contents

List of Illustrations

Abbreviations

Bagford	*The Bagford Ballads: Illustrating the Last Years of the Stuarts*, ed. Joseph Woodfall Ebsworth (Hertford: Printed for the Ballad Society by S. Austin, 1878, repr. New York: AMS Press, 1968)
Bodleian	Bodleian Library, Oxford, ballad collections, including Wood, and Douce
EETS	Early English Text Society
Pepys	*Catalogue of the Pepys Library at Magdalene College Cambridge: The Pepys Ballads Facsimile*, ed. W. G. Day (Cambridge: D. S. Brewer, 1987)
Roxburghe	*The Roxburghe Ballads* (1869; repr. New York: AMS Press, 1966)
STC	*A Short-Title Catalogue of Books Printed in England, Scotland, and Ireland and of English Books Printed Abroad, 1475–1640*, ed. Alfred W. Pollard and G. R. Redgrave (London: Bibliographical Society, 1926)
STC2	*A Short-Title Catalogue of Books Printed in England, Scotland, and Ireland and of English Books Printed Abroad, 1475–1640*, ed. Alfred W. Pollard and G. R. Redgrave, 2nd edn. (London: Bibliographical Society, 1991)
Thomason	*Catalogue of the Pamphlets, Books, Newspapers, and Manuscripts Relating to the Civil War, the Commonwealth, and Restoration. Collected by George Thomason, 1640–1661* (Ann Arbor: University Microfilms International, 1981)
Wing	*Short-Title Catalogue of Books Printed in England, Scotland, Ireland, Wales, and British America, and of English Books Printed in Other Countries, 1641–1700*, ed. Donald Goddard Wing (New York: Index Society, 1945–51)
Wing2	*Short-Title Catalogue of Books Printed in England, Scotland, Ireland, Wales, and British America, and of English Books Printed in Other Countries, 1641–1700*, ed. Donald Goddard Wing, 2nd edn., rev. and ed. John J. Morrison and Carolyn W. Nelson (New York: Modern Language Association of America, 1994–)

Introduction

Women's bodies are the stuff of history. In early modern England, those bodies gave birth to babies, nursed them, cooked the dinners, milked the cows, and spun the yarn. This book argues that women's bodies are the stuff of history in a second way. Men's bodies, after all, plowed the fields, ground grain into flour, and sheared the sheep. But only women's bodies had the power to make new life. Such power was the source of much speculation. Sixteenth- and seventeenth-century people had no sex-education diagrams, no ovulation-predictor test kits, no ultrasound scans. Many facts we take for granted were open to debate: did women always need men to make babies? why did children often (but not always) look like their parents? could a fetus change its sex within the womb?

Since little was certain about the mysteries of reproduction, the topic lent itself to a rich array of theories. The insides of women's reproductive bodies provided a kind of open interpretative space, a place where many different models of reproductive processes might be plausible. These models were profoundly shaped by cultural concerns; they afforded many ways to discuss and make sense of social, political, and economic changes. And early modern English men and women experienced wrenching changes, such as the Protestant Reformation and the Civil War. Both of these, I argue, made their mark on ordinary people's ideas about women's reproductive bodies. It is not just that models of the body reflect historical change. Rather, men and women thought through the body, using ideas about reproduction as a kind of imaginative resource to understand and to justify their changing circumstances.

This book explores the richness of ordinary people's ideas about the body by analysing cheap print—those small books, pamphlets, and broadsides available to even the poorest of England's readers. The sixteenth and seventeenth centuries saw a huge increase in literacy and in books aimed at novice readers. Ballads, works of devotion, pamphlets, and newspapers began to proliferate. So too did popular medical books, those which proclaimed themselves to be for 'the use of families' or 'the meanest capacity' rather than for physicians and surgeons. Very few English men and even fewer women ever read a Latin anatomical text, but almost everyone encountered models of the body in the ballads, jokes, religious works, and popular medical books at the centre of this study. Even those who could not read heard jokes and sang ballads. I call these models of the body 'vernacular' because they were newly available in small cheap printed books that came to circulate far more widely than had manuscripts or than did books for learned readers.

I joke with friends that I always know which stack of books is mine in a research library—they are the small grubby ones, bound in plain well-worn brown leather. Often a single book has several pamphlets bound in it. These are the lowest common denominator of print, and as such they offer historians models of the body that were very widely available. Such sources need to be read carefully—they are not simple mirrors of everyday beliefs. Instead, as we shall see, different genres, such as murder pamphlets, newsbooks, ballads, and prayerbooks, call for specific interpretative strategies and careful attention to patterns of reading and genre conventions. But such care is more than repaid by stories in these small books—witches nursing ferrets and toads as if they were babies, thousands of women marching on Parliament, men worrying about the paternity of their babies born five months after the wedding, preachers trying to persuade their flocks about how exactly Jesus was conceived in Mary's womb, and many more. It was by means of stories such as these that ordinary people made sense of their bodies.

Historians have long known that bodies and politics were connected—we need only think of the very common early modern analogy in which the king is like the head or heart and the peasants like the feet. Putting women's bodies at the centre of my analysis brings something new to both bodies and politics. Reproduction (most but not all of which was understood to take place within the female body in the sixteenth and seventeenth century) was central to ordinary people's political imaginations because of the pivotal role of gender relations in the early modern period. All relations of power—between a monarch and his/her subjects, a bishop and his flock—were analogous to the relations between a man and the family he headed. A husband who could not maintain good order in his household would not be able to govern any other community effectively. In other words, at the heart of relations of power was man and wife.

At the same time that the family was politics writ small, it was reproduction writ large. Imagining conception as a contest of strength between male and female seeds, or imagining childbirth as a baby fighting his way (and popular medical books do make the baby male) out of the prison of the maternal body—or any of the other images I explore—made the female reproductive body a microcosm of relations between men and women. Gender relations, in other words, were the hinge that connected body and politics and made the female reproductive body a powerful symbol.

My story opens with the tumult of the Protestant Reformation. English women had long been taught to identify with the Virgin Mary when they were pregnant, and had engaged in many devotional practices that underlined and reinforced that connection. With the coming of reform in the 1540s, those links were broken. No longer were women permitted to clutch a relic of the Virgin while in labour, or to make thank-offerings at her statue in their local church after delivery. It was not just childbirth practices that were under attack; ideas about conception and the relation between the Virgin's pregnancy and those of ordinary women were also controversial. A welter of ideas about the mechanics of conception and the extent to which the fetus develops from the mother's body were explored in a controversy about the nature of Mary's conception of Christ. These were not abstruse theological debates. A woman who disputed the nature of the Incarnation (Christ's taking bodily form in Mary's womb) was put on trial and eventually burnt at the stake for heresy in 1550. Her beliefs were far from mainstream, but the very public nature of her trial and execution, and the sermons and pamphlets written about her, made the mechanics of conception, like the devotional practices associated with childbirth, into politically sensitive topics.

Practices were reformed more quickly than were ideas. Before the Reformation, conception and fetal development were understood in wondrous terms: every pregnancy echoed, in some small way, the miracle of Christ's taking human form. The womb was central to these ideas; it was the womb that actively transformed and developed tiny amounts of male and female seed into a new person. In the early seventeenth century, ideas about the womb began to change. Its wonderful powers sometimes became terrible ones, threatening the life of the mother or breeding monsters rather than babies. None of these ideas about the functions of the womb were new. Rather, popular medical writers took ideas from classical antiquity and medieval scholarship that resonated with ideas about gender relations at a particular time. Good and bad depictions of the womb could be found in many sources, and the shift from one to the other in popular books reflects changing patterns of appropriation rather than the creation of novel ideas. The development of the bad womb is also related to a flood of cheap print in the later sixteenth century that depicted bad mothers. Witches who harmed children and mothers who murdered their babies became stock characters in a newly emergent print marketplace. Their stories, told in small eight- or sixteen-page pamphlets, created a repertoire of dangerous mothers, and since the womb was motherhood writ small, it too became capable of harm as well as good.

Cheap pamphlets about witchcraft and infanticide that offered readers stories about motherhood gone wrong were just the beginning. The advent of print had unexpected consequences for ideas about women's bodies. At the outset, books about women's reproductive bodies were apologetic about their topic, worried about male readers' responses to what had formerly been largely female knowledge. However, as the market for cheap print expanded, ways of talking about women multiplied, and by the middle of the seventeenth century, men began to write about the insides of women's bodies without any apology or hesitation. The proliferation of men's writings about women's bodies helped to freight those bodies with political significance.

The events of the 1640s both exploded the print marketplace and remade gender relations. In 1641 state control of the print trade lapsed with the closure of the Court of Star Chamber, where violators of the rules about printing had been tried. At the same time, political unrest fuelled both the supply and the demand for cheap print about current events. That same unrest led to the unprecedented spectacle of women engaging in massive political protests—thousands of women marching through London to present their petitions to Parliament. At the same time, women were preaching and prophesying in public, and their doings were quickly translated into cheap print. 'The world turned upside down', as contemporaries called the upheavals that culminated in civil war and regicide, was a moment when all kinds of relations of authority were called into question, and none more potently than those between man and woman.

At the same time, making women's bodies into models of gender relations was not accomplished easily. I look closely at the story of one female prophet of the 1640s, Sarah Wight, and the minister Henry Jessey's struggles to tell her story. The witness of the body was supposed to underwrite religious truth, but Jessey had a hard time asserting that Wight had not eaten for weeks yet survived, or that she was deaf to worldly sounds but heard the divine. Wight was 15 at the time of her troubles, so hers was not yet a reproductive body. Instead, she wrestled with her role as a daughter, often testing the limits of her female role while highlighting the usual expectations for female bodies.

Women's reproductive bodies became the stuff of political ideas in cheap print largely through the agency of Nicholas Culpeper, a radical London apothecary and medical writer. His germinal 1651 midwifery manual offered a new way to write about making babies. First, he wrote without shame and without worrying about the potential for corrupting male readers. Instead, he wrote gleefully, joking with male and female readers. Second, he tried to ground social relations in the body itself. He was the first vernacular midwifery writer to talk about male bodies as well as female ones in print. Talking about men as well as women became a way of making female bodies inferior to male ones in Culpeper's account. He belittled women's own ideas about their bodies and instead urged his readers to place their faith in the male science of anatomy. This combination of anatomical and epistemological inferiority can be understood as a response to the gender upheavals of the 1640s; if gender hierarchies were not reproduced socially, perhaps they could be enacted within the theatre of the body. Perhaps the body could provide the blueprint for society.

Culpeper's radical reworking of the relationship between body and society was eagerly adopted by other writers; more popular midwifery books were published in the decade of the 1650s than in the previous century. At the same time, the institution of the family was under new pressures, and so writers and printers tried out different ways in which the female body might emblematize appropriate gender relations. On the one hand, the parliamentary government reworked some of the ceremonies central to family formation and reproduction: they tinkered with baptism and marriage, and made new laws against adultery and incest. On the other, readers encountered a wild variety of sexual and familial relations in cheap print that described the new religious radicals— these were people who had sex with whomever they wanted, or attended church naked, or engaged in parodies of the marriage ceremony. Many of these texts were probably fiction, but fiction eagerly consumed. At the same time, midwifery writers tried to make the female body into a miniature of family relations. Pregnancy was described, not so much as a feature of a female body, but with great attention to the roles of the father at conception and the fetus (always male) at birth. The very institution of the family seemed to be embodied in pregnant women.

The vast social experiment of the 1650s ended, not with a bang, but with a return to monarchy. Charles II was crowned in 1660, and the country tried to return to things as they had been. But the past could not be so easily forgotten; the threat of a return to revolution haunted the political imagination of the Restoration. When Charles II failed to produce a legitimate heir, the issue of succession provoked a crisis in masculinity. In ballads and in midwifery manuals, writers worried about paternity and the age-old question of how a father could know that his children were truly his own. The female body had become another space within which political issues could be imagined and worked through. With the so-called warming-pan baby scandal of 1688, it was as if the stories in ballads became reality—was the heir to the throne really the heir, or some suppositious babe? My story has come full circle—from stories about reproduction becoming suffused with political meaning to high politics becoming, momentarily, about reproduction.

My story speaks to three different groups of readers: historians of medicine, historians of early modern England, and those interested more generally in issues about women's bodies and reproduction. What is obvious for one group will be news to another, and so I beg a reader's indulgence when he or she meets a basic explanation of, say, the Levellers, or of the Hippocratic model of conception, that is common knowledge in his or her discipline—it is not so for other readers.

First, I am writing for members of my own discipline—the history of medicine. Here, the centre of my story is about what we make of popular knowledge. Often when I talk about this project, I am asked about the scientific advances that my questioner assumes underlie the changes I describe. They ask, 'What about William Harvey? Didn't he write something about reproduction?' He did, but here I want to uncouple vernacular knowledge from the assumption that it is trickle-down science. As I have said elsewhere, too often our image of scientific knowledge is like a fried egg, sunny side up.[1] The good stuff is in the middle, where new knowledge is made. The transmission of that knowledge outwards is, in this model, always imperfect and corrupting. By the time you get to the crispy brown edge of a well-done fried egg, it bears no resemblance to the yolk and not much to the rest of the white. This model is particularly inappropriate for the early modern period, when the rediscovery of ancient knowledge was often more highly valued than the creation of new knowledge, and when the makers of new knowledge lacked the kinds of social authority that they were later to acquire. Nor does this model help us to understand the work of transmuting one kind of knowledge into another.

Instead, I draw upon models taken from cultural history, seeing vernacular knowledge as a cultural artefact in its own right. Rather than focusing on the gradual transmission of new anatomical or physiological knowledge from Latin texts to vernacular ones, I am interested in how popular writers appropriated bits of knowledge and remade them into something else.[2] Most of what early modern writers wanted to say about women's bodies could be found in one classical authority or another, or in the learned writings of the previous centuries. What matters to me is when and why these writers selected the pieces that they did, given that many of those pieces had long been available. While some choices may reflect the exigencies of the printshop—a printer did not want to commission a new woodblock, so an older one was employed—many are more complex. Writers put together versions of female reproductive bodies that contained claims about maleness and femaleness that seemed useful or appropriate or simply true at that particular moment.

This book also speaks to those historians of medicine who have been exploring the consequences of print for obstetrics and gynecology. The story is not a

[1] Mary E. Fissell and Roger Cooter, 'Exploring Natural Knowledge: Science and the Popular in the 18th c.', in *Cambridge History of Science*, iv: *Science in the 18th c.*, ed. Roy Porter (Cambridge: Cambridge University Press, 2003), 145–79.
[2] Roger Chartier, 'Culture as Appropriation: Popular Cultural Uses in Early Modern France', in Steven L. Kaplan (ed.), *Understanding Popular Culture: Europe from the Middle Ages to the 19th c.* (Berlin: Mouton Publishers, 1984), 175–91.

simple one, and it is still in the making. Monica Green and Helen King have suggested that the advent of print, rather than broadening medical discourse about women's reproductive bodies, actually limited it.[3] Far fewer texts (albeit in many more copies) were available in the first century of print than were available in manuscript a century before. Of course, manuscripts continued to be read and copied, but Green and King's views are a valuable corrective to our assumptions about the impact of print. In a similar way, Patricia Crawford argues that there was a change over the sixteenth and seventeenth centuries in the mode of transmission of sexual knowledge, a shift away from women's orally shared sexual knowledge towards a privileging of textual forms of that knowledge. Drawing upon different materials, Robert Martenson also suggests a shift away from women's knowledge, in this case a privileging of anatomical textual knowledge.[4]

Print did tilt the playing field, but in a broader sense than these historians have yet argued. A man or a woman in 1620 who read a popular medical book probably also read a number of other books, pamphlets, and broadsides. While I can never hope to re-create an early modern reader's experience in full, I have tried to draw on those kinds of printed works that were the most accessible, those which historians have come to call 'cheap print'.[5] The cheapness of the works, however, should not be taken to mean that their readers were necessarily of the poorer classes. People at all social levels read cheap print.[6] Rather, my choice of cheap print is intended to recover models of the body that were the most widespread, the most available in printed form. By the end of my story, perhaps half of all English men and at least a third of all English women could read.[7] As recent scholarship has shown, however, the barrier between the

---

[3] Monica H. Green, 'Obstetrical and Gynecological Texts in Middle English', *Studies in the Age of Chaucer*, 14 (1992), 53–88; ead., 'From "Diseases of Women" to "Secrets of Women": The Gynecological Literature in the Later Middle Ages', *Journal of Medieval and Early Modern Studies*, 30 (2000), 5–39. Helen King and Monica Green, session at 'Attending to Early Modern Women', conference at University of Maryland, College Park, Nov. 2003.

[4] Patricia Crawford, 'Sexual Knowledge in England, 1500–1750', in Roy Porter and Mikulas Teich (eds.), *Sexual Knowledge, Sexual Science: The History of Attitudes to Sexuality* (Cambridge: Cambridge University Press, 1994), 82–106. Robert Martenson, 'The Transformation of Eve', in Porter and Teich, *Sexual Knowledge, Sexual Science*, 107–33.

[5] The term is originally Tessa Watt's. Tessa Watt, *Cheap Print and Popular Piety, 1550–1640* (Cambridge: Cambridge University Press, 1991). See also Margaret Spufford, *Small Books and Pleasant Histories: Popular Fiction and its Readership in 17th-c. England* (Cambridge: Cambridge University Press, 1981).

[6] For this reason, I prefer the term 'vernacular' to 'popular' to describe the medical books at the heart of this study. Too often, 'popular' has been taken to mean 'of the poorer classes'.

[7] David Cressy's work remains foundational in studies of early modern English literacy. David Cressy, *Literacy and the Social Order: Reading and Writing in Tudor and Stuart England* (Cambridge: Cambridge University Press, 1980). But see also Thomas Laqueur, 'The Cultural Origins of Popular Literacy in England, 1500–1850', *Oxford Review of Education*, 2 (1976), 255–75; Margaret Spufford, 'First Steps in Literacy: The Reading and Writing Experiences of the Humblest 17th-c. Spiritual Auto-

literate and the non-literate was smaller than we may have imagined.[8] Much reading was reading aloud, and many of the materials I analyse, such as the pamphlets in Chapter 3 and the broadside ballads in Chapter 7, were designed to be read aloud or, in the case of ballads, sung. It is in this larger matrix of cheap print that ideas about women's bodies were both constrained and expanded. Printed texts did provide a new kind of authoritative voice about women's bodies, but they also offered a cacophony of conflicting ideas, especially after the lapse of state controls on printing in 1641.

By the 1650s, English medical writers were producing home-grown books for English readers, complementing the rich local literature of pamphlets, ballads, newsbooks, and broadsides. Before that, English readers learned about the reproductive body from books originally written in Latin, German, or French. These books were not merely translated, however. They were transmuted, changed into works tailored for English audiences. While a small group of scholarly European men (and even a few women) undoubtedly shared a model of the body engendered in Latin texts, I am interested in something both larger and smaller. The readers of popular books were much more numerous than those of scholarly texts, but they were also much more bound by location and language. It is in those local and particular works that I have found local and particular bodies.

Thus my story is also one about the consequences of print technology in the broadest sense of the term. The development of cheap print and its cousin, the public sphere, had unexpected consequences for the ways in which early modern people might imagine bodies and society. I do not wish to make a narrow argument about technological determinism and the invention of movable-type printing, saying, for example, that the technology produced new ideas about the female body in any simple or direct way. Rather, I am interested in what historians used to call 'popular culture' and its relation to a culture of print, by which I mean a complex and interconnected system of printing, increased literacy, shifting patterns of censorship, and evolving styles of storytelling. The intersections of that culture of print and the wrenching changes of religion and civil war created new ways to imagine the relationship between body and gender, new in both their details and in their modes of articulation.

While working on this project, I have worried many times that my use of the term 'cheap print' was just an easy way around the vexed term 'popular culture'—a substitute that seems to avoid theoretical difficulties while merely

biographers', *Social History*, 4 (1979), 407–35. The very nature of reading, a process that happens at many levels of proficiency and leaves few historical traces, suggests that we will never be able to pinpoint levels of literacy in the past.

[8] See especially Adam Fox, *Oral and Literate Culture in England, 1500–1700* (Oxford: Clarendon Press, 2000).

obscuring them. Cheap print is a useful category for this study because it does not presume a particular readership or social location; it merely describes a form of printed work. However, if 'cheap print' is to be more than a polite circumlocution, we need to continue to develop interpretative strategies for its use. Inferring patterns of gender relations from reading a handful of ballads ignores the richness of cheap print and the subtleties of its readers and manufacturers. I have read a great deal of cheap print, while paying close attention to rhetorical devices (which provide clues about patterns of intended readings), genre conventions, and their appropriations across genres. I have also grounded the analysis in the material particulars of the print marketplace. In other words, I am advocating that we read cheap print with as much sophistication and care as we have read other texts.

For historians of early modern England, my story has additional meanings. Having come of age as a social historian, I am now revisiting some of the themes of that earlier work, but as a cultural historian. One of the grand accomplishments of social history was to put ordinary people into history, to insist that factory hands, dairymaids, agricultural labourers, hospital patients, and the like were part of history too. For sixteenth- and seventeenth-century England, social historians rewrote the English Civil War as a revolution, a radical moment that engaged the hearts and minds of many Englishmen (though little was said about Englishwomen). Subsequent revision has portrayed the events of the 1640s as contingent, not as the clash of ideologies but the local and particular working-out of allegiances and hostilities.[9] My story draws more on the post-revisionists, who are coming to re-emphasize the impact of the revolution.[10] I share with these scholars a commitment to thinking about the cultural consequences of 'the world turned upside down'. Like others, I am less concerned with the vexed questions about how England came to war than with the meanings men and women made of that crisis. By putting the body and gender relations into the story of the Civil War, I am suggesting

[9] For the older social-history perspective, see Christopher Hill, *The World Turned Upside Down: Radical Ideas during the English Revolution* (London: Maurice Temple Smith, 1972); Brian Manning, *The English People and the English Revolution* (London: Heinemann, 1976). For paradigmatic studies that emphasize the local and contingent nature of the Civil War, see John Morrill, *The Revolt of the Provinces* (London: Unwin and Allen, 1976); David Underdown, *Revel, Riot and Rebellion: Popular Politics and Culture in England, 1603–1660* (Oxford: Clarendon Press, 1985).

[10] See e.g. Ann Hughes, 'Women, Men and Politics in the English Civil War', Inaugural Lecture, 8 Oct. 1997 (Keele: University of Keele, 1997); ead., 'Gender and Politics in Leveller Literature', in Susan D. Amussen and Mark A. Kishlansky (eds.), *Political Culture and Cultural Politics in Early Modern England: Essays Presented to David Underdown* (Manchester: Manchester University Press, 1995), 162–88; David Cressy, 'The Protestation Protested, 1641 and 1642', *Historical Journal*, 45 (2002), 251–79; Patricia Crawford, 'The Challenges to Patriarchalism: How Did the Revolution Affect Women?', in John Morrill (ed.), *Revolution and Restoration. England in the 1650s* (London: Collins and Brown, 1992), 112–28. More generally on the impact of warfare, see Charles Carlton, *Going to the Wars: The Experience of the British Civil Wars, 1638–1651* (London: Routledge, 1992).

that the events of the 1640s mattered to ordinary people very deeply because the questioning of authority on the grand scale also meant its interrogation in relations between men and women.

The narrative of the Protestant Reformation I tell here can also be understood as a kind of cultural-history revisiting of social themes. Historians have counted the forms of words in wills, tallied parish spending on devotional objects, and combed through church court records, creatively pursuing the question of when England became a Protestant nation. Recently, historians have attempted to move beyond this double axis of fast/slow and 'reform from above'/'reform from below'. Like these scholars, I am less concerned with when England became Protestant than with how it did so, with the processes of accommodation and appropriation that eventually changed beliefs and practices.[11] I suggest that putting the body into that mix of beliefs and practices can help us understand the magnitude of the transformation from late medieval Christianity to early modern Protestant identity. Women's reproductive bodies were an important topic through which aspects of the Protestant Reformation were realized, however imperfectly. Because late medieval pregnancy and childbirth were understood in deeply religious terms, changes in one part of the equation, religion, meant changes in the other—reproduction. Or, to look at the relationship the other way, late medieval Christianity was often interpreted and performed in very bodily ways, and it should not come as a surprise to us that it was difficult for reformers to undo those habits of thought and feeling enacted through the body.

To say that the Reformation and the Civil War reshaped women's bodies is not quite right. Changes in the representations of reproduction were part of these larger events, not merely the results of them. I say this because I see images of the body as a crucial way of talking about gender relations that lay at the heart of these crises. Part of the resolution of the turbulence of the 1640s was the reassertion of men's authority over women, a reassertion accomplished by means of new ideas about the relationship of men's and women's bodies. Similarly, becoming Protestant was a process that crucially involved reworking images of the female reproductive body. Although I did not envision this conclusion at the outset of my research, I have come to argue that understandings of the body were crucial to social and political change in early modern England.

---

[11] Paradigmatic studies include Watt, *Cheap Print and Popular Piety*; Ronald Hutton, 'The English Reformation and the Evidence of Folklore', *Past & Present*, 148 (1995), 89–116. On the (continued) vitality of Catholicism, see Eamon Duffy, *The Stripping of the Altars. Traditional Religion in England 1400–1580* (New Haven: Yale University Press, 1992); Alexandra Walsham, ' "Domme Preachers"? Post-Reformation English Catholicism and the Culture of Print', *Past & Present*, 168 (2000), 72–123.

The chronology I present here also offers new ways of outlining women's history and the history of the body. Much of women's history has quite rightly interrogated customary chronologies, exploring, for example, the persistence of patriarchal forms or the very gradual shifts in women's waged work, but here the grand events of 'men's' history matter for women's history.[12]

Other historians have described a 'crisis' in gender relations that extended from the latter part of the sixteenth century well into the seventeenth.[13] My understanding of this crisis derives in part from Laura Gowing's work, in which she argues that gender relations, like any other relations of power, are always unstable and therefore always being acted out, tested, represented, and rearticulated. In her most recent book, she depicts some long-term continuities in the ways that women reproduced the gender order through day-to-day body practices.[14] Some of the practices that Gowing traces were structured by the tensions inherent in the deeply patriarchal system that governed gender relations in early modern England. It was never an easy or uncontested way to organize social life. Historians of early modern England have been fascinated with the theme of order, and I am suggesting that if order was such an important theme in that culture, that theme was often rehearsed and experienced through gender relations. However, within this ongoing exploration of the limits and meanings of gender roles, there were moments of particular stress. I argue that the Reformation and the Civil War, whether we call them crises or not, made for gender trouble. I am also suggesting that we pay careful attention to the different forms and genres though which gender relations were articulated. Bodies are good to think with, but they are also embedded in social practices. Some aspects of patriarchy can become problematic while others persist, and our task is to understand both continuities and changes.

[12] Judith M. Bennett, 'Confronting Continuity', *Journal of Women's History*, 9 (1997), 73–94; Phyllis Mack, 'The History of Women in Early Modern Britain: A Review Article', *Comparative Studies in Society and History*, 28 (1986), 715–22. On women in early modern England, see the invaluable synthesis by Sara Mendelson and Patricia Crawford, *Women in Early Modern England* (Oxford: Oxford University Press, 1998).

[13] David Underdown, 'The Taming of the Scold: The Enforcement of Patriarchal Authority in Early Modern England', in Anthony Fletcher and John Stevenson (eds.), *Order and Disorder in Early Modern England* (Cambridge: Cambridge University Press, 1985), 116–36. Underdown's findings are disputed in Martin Ingram, ' "Scolding Women Cucked or Washed": A Crisis in Gender Relations in Early Modern England?', in Jennifer Kermode and Garthine Walker (eds.), *Women, Crime, and the Courts in Early Modern England* (Chapel Hill: University of North Carolina Press, 1994), 48–80.

[14] Laura Gowing, *Domestic Dangers: Women, Words, and Sex in Early Modern London* (Oxford: Clarendon Press, 1996). Gowing draws upon the theoretical insights of Judith Butler, *Gender Trouble: Feminism and the Subversion of Identity* (London: Routledge, 1990). Anthony Fletcher offers a third chronology, in which crucial changes in gender relations occur in the late 17th c. I emphasize changes throughout the 17th c. Anthony Fletcher, *Gender, Sex and Subordination in England, 1500–1800* (New Haven: Yale University Press, 1995). Laura Gowing, *Common Bodies: Women, Touch and Power in 17th-c. England* (New Haven: Yale University Press, 2003).

The original inspiration for this study was Emily Martin's exploration of women's ideas about their bodies in contemporary Baltimore, in which she showed how women used images drawn from industrial processes to understand reproduction.[15] For readers who come to this book with similar interests and concerns, I wish to explore how bodies have histories, and how women's bodies, in particular, came to bear certain kinds of meanings in the sixteenth and seventeenth centuries. The grand narratives of the history of the early modern body emphasize the formation of the nation-state and in their various ways trace that process through reworkings of a body whose sex is not much addressed. However, the male body is usually paradigmatic in these analyses. For example, in Norbert Elias's germinal account of the process by which bodily precepts of politeness became internalized in court culture, the examples are usually about men.[16] Similarly, Michel Foucault's analysis of an analogous process of internalization draws upon examples such as soldiers drilling in formation.[17] It is not that these accounts are wrong or unhelpful, just that their scale is different than mine. By looking at a single country, and focusing on cheap print, my analysis reveals the volatility of images of the body. Were my focus male bodies, perhaps my story would more closely resemble these other analyses of the development of a kind of interiority. But women's bodies, in particular women's reproductive bodies, were put to more local and contentious uses, in part because they were so fruitful a site for imagining gender relations.

The other big narrative of the body is that constructed by Thomas Laqueur in his *Making Sex: Body and Gender from the Greeks to Freud.*[18] Laqueur argues that early modern writers employed a one-sex model of the body, derived from classical antiquity. In this model, male and female were differences of degree, not kind. Only in the late eighteenth century, with the political upheavals that produced the modern political subject, did a two-sex model develop, in which male and female were categorically different. Laqueur's model has been very influential for historians of gender, but my story is more particular, and in this case, a smaller canvas is a messier canvas.[19] In cheap print, multiple stories were always being told about women's bodies. Women's bodies were sites of contest, places that people argued about and through which they tried to construct

[15] Emily Martin, *The Woman in the Body* (Boston: Beacon Press, 1987).

[16] Norbert Elias, *The Civilizing Process*, trans. Edmund Jephcott (New York: Pantheon Books, 1982).

[17] Michel Foucault, *Discipline and Punish: The Birth of the Prison*, trans. Alan Sheridan (New York: Pantheon Books, 1977).

[18] Thomas Laqueur, *Making Sex: Body and Gender from the Greeks to Freud* (Cambridge, Mass.: Harvard University Press, 1990).

[19] For Laqueur's influence see e.g. Fletcher, *Gender, Sex and Subordination in England*; Elizabeth Foyster, *Manhood in Early Modern England: Honour, Sex, and Marriage* (London: Longman, 1999).

themselves as authoritative. Where Laqueur focuses on all kinds of medical texts, mixing anatomical works meant for a relatively learned audience with cheaper books intended for a vernacular audience, I create a different mix by looking at small cheap books that address both body and gender. I agree with Laqueur that our divide between sex and gender—between physical bodily difference and social precepts about difference—makes little sense for the early modern period. But I am not sure that the divide is ever so neat. Talking about sex is always talking about gender, in the sense that scientific or medical knowledge is always made in a social context. Such knowledge always bears the traces, however faint, of the world in which it was made. The kind of knowledge that is at the heart of this book, however, is even more social. It is knowledge made to sell to a broad audience, intended, as my writers would have it, 'for the meanest capacity'.

From a broader perspective, I suggest that an analysis of the workings of women's bodies in early modern England can be placed alongside anthropologists, and historians' accounts of the ways that gender and bodies get connected in different cultures. Francesca Bray's analysis of what she calls 'gynotechnics' (in this case, the technologies of fabric production and of reproduction) or Charlotte Furth's interpretation of women's medicine in early modern China show us how social change remade images of the female body. For Bray, the reworking of patriarchy in late imperial China hinged on a shift in market relations that made women less and less likely to be economically productive. Instead, moralists defined womanhood around reproduction.[20] Furth, dealing with roughly the same time period, illustrates how printing remade ideas about women's reproductive bodies and who ought to provide health care for them.[21] In each case, historical changes seemingly distant from women's bodies turn out to have significance for gender and bodies. To say that our bodies are marked by history is a kind of shorthand for the complex relationship between our physical selves and our perceptions and understandings of them. The ways that we imagine our bodies influence how we feel about them and what we do about them. In particular, ideas about women's reproductive bodies are often maps of gender relations. In this sense, women's bodies are 'about' men as well as women.

[20] Francesca Bray, *Technology and Gender: Fabrics of Power in Late Imperial China* (Berkeley: University of California Press, 1997).
[21] Charlotte Furth, *A Flourishing Yin: Gender in China's Medical History, 960–1665* (Berkeley: University of California Press, 1999).

1

Reforming the Body

In 1540 Thomas Raynalde published the first printed book in English about pregnancy and childbirth.[1] Five years later he published another edition, with a new section that explained the anatomy of women's reproductive parts and the processes of conception. Called *The Birth of Mankind or The Womans Book*, this small text gave anyone who could read the rudiments of midwifery and offered advice on pregnancy and the care of the newborn. The work was, in part, a translation of a 1513 German text that was already becoming a bestseller. The English book became similarly popular, going into at least a dozen editions over the next century.

In the 1540s, writing about women's reproductive bodies was a politically charged act. The literal subject of the book—how women get pregnant and give birth—was the stuff of intense religious and political disputes. These arguments were not just at the level of high theological debate. As we shall see, they were the stuff of popular protest and Royal proclamation. *The Birth of Mankind* is a guide for women about pregnancy, but it is also a vision of women's reproductive bodies constructed and consumed in a moment when ideas about conception and childbirth practices were the targets of religious reform.

Religious reformers worried about the female body because the central narrative about reproduction in late medieval England was a sacred one: the story of Mary's miraculous conception of Christ. Women were encouraged to identify with the Virgin Mary while pregnant and used saints' relics and items associated with her to try to ensure a safe delivery. Early sixteenth-century women in labour employed a wide range of sacred objects to help them. Often these items represent a kind of sympathetic magic, the transfer of sacred power by means of a material object. One of the most popular practices was for a woman in labour to wear a girdle or sash around her body that had previously been wrapped around the statue of the Virgin Mary in her local church. In 1503 Henry VII's wife Elizabeth of York paid 6*s*. 8*d.* to a monk who brought her the

---

[1] Manuscript books had existed for centuries. See Green, 'Obstetrical and Gynecological Texts in Middle English'. In what follows, I modernize spelling by changing y and j to i in quotes where appropriate.

girdle usually wrapped around a cult statue of the Virgin in order to protect herself during childbirth.[2]

Other relics and sacred objects were similarly employed. When Thomas Cromwell directed a survey of the smaller monasteries and convents in 1535, his visitors uncovered a rich array of sacred objects associated with childbirth. In the north of England, institutions at Haltemprice, Calder, Conishead, Dale, and Kirkham owned girdles of the Virgin Mary herself for labouring women to borrow. Selby, Fountains, Jervaulx, Shelford, Arthington, and Blanchland also had girdles of the Virgin Mary, although the visitors neglected to specify whether these were loaned out for childbirth.[3] Meaux, Newburgh, Rievaulx, Chester, Pontefract, Holy Trinity York, Kirkstall, Coverham, and Newminster had girdles associated with saints such as St Francis, St Bernard, and St Werburgh that were loaned to lying-in women to aid in their deliveries. The Bendictine nuns of St Mary's, Derby had St Thomas's shirt; Holme Cultram had a necklace known as an *agnus dei*; the Cistercian nuns at Keldholme had a finger of St Stephen, those at Sinningthwaite had St Bernard's tunic, and Durham Priory had St Margaret's cross, all given out to assist pregnant women.[4] Sometimes there was a local link, such as at Chester, where St Werburgh was buried, or York, where the girdle was that of a former prior. Cromwell's visitors were much more interested in the misbehaviour of the nuns and monks than in relics and what they called superstition, so this rich list of childbirth relics in the north of England must be considered only a small fraction of what was available.

The North was not unusual; all over England, convents and monasteries owned relics used in childbirth. The abbey in Bruton, Somerset was fortunate to possess both the girdle of the Virgin Mary, in red silk, and that of Mary Magdalene, in white silk, used by labouring women.[5] Women in Burton-on-Trent leaned upon the staff of St Moodwyn while in labour.[6] In Norwich,

---

[2] Keith Thomas, *Religion and the Decline of Magic* (New York: Charles Scribner's Sons, 1971), 28.

[3] *Letters and Papers, Foreign and Domestic, of the Reign of Henry VIII*, ed. James Gairdner (London: Printed for Her Majesty's Printing Office by Eyre and Spottiswoode, 1887), x. 138–43. Hereafter cited as *Letters and Papers*. On the *agnus dei*, see John Cherry, 'Healing through Faith: The Continuation of Medieval Attitudes to Jewellery into the Renaissance', *Renaissance Studies*, 15 (2001), 154–71, esp. 157–60. On late medieval childbirth, see Gail McMurry Gibson, 'Scene and Obscene: Seeing and Performing Late Medieval Childbirth', *Journal of Medieval and Early Modern Studies*, 29 (1999), 7–24; Fiona Harris Stoertz, 'Suffering and Survival in Medieval English Childbirth', in Catherine Jorgenson Itnyre (ed.), *Medieval Family Roles: A Book of Essays* (New York: Garland, 1996), 101–20.

[4] *Letters and Papers*, 138–43.

[5] *Visitation Articles and Injunctions of the Period of the Reformation*, ed. Walter Frere with the assistance of William Kennedy, ii, Alcuin Club Collections, 15 (London: Longmans, Green, 1910), 58; *Three Chapters of Letters Relating to the Suppression of the Monasteries, edited from the originals in the British Museum*, ed. Thomas Wright, Camden Society, 26 (1843), 58–9.

[6] Duffy, *Stripping of the Altars*, 384.

women borrowed St Ethelrede's ring to help them in childbirth.[7] Nor were such items owned solely by religious communities. In 1530 Sir William Clopton of Long Melford, Suffolk, bequeathed to his son a relic of the true Cross—but only on the condition that the son loan it out to honest women of the parish to aid them in childbirth.[8]

As such lists of relics suggest, late medieval English women could draw upon a wealth of saints, mostly but not all female, to help them in pregnancy and childbirth. St Margaret was perhaps the best known of these. In John Mirk's book of sermons, intended for use by parish priests, he tells the faithful of St Margaret's powers on her feast day. Women who call on her while in labour will be granted a speedy delivery and a good Christian child.[9] A fifteenth-century English poem about St Dorothy assures its hearers that no house in which the saint is honoured will be struck by lightning, nor will any of its women miscarry while pregnant.[10] Somewhat paradoxically, many of the virgin saints so revered in late medieval England were also known for their help in childbirth, St Margaret being the paramount example.[11]

The most important help for pregnant and labouring women, however, was the Virgin Mary herself. The late medieval church suggested that women in labour pray to the Virgin specifically to intercede for them and grant them an easier delivery.[12] The church offered special Masses for the same purpose, and it was widely believed that gazing at the host during the elevation could also ensure safe delivery.[13] God directed the early fifteenth-century mystic and visionary Margery Kempe, who bore fourteen children, to reflect upon and imagine the birth of the Virgin as well as that of Christ.[14] Childbirth was thus

---

[7] *Letters and Papers*, x. 143. It is not clear which institution owned this relic since this record is just a fragment. Threads from the wimple of St Ethelrede were offered for sore throats and the wimple of St Audrede [another name for Ethelrede] for sore breasts by the same institution, possibly St Olave's, Norwich.

[8] Gail McMurry Gibson, *The Theater of Devotion: East Anglian Drama and Society in the Late Middle Ages* (Chicago: University of Chicago Press, 1989), 61; Duffy, *Stripping of the Altars*, 490.

[9] John Mirk, *Mirk's Festial: A Collection of Homilies, by Johannes Mirkus (John Mirk)*, ed. Theodore Erbe, part 1, EETS e.s. 97 (London: Kegan Paul Trench Trubner, 1905), 202.

[10] Osbern Bokenham, *Legendys of Hooly Wummen*, ed. M. J. Serjeantson (London, EETS, by H. Milford, for Oxford University Press, 1938), 134. On the importance of female saints and their connection to patterns of female devotion, see Eamon Duffy, 'Holy Maydens, Holy Wyfes: The Cult of Women Saints in 15th- and 16th-c. England', in W. J. Sheils and Diana Wood (eds.), *Women in the Church: Studies in Church History*, 27 (1990), 175–96.

[11] Duffy, 'Holy Maydens'.

[12] Thomas, *Religion and the Decline of Magic*, 28, 73, 188.

[13] Ibid. 34; Duffy, *Stripping of the Altars*, 100.

[14] Gibson, *Theater of Devotion*, 49–52. While no one would call Kempe typical, Gibson makes a good case for understanding her as typifying many aspects of 15th-c. devotions. For example, she traces many of Kempe's visions to Nicholas Love's wildly popular English version of Pseudo-Bonaventure's *Meditations on the Life of Christ*. So too, she links Kempe's visions to local mystery plays which focused on the life of the Virgin.

like many other hazardous undertakings: an event for which the church offered specific help. The Sarum Missal, the most commonly used in England, included specific prayers or Masses for a time of murrain (a cattle plague), for those going on a journey, and for those at sea, as well as for a woman with child.[15]

Most late medieval visual images of pregnancy and childbed in England were religious in origin, although few survived sixteenth- and seventeenth-century waves of iconoclasm. Women might see the Annunciation depicted in stained-glass windows, as in the rare surviving example in St Peter Mancroft, Norwich (see Fig. 1.1).[16] Here we see a very bodily rendition of the theme—a tiny Christ Child, bearing a cross, descends towards Mary in a beam of light. In St Mary's, Bury St Edmunds, there was a carving of an obviously pregnant Virgin (Fig. 1.2).[17] St Elizabeth shows Mary her pregnant belly in a church window in Sts Peter and Paul, East Harling (Fig. 1.3). In Holy Trinity, Long Melford, there was an alabaster panel depicting the Virgin Mary in childbed, attended by an (apocryphal) midwife. The history of this panel reminds us that images such as these, extant today, are but a tiny fraction of those which decorated churches before the Reformation. This panel survived the iconoclasms of the Reformation and the Civil War because it was hidden under the chancel floor, and discovered accidentally by eighteenth-century workmen.[18]

These same images were translated into vernacular print when primers were published in English for the first time in the 1530s. Often these small works of popular devotion emphasized Mary's story. In a 1538 text, readers saw the Annunciation (Fig. 1.4), shown as a dove descending, and Mary's visit to her pregnant cousin Elizabeth (Fig. 1.5). The Nativity is framed by a picture of a rosary or paternoster, making the link between veneration of the Virgin and a specific devotional object (Fig. 1.6). The narrative thrust of the images in this book is Mary's motherhood: readers also saw pictures of the Adoration of the Magi; Christ's circumcision; the flight into Egypt; and Mary's assumption into heaven. Even the title page of the book is an image of Mary (Fig. 1.7) that alludes to her own immaculate conception.[19] Stories about the Crucifixion also linked Mary to all women's suffering in childbirth. According to late medieval belief Mary did not experience labour pains when she gave birth to Jesus, but

[15] *The Sarum Missal in English* (London: The Church Press, 1867), esp. 546, 547, 566, and 567.
[16] Gibson, *Theater of Devotion*, 147.
[17] Ibid. 175.
[18] Ibid. 62; Sir William Parker, *The History of Long Melford* (London: Wyman & Sons, 1873).
[19] *Here after foloweth the Prymer in Englysshe sette out alonge, after the vse of Sarum* ([Newly imprynted at Rown: by Nycholas le Roux, for F. Regnault, 1538]), STC 16004. Although published in Rouen, this text, like others published by Regnault, was in English and Latin and clearly intended for the English market. Annunciation: sig. Eiii'; Visitation: sig. Fi'; Nativity: sig. Giii'; Circumcision: sig. Hii'; Adoration: sig. Hv'; Flight: sig. Hviii'; Assumption: sig. Iiiii'.

Fig. 1.1. (*right*) Stained-glass window
of the Annunciation, showing
impregnation of the Virgin by a tiny
Christ Child. St Peter Mancroft,
Norwich. © Crown Copyright.
Courtesy National Monuments Record

Fig. 1.2. (*below left*) Carving of an
obviously pregnant Virgin. St Mary's,
Bury St Edmunds. By permission of the
Churchwarden, St Mary's Church, Bury
St Edmunds

Fig. 1.3. (*below right*) Stained-glass
window of the Visitation. Sts Peter and
Paul, East Harling. Reproduced by
permission of English Heritage.
National Monuments Record

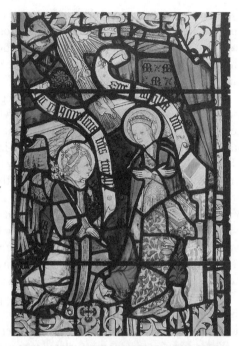

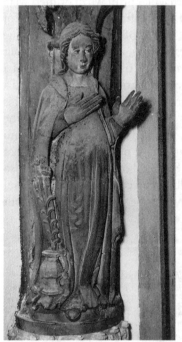

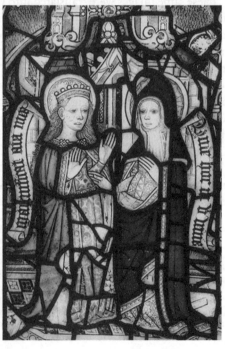

Fig. 1.4. The Annunciation, from a
1538 primer, *Here after foloweth the
Prymer in Englysshe.* Courtesy of the
Folger Shakespeare Library

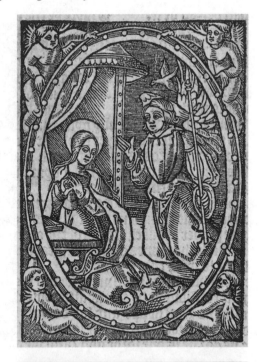

Fig. 1.5. The Visitation, from a 1538
primer, *Here after foloweth the Prymer
in Englysshe.* Courtesy of the Folger
Shakespeare Library

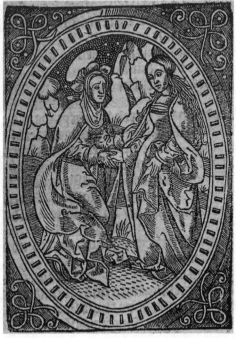

Fig. 1.6. The Nativity, with devotion to Mary linked to the paternoster or rosary—also a source of teething beads. *Here after foloweth the Prymer in Englysshe* (1538). Courtesy of the Folger Shakespeare Library

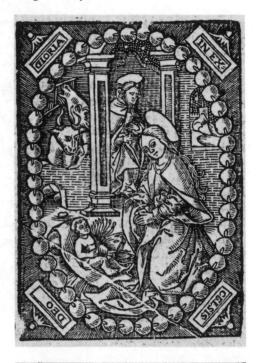

Fig. 1.7. The title page from the 1538 primer makes Mary the centre of the story. *Here after foloweth the Prymer in Englysshe*. Courtesy of the Folger Shakespeare Library

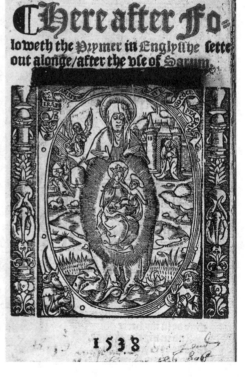

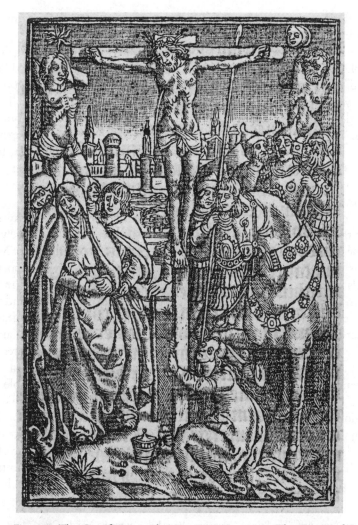

Fig. 1.8. The Crucifixion, with Mary swooning away. *This Primer of Salysbury use is set out a long Latin* (1531). Courtesy of the Folger Shakespeare Library

suffered cognate pains at his crucifixion, as she, in effect, gave birth to the salvation of mankind. She was often depicted next to the Cross, overwhelmed by bodily suffering, as in an image from a 1531 English primer (Fig. 1.8).[20] As in many other instances, women were taught that Mary was both unlike them (in

[20] *This Primer of Salysbury vse is a set out a long Latin* (Parys: venudatur a F. Regnault, 1531), STC 15971, fo. Xciii[v]. (Like the above, this work was produced in France for the English market.) On this

not suffering in giving birth) and like them (in suffering those pains, albeit under unusual circumstances).

Central to the veneration of Mary was the mystery of Christ's conception. As one scholar explains, 'The incarnational preoccupation of the late Middle Ages tended to make the Virgin Mary—perhaps even more than Christ himself— the very emblem of Christian mystery.'[21] The fifteenth-century poem 'I syng of a mayden' expresses wonder at Mary's corporeal status as both mother and virgin: 'Moder & mayden was never none but che'.[22] Another such expressed the paradox of a virgin mother by alluding to 'maydens mylke' that fed the infant Christ.[23] Veneration of the Virgin Mary emphasized wonder and mystery: she was an ordinary woman and yet the mother of God; she was both a virgin and a mother.

Women and men in the early sixteenth century heard, read, and saw stories about the Nativity that were richer and more corporeal than the purely scriptural account, full of juicy details about the miraculous conception of Mary as well as that of Jesus. Sermons, poems, and plays, based on the apocryphal gospels of James and proto-Matthew, offered late medieval English men and women all kinds of body stories. Mystery plays, performed in cities and towns, gave viewers and participants a rich array of details about Mary's miraculous motherhood.[24] In the York plays about the Annunciation and the Nativity, a lengthy scene is devoted to Joseph's doubts about his young wife's pregnancy, and in the Coventry cycle, an entire play is devoted to the subject. In an East Anglian play, Mary describes the moment of conception in pleasurable bodily terms, 'I cannot telle what joy, what blysse, Now I fele in my body!' The stage directions suggest that three beams of light were directed at Mary's body, and she says 'A, now I fele in my body be Parfyte [perfect] God and parfyte man'.[25] A scholar has described this cycle of plays as centred on 'the pure womb of Mary (and that of her own mother, Anne)'.[26] At the same time, these accounts stress Mary's pregnant body, like that of any other woman, and they affirm her con-

---

theme, see Amy Neff, 'The Pain of *Compassio*: Mary's Labor at the Foot of the Cross', *Art Bulletin*, 80 (1998), 254–73.

[21] Gibson, *Theater of Devotion*, 137.

[22] Duffy, *Stripping of the Altars*, 256–7; the poem is cited from *Religious Lyrics of the XV Century*, ed. Carleton Brown (Oxford: Clarendon Press, 1939), 119.

[23] Duffy, *Stripping of the Altars*, 258.

[24] The literature on mystery plays is substantial. The most helpful studies for this work focus on the relationship of the text to its context. See Sarah Beckwith, *Signifying God: Social Relation and Symbolic Act in the York Corpus Christi Plays* (Chicago: University of Chicago Press, 2001); David Mills, *Recycling the Cycle: The City of Chester and its Whitsun Plays* (Toronto: University of Toronto Press, 1998). See also Elizabeth A. Witt, *Contrary Marys in Medieval English and French Drama* (New York: Peter Lang, 1995).

[25] *The Mary Play from the N-Town Manuscript*, ed. Peter Meredith (Exeter: University of Exeter Press, 1997), 76, 77.   [26] Gibson, *Theater of Devotion*, 166.

tinued virginity even after birth. Often the stories tell of Joseph, desperately looking for a midwife and returning (usually too late) with two of them. One doubts her post-partum virginity and examines her, whereupon her hand shrivels. Only when she begs pardon of Mary and touches the garment of the baby Jesus is her hand restored to health.[27]

In these accounts, Mary was also the result of a miraculous conception, being born to St Anne after she suffered twenty years of barrenness with her husband Joachim. Anne went on to marry two further husbands and bear two more daughters named Mary. These Marys bore six of the Apostles, and with Elizabeth's son John the Baptist, form a kind of extended family for Jesus, known as the Holy Kindred, often portrayed in churches.[28] In the parish church at Ranworth, the screen in front of the south altar has paintings of the three Marys with their children, including a child apostle with a tiny pipe for blowing bubbles and another toddler holding a toy pinwheel. Included in the midst of this display of fecundity is St Margaret, virgin and patron of child-birth. As Eamon Duffy has suggested, the tensions we might see between a virgin saint and the mothers and children so lovingly portrayed were not the key to these paintings. Instead, local women revered Margaret for the power her virginity afforded her, while also identifying with the touching domestic details of the three Marys and their children. It was at this altar that women offered a candle when they came to church to offer thanks after a safe delivery.[29]

Women who could afford it offered more than just candles after childbirth. The wax seals, imprinted with the *agnus dei* (the lamb of God), or other religious images, used as amulets to ensure a safe delivery, might later be pinned to a statue of the Virgin Mary as thank-offerings. Wealthier parishioners made these offerings in silver, and in some places there were enough of such offerings to fashion a pair of silver shoes for the statue of the Virgin. The statue of the Virgin in the Lady Chapel at Long Melford, Suffolk, for example, had many offerings associated with it. According to a list compiled in 1529, Alice Tye and Mrs Brooke had each given lavish girdles of the sort loaned out to women in childbirth. On the apron of the statue were pinned nine rings (silver or gilt); fifteen silver buckles; a silver spoon; silver, coral, and jet beads that could be used for rosaries; a number of stones set in silver; an *agnus dei* set in silver; and

---

[27] *Ludus Coventriae; or, the Plaie called Corpus Christi*, ed. K. S. Block, EETS e.s. 120 (Oxford: Oxford University Press, 1922), 144 (l. 291); *The Middle English Stanzaic Versions of the Life of Saint Anne*, ed. Roscoe Parker, EETS o.s. 174 (London: Milford, for Oxford University Press, 1928), 27; Mirk, *Mirk's Festial*, 23.

[28] On Anne, see Jacobus de Voragine, *The Golden Legend*, trans. William Granger Ryan (Princeton: Princeton University Press, 1993), ii. 149–58; on English devotions to her, see Duffy, 'Holy Maydens', 191–3; Nicholas Orme, 'Church and Chapel in Medieval England', *Transactions of the Royal Historical Society*, ser. 6 (1996), 75–102 at 89–90. Thanks to Diarmaid MacCulloch for this last reference.

[29] Duffy, 'Holy Maydens', 194–6.

a variety of other valuables. The statue was outfitted with clothes, such as a coat in crimson velvet, or one in white damask with green velvet trim. There were matching miniature coats for the infant Jesus.[30] Domestic and devotional worlds intersected in such objects. Coral beads were well-known teething remedies as well as rosary beads. Baby clothes for the statue of the infant Jesus were fancier versions of those worn by local babies.

These elaborate costumes, coordinated with altar cloths, are reminiscent of the baby Jesus dolls given as wedding gifts to young Italian women, both to those who married men and those who, as nuns, symbolically married the Lord. Christiane Klapisch-Zuber has suggested that these dolls, and their elaborate clothing, were intended to promote appropriate maternal feelings in their recipients, and even to function as objects of 'visual impregnation', a sort of fertility charm.[31] The dolls discussed by Klapisch-Zuber are a kind of mirror image of the English statues; they move the sacred into domestic space, while the English church statuary puts fragments of the domestic (spoons, baby clothes) into sacred space. These offerings made women's travails in childbirth part of the fabric of the church. The list-maker in Long Melford carefully noted which women had given which objects.

These small votive objects, the relics loaned out by monasteries and convents, the church paintings and statues, sermons, prayers, and mystery plays all point to the way in which pregnancy and childbirth were understood in relation to stories of the Nativity and of helper saints. English women in the early sixteenth century were offered a rich array of religious meanings for their travails in reproduction. To judge by lists of benefactions, it seems that many women responded to these meanings, incorporating and appropriating aspects of these beliefs into their own lives.

Not all women, however, liked these religious beliefs and practices. A tiny but vocal minority of English men and women contested these meanings of conception and childbirth, grounding their objections in their readings of Scripture. Lollards were a group of believers who drew on some of the criticisms of the church formulated by John Wyclif (*c.*1328–84). They challenged many aspects of the later medieval church, and have been described as a kind of premature reformation because many of their beliefs foreshadowed those of

[30] Parker, *History of Long Melford,* 78–9, 81. See also the recent transcription, David Dymond and Clive Paine, *The Spoil of Melford Church: The Reformation in a Suffolk Parish* ([Bury St Edmunds]: Salient Press [Suffolk County Council], 1992).

[31] Christiane Klapisch-Zuber, 'Holy Dolls: Play and Piety in Florence in the Quattrocento', in her *Women, Family, and Ritual in Renaissance Italy,* trans. Lydia Cochrane (Chicago: University of Chicago Press, 1985), 310–29. See Gibson, *Theater of Devotion,* 63, for a discussion of this practice in relation to Margery Kempe. See Jacqueline Marie Musacchio, *The Art and Ritual of Childbirth in Renaissance Italy* (New Haven: Yale University Press, 1999), for a fascinating discussion of the many material objects connected with childbirth that survive from Renaissance Italy.

Protestant reformers.[32] They remain a shadowy group, revealed in sudden snapshots when arrested and tried for heresy but otherwise hard to find in the historical record.

Lollards and other free thinkers did not like the usual accounts of the conception of Christ and said so in colourful and emphatic terms. What has come down to us is a series of fragments in which women and men disparaged Mary's role in the conception of Christ. In 1511, Simon Piers, who may have been a Dutchman, asserted that Christ took no humanity from Mary. In 1520, one John Morress said that the Virgin was but a sack. In Yorkshire in 1534, a priest stated that the Virgin was like a pudding when the meat was taken out. Two years later, a preacher in Kent is supposed to have said that the Virgin was not the queen of heaven but the mother of Christ; and that she could do no more than any other woman, comparing her to a saffron bag. The image of the Virgin as a saffron bag must have had wide circulation, for it was one of the specific heresies forbidden by the Church in 1536. The wording of the forbidden belief helps to explicate this curious idea: 'a bag of saffron or pepper when the spice was out'.[33] In other words, the Virgin was just a container, and her son had no necessary connection with her, merely residing in her body. This image of a saffron bag must have had special relevance in the south of England, where saffron was grown. Saffron was fantastically expensive, because it was painstakingly harvested from the stamens of a particular type of crocus—and it took many such tiny stamens to make even a small bag of the spice. A saffron bag would have become coloured by the yellow spice inside it—but the bag conveyed none of its essence to the spice.

By the late 1530s, the idea that the Virgin contributed nothing but houseroom to her son may also have had Continental origins. Anabaptists of various kinds had been reformulating ideas about the body of Christ, asserting that Christ did not have a human body, or that his human body came from heaven and was not made from Mary's flesh.[34] After Continental persecutions, many Anabaptists fled to England, and there is an intriguing suggestion that English

[32] On the Lollards, see Margaret Aston, *Lollards and Reformers: Images and Literacy in Late Medieval Religion* (London: Hambledon, 1984); ead., *England's Iconoclasts* (Oxford: Clarendon Press, 1988), esp. 130–9; Anne Hudson, *The Premature Reformation: Wycliffite Texts and Lollard History* (Oxford: Clarendon Press, 1988); Shannon McSheffrey, *Gender and Heresy: Women and Men in Lollard Communities, 1420–1530* (Philadelphia: University of Pennsylvania Press, 1996).

[33] Piers: Lambeth Palace Library, Register Warham, iii, fo. 175ʳ, cited in John Davis, 'Joan of Kent, Lollardy and the English Reformation', *Journal of Ecclesiastical History*, 33 (1982), 225–33 at 231; Moress: Rochester Diocesan Registry, Rochester Registers iv (Fisher), fo. 41ᵛ, cited in Davis, 'Joan of Kent', 231; pudding: A. G. Dickens, *Lollards and Protestants in the Diocese of York, 1509–1558* (Oxford: Oxford University Press, 1959), 75; saffron bag: John Strype, *Ecclesiastical Memorials*, in *Strype's Works* (Oxford: Clarendon Press, 1822), i, pt. 1, 442; *mala dogmata*: ibid., pt. 2, 260, item XL.

[34] George Hunston Williams, *The Radical Reformation* (Philadelphia: The Westminster Press, 1962), esp. 325–37 and 401–3.

Anabaptists published their own discussion of the Incarnation of Christ some-time in the 1530s, a text that has not survived.[35]

Linked to the issue of Christ's conception was the nature of the Eucharist. Lollards had long maintained that the host was not transformed into the literal body and blood of Christ, but rather was a symbol or commemoration of Christ's body. Concerns about the physical nature of Christ at his concep-tion were easily connected to those about his physical nature in communion. A group of heretics in Kent in 1511 denied that the bread of communion was transformed into Christ's body, believing instead that it was 'only material bread in substance'. A few decades later, a large number of men and women abjured—denied their heretical beliefs—in London. They form an intriguing catalogue of plebeian independent thinkers. Many disliked the worship of images, going on pilgrimages, and transubstantiation. Henry Tomson, a tailor, Grace Palmer, Thomas Eve, a weaver, Lawrence Maxwell, a tiler, and others denied that bread was transformed into Christ's body in the Eucharist. Others criticized beliefs in the Virgin Mary's powers. Grace Palmer said that her neighbours should not go on pilgrimages to 'a piece of timber painted' and regretted that she had ever lit a candle before an image. Margaret Bowgas told her interrogator that 'I believe in God, and he can do me more good than our Lady, or any other saint.' By the late 1520s, some of these men and women were reading Luther and other Conti-nental reformers, so that home-grown beliefs were augmented by new Protestant thought.[36] We may never be able to trace the strands of influence—Lollard, Anabaptist, or other—that shaped some English people's critique of Mary's miraculous motherhood of Christ. What comes through in the frag-mentary testimony of those who found themselves in trouble for heretical statements is the variety of ways in which men and women disputed with a late medieval emphasis on the bodily-ness of Christ's story and the importance of Mary his mother. Thomas Dawby, who said that the Virgin was but a sack, also broke a statue of her in his church, saying that it was but an idol. When Joan Sampson, a Lollard woman in labour, was urged to pray to the Virgin Mary, she indicated her scorn for the practice by spitting. Her attendants were

[35] Williams, *Radical Reformation*, 402.
[36] John Foxe, *The Acts and Monuments*, ed. George Townsend (New York: AMS Press, 1965), v, Kent, 1511: 648–53; Tomson: 32; Palmer: 33; Eve: 38; Maxwell: 29; Bowgas: 39; reading Luther, etc.: 28, 29, 33, 38, 39. On the contexts of these various beliefs see Hudson, *Premature Reformation*, 446–507, and Susan Brigden, *London and the Reformation* (Oxford: Clarendon Press, 1989), 82–128. On the larger issues of the relationship between Lollardy and Protestantism, see the recent essay by Patrick Collinson, 'Night Schools, Conventicles and Churches: Continuities and Discontinuities in Early Protestant Ecclesiology', in Peter Marshall and Alec Ryrie (eds.), *The Beginnings of English Protes-tantism* (Cambridge: Cambridge University Press, 2002), 209–35 for an introduction to this con-tested topic.

appalled.[37] An earlier Lollard poem criticized women who tied the strings from the Virgin's smock around their belly while in labour, a practice analogous to the use of the Virgin's girdle.[38] Elizabeth Sampson, perhaps a relative of Joan, admitted that she had called Our Lady of Willesden (a popular pilgrimage site) 'a burnt-arse elf'. 'Burnt-arse' meant afflicted with venereal disease, usually associated with prostitutes. Sampson could hardly have chosen a more offensive remark—comparing the Virgin to a poxed whore—and she probably knew full well the import of her words.[39]

Nor was Mary's motherhood of Christ uncontentious within the conservative parts of the church. Robert Serles, a preacher at Canterbury Cathedral, was accused of teaching that Mary had fully conceived Christ when she was only 14 years old, and that she nourished him, not with real milk, but with milk that came from heaven, because only a woman who had known a man could make real milk. Serles was a conservative (despite his appointment as a preacher) and was preaching on the Feast of the Assumption, so his statement is probably best understood as a reflection of traditional aspects of the worship of Mary.[40] These varied beliefs about the corporality (or lack of it) of Mary's motherhood, expressed by Lollard, reformer, or conservative, suggest that the conception of Christ was an issue that could evoke strong feelings in English men and women.[41] It was not a neutral or trivial topic.

By the time that many of these comments were made, however, the forces of change were already set in motion. When Henry VIII broke with Rome in the 1530s, some of his countrymen were already reading the works of Martin Luther and other Continental reformers, but Henry's church was more like a Catholic one severed from papal authority than any in Calvin's Geneva or Bullinger's Zurich. Henry abolished monasteries and convents, ordered that the Bible in English be placed in every parish church, attacked idolatrous worship and the use of relics, and clamped down on pilgrimages.

[37] Brigden, *London and the Reformation*, 96; the original source is Foxe's *Acts and Monuments*, iv. 206.

[38] *Pierce the Plowman's Crede*, ed. Walter W. Skeat, EETS o.s. 30 (London: N. Trubner, 1873), 4; lines 77–9.

[39] Dawby: *Letters and Papers*, xviii, pt. 2, no. 546, 315; Elizabeth Sampson: Foxe, *Acts and Monuments*, iv. 175.

[40] *Letters and Papers*, xviii, pt. 2, no. 546, 303–4. On the larger topic of Mary, see Jaroslav Pelikan, *Mary through the Centuries: Her Place in the History of Culture* (New Haven: Yale University Press, 1996); Marina Warner, *Alone of All Her Sex: The Myth and Cult of the Virgin Mary* (New York: Vintage Books, 1976); Donna Spivey Ellington, *From Sacred Body to Angelic Soul: Understanding Mary in Late Medieval and Early Modern Europe* (Washington, DC: Catholic University of America Press, 2001).

[41] Anne's conception of Mary was also hotly contested at this time, especially between the Franciscans and the Dominicans. In mystery plays and other late medieval sources, the two conceptions are often tightly linked, and dispute about one may have coloured debates about the other.

As a part of his reforms of the excesses of the Church, Henry VIII's bishops addressed so-called 'superstitious' practices around childbirth. Many relics loaned out to labouring women were destroyed when monasteries and convents were dissolved, but reforms went further. Bishops had long been concerned that midwives should be able to baptize a newborn baby at risk of dying. In 1537, for example, Rowland Lee, a very traditional bishop of Coventry and Lichfield, ordered his parish priests to teach their flocks the form of baptism in English at least twelve times a year, so that a midwife could baptize properly. He also told his priests to 'command' all labouring women to have a vessel of clean water at the ready when they went into labour, just in case an emergency baptism was needed.[42]

The following year, Nicholas Shaxton, the evangelical Bishop of Salisbury, tried to reform childbirth practices. He ordered that no statues or images were to be adorned with gold, silver, or clothes; nor could people offer candles to them. This proscription went to the heart of the popular practice of making votive offerings to a saint, usually the Virgin, in thanks for a successful delivery. Shaxton, like his predecessors, ordered his priests to ensure that midwives knew the correct form of words for an emergency baptism, but then he intervened more directly in the birthing room:

charging also the said midwives, to beware that they cause not the woman, being in travail [labour], to make any foolish vow to go in pilgrimage to this image or that image after her deliverance, but only to call on God for her help. Nor to use any girdles, purses, measures of our Lady, or such other superstitious things to be occupied about the woman while she laboureth, to make her believe to have the better speed by it.[43]

Shaxton thus tried to make midwives into shock troops of reform, insisting that they forbid their clients to use customary measures to ensure a safe and speedy delivery—no girdles of the Virgin, no promises to go on pilgrimage, and no pleading with the Virgin Mary as intercessor. Instead, women were only allowed to call on God himself. Shaxton inveighed against the use of relics in colourful language, listing 'stinking boots, mucky combs, ragged rochets, rotten girdles, pyld purses, great bullocks' horns, locks of hair, and filthy rags, gobbetts of wood, under the name of parcels of the holy cross, and such pelfry beyond estimation'.[44] Shaxton ordered his priests to bring all their relics to his house in Ramsbury, where he would decide which ones might be returned to churches and which ones were mere idolatry. He was at this point one of the hotter sorts of reformers, much more radical than many of his flock or his King.

In 1539 King Henry VIII put the brakes on further reformation by issuing the Six Articles. First and foremost of these was that 'the natural body and

---

[42] *Visitation Articles*, ii. 23.   [43] Ibid. 58–9.   [44] Ibid. 57, 58–9, 59–60.

blood of our Saviour Jesus Christ, conceived of the Virgin Mary' was really present in the bread and wine of communion.[45] Christ's real body, conceived in human form in Mary's womb, was the substance of the consecrated bread and wine. This first article was enforced much more fiercely than the other five. Anyone who denied transubstantiation (the technical term for the mode by which Christ becomes truly present in the bread and wine) would be burned as a heretic and forfeit all his or her property, impoverishing his or her children. Usually, a heretic could avoid execution if he or she would abjure or repent of the heretical belief, but Henry refused to allow any such escape clause for those who denied transubstantiation. Leading reformers such as John Hooper fled to the Continent, Nicholas Shaxton and Hugh Latimer resigned their bishoprics, and over 500 Londoners were rounded up for questioning.

A year later, when Richard Jonas translated the *Birth of Mankind* from Latin into English, and Thomas Raynalde published it, they understood their project as a part of radical reform. Raynalde's career as a printer and publisher makes his sympathies clear: he was an advocate for English and Continental reformers. He and/or his son published works by English reformers such as George Joye, John Hooper, and Miles Coverdale, and Continental ones such as Heinrich Bullinger and Huldrich Zwingli.[46] Although we know nothing of Jonas's life, his preface to his translation suggests that he understood his project in relation to currents of religious reform. He dedicated his book to Queen Katherine (Katherine Howard), who married Henry VIII in July 1540, saying

Where as of late (most excellent vertuous Quene) many goodly and proper treatise, as well concerninge holye scripture, wherein is conteyned the onely comforte and consolation of all godlye people: as other prophane artes and sciences right necessary to be knowen have ben . . . set forth in this oure vulgare Englisshe tunge.[47]

The phrase describing Scripture as 'the only comfort and consolation of all godly people' is a clear statement of Jonas's religious politics. Only Scripture, not saints, or pilgrimages, or prayers for the dead, or good works matter to the godly.

Jonas was keenly aware of the novelty of his project, and kept emphasizing the importance of the vernacular. He noted that the translations of religious and scientific works have enriched 'our mother tongue', and specified that his translation was from the Latin edition of Eucharius Rösslin's 1513 German

[45] *Documents of the English Reformation*, ed. Gerald Bray (Cambridge: J. Clarke, 1994), 224.
[46] All references are to the second, revised edition of the STC. Joye: STC2 14825; Hooper: STC2 13755; 13762; Bullinger: STC2 5189.7; Redman: STC2 20827. There were two Thomas Raynaldes, father and son, and it is not possible to distinguish fully when the son takes over from the father. The 1540 edition was published by the father, as was the 1545, but subsequent editions are less clear. Many thanks to Peter Blayney for his help on this topic.
[47] *The Byrth of Mankynde* (Imprynted at London by T.R., 1540), STC2 21153, sig. ABii^r.

text, but originally it was written by a physician 'in his owne mother tunge, that is beyinge a Germayn, in the Germayne speche'.[48] To us, the phrase 'mother tongue' is hackneyed, but in 1540 it was fresher. Thomas Cranmer, Archbishop of Canterbury, used the same phrase in the same year in his so-called 'Great Bible', noting 'The Saxones tonge whiche at that time was oure mothers tonge'. The phrase was even more resonant in a book about motherhood.

Jonas's use of 'mother tongue' points both to his awareness of the political and religious implications of publishing in the vernacular and his curious status as a man writing about women's work. Delivering babies was the task of a midwife, not a surgeon, and the birthing room was full of other women who supported the mother-to-be during labour. Men had no place there. Perhaps unconsciously, Jonas dealt with the incongruity of his role by comparing the work of translation to the pains of labour. He asks the Queen and noble readers to accept his 'paynes', and suggests that he will undergo more pains in the future when he revises the book. He continues: 'I have judged my labor and paynes in this behalf right well bestowed' if his readers find light and comfort in its pages. Like subsequent male writers on midwifery, Jonas worried about male readers who might read the book for the wrong reasons. In his admonition to the reader, he calls on men to eschew all ribald and unseemly comment, and warns them that God will call them to account for all idle words, let alone lewd or uncharitable ones.[49]

Jonas's book, unlike its German antecedent, did not attempt to create new roles for men in pregnancy and childbirth. The 1513 German text has an introductory prologue in verse that emphasizes the importance of men in reproduction. In the poem, called an 'Admonition to Pregnant Women and Midwives', Eucharius Rösslin stresses connections to a male God, saying that God made souls in his image. Like any father, 'Who tears apart both body and land / At seeing his child in danger's hands', God suffered in order to ensure the safety and comfort of his children. Midwives are particularly at fault; Rösslin describes how, 'through neglect and oversight / They destroy children far and wide', and he threatens midwives that God will call them to account. He belittles midwives' learning: 'And since no midwife that I've asked / Could tell me anything of her task / I'm left to my medical education.'[50] In the prologue, Rösslin transforms midwifery into a male science. He describes how God had

---

[48] *Byrth* (1540), sig. ABiiᵛ. On the next page he again emphasizes that he is translating the text into English for the English people.   [49] Ibid. sigs. ABiiiʳ; ABiiiᵛ; ABiᵛ.

[50] Eucharius Rösslin, *When Midwifery became the Male Physician's Province: The 16th-c. Handbook, The Rose Garden for Pregnant Women and Midwives, Newly Englished*, trans. Wendy Arons (Jefferson, NC: McFarland & Co., 1994), 33, 34, 35. Hereafter cited as 'Arons'. On German popular medical books and religious themes, see Kathleen M. Crowther-Heyck, ' "Be Fruitful and Multiply": Genesis and Generation in Reformation Germany', *Renaissance Quarterly*, 55 (2002), 904–35.

given man reason and sense, so that men have discovered the breadth of the seas and the earth, measured the heavens, observed the stars and the planets, and determined the course of the sun and the moon. He continues by describing how Galen, Rhazes, Avicenna, and Averroes, through divine grace and hard work, learned how the human body worked and how to heal it. Then Rösslin turns to the art of midwifery, having given it the preceding all-male pedigree.[51] In other words, in the German version of the text, men were positioned as the most important players in midwifery, while in the English version, female midwives became the key to successful childbirth. Jonas faults bad midwives, but he emphasizes that there are many good ones, saying 'there be many of them right expert, diligent, wise, circumspecte, and tender'.[52] Instead of insisting on the importance of men, Jonas expresses concern about the wrong kind of man reading his book.

In his 1545 version of the book, Raynalde likewise places human conception in a religious framework, saying that 'There is nothinge under heaven which so manifestly & plainly doth declare & shew the magnificent mightinesse of the omnipotent living god' than the generation and conception of living things. God has given mortal beings the power to 'ingender and produce other like things unto themselves', without which 'all manner of things would soon perish and come to an ende'. He continues: 'As ye may evidently see in the sowing of Corn, and all other manner of seed.'[53] 'Corn' here means all sorts of grain, such as wheat and rye—the very stuff of life itself, the basics of every ordinary person's daily diet. In a time when famine and bad harvests made many go hungry, the hand of God seemed very direct in the affairs of men and women. It made sense that both kinds of God-given life—nourishment and reproduction—happened in the same way.[54]

Raynalde continues by comparing the earth to a mother, making both the land and the female body powerfully generative of new life: 'The earth unto all seades, is as a mother and nource containing, clippinge, and enbrasinge them in her wombe, feadinge and fosteringe them as the mother doth the childe in her belly or matrice.'[55] Whether plants or people, the process is the same; as Raynalde says, 'Every thing, then, the which doth encrease in his kinde, must firste be conceaved in the wombe and matrice of the mother.'[56] Women who

[51] Arons, 38.   [52] *Byrth* (1540), sig. ABiii^v.
[53] Thomas Raynalde, *The Byrth of Mankynde, otherwyse named the Womans booke* (London: Tho. Ray. [1545]), STC 21154, fos. 136^r–137^r. I have changed the first two 'ye's to 'the's for clarity.
[54] These themes are common to many medieval and early modern works on reproduction. See e.g. *The Knowing of Women's Kind in Childing: A Middle English Version of Material Derived from Trotula and Other Sources*, ed. Alexandra Barratt (Turnhout: Brepols, 2001), 40–1; *The Trotula: A Medieval Compendium of Women's Medicine*, ed. Monica H. Green (Philadelphia: University of Pennsylvania Press, 2001), 71.
[55] Raynalde, *Byrth* (1545), fo. 137^v. 'Clipping' here means clasping or embracing.
[56] Ibid. fo. 138^r.

had difficulties conceiving were like fields that did not yield good harvests: 'The earth may be over waterish, dankisshe, or over hote and dry, or elles full of stones, gravell, or other rubrish, or full of ill weedes . . .'[57] For sixteenth-century English men and women, these images of seeds and earth echoed biblical parables that they were hearing in church, and, for the first time, reading in English Bibles. Luke 8: 4–15 is the story of a man who sows seed on different types of land:

some fell by the wayside; and it was trodden down, and the fowls of the air devoured it. And some fell upon a rock; and as soon as it was sprung up, it withered away, because it lacked moisture. And some fell among thorns; and the thorns sprang up with it, and choked it.

Only the seed that falls on good ground flourishes, as God's word planted and tended in a receptive listener would bear the fruit of salvation.[58]

In one of his very few allusions to the male body, Raynalde admits that the fault may be with the man: 'The sowar may unordinatly strewe and caste the seade on the earth.'[59] The comparison between seeds growing in the earth and babies growing in their mothers' wombs provided a test for fertility that acknowledged that a problem might lie in the man or the woman. The man and woman were each to take seven seeds of wheat, barley, and beans, and soak them in their respective urines for twenty-four hours. Then each planted his or her seeds in a pot, and watered the pot with his or her urine. 'Marke whose potte dothe prove, and the seades therin contained doth growe, in that party is not the lacke of conception', explains Raynalde, although he also warns 'but truste not much this farfet experiment'.[60] The number seven had magical properties, but the rest of the procedure relied on the commonplace analogy between grain-growing and human reproduction.

While the exact process by which a seed became a plant was mysterious, plowing and sowing seed was familiar to almost every man and woman in early modern England, a profoundly rural society in this period. The material realities of day-to-day existence provided a convenient and persuasive analogy for the human body that was underwritten by biblical analogy. Once conception had occurred, the fetus was imagined as a sort of guest within the mother's body, and it was her job to provide appropriate hospitality to it, just as she would in her own home. It was believed that the fetus was nourished by maternal blood—specifically, by blood that no longer was discharged as menses. As Raynalde describes,

[57] Raynalde, *Byrth* (1545), fo. 137ᵛ.
[58] See also Matthew 13 for this parable and two others about seed. I suspect that the religious contexts for medical and body imagery are far more significant than many historians have suggested.
[59] Raynalde, *Byrth* (1545), fo. 137ᵛ.   [60] Ibid. fo. 141ʳ.

Prudent lady nature ful wisely hath provided that there shulde be always pres[en]t and ready, a continual course and resort of blud in the vaines of the matrice as a very natu-rall source, spring, fountaine, or wel[l] evermore redy to arrouse, water and nourishe the feature [the fetus] so sone as it shal be conceaved.[61]

Like a good housewife, the womb was always ready for a guest. Even if the woman never conceived, or never even had sexual relations, 'yet is ther no faut in nature, who hath prepared place and foode to be at all times in readinesse'.[62] The idea that women's bodies were naturally welcoming and generous fitted well with contemporary notions of hospitality.[63] Despite the grinding poverty in which many people existed, hospitality was widely recognized as a virtue. Folk tales, for example, describe how a couple shares their meagre meal with an unknown traveller, and are rewarded with riches. Similarly, the Bible is full of stories about hospitality, such as when Abraham welcomes three guests, one of whom is God, who promises that Sarah will have a child despite her age (Genesis 18), or when Rebecca welcomes Abraham's servant and then becomes Isaac's wife (Genesis 24). In each of these tales, it is the woman who provides food for the guests, and who subsequently bears a son or, in Rebecca's case, twin sons.

The idea that women's reproductive bodies are hospitable and generous is very different from our contemporary notions. As Emily Martin has shown, medical textbooks of our own day depict women's reproductive cycles as spendthrift—producing an egg and a uterine lining for a potential baby every month is described as wasteful. Male production of billions of sperm, however, is represented as marvellous or wonderful.[64] Five centuries ago, different values could make women's monthly cycles a virtue rather than a waste. Although menstrual blood has been associated with profound taboos from ancient times, Raynalde argued that it must be good, because it nourished the fetus. The image of a woman's body as a hospitable home made menstrual blood 'pure and holsum', in Raynalde's words. He criticizes those authors who depict menstrual blood as 'venemous and daungerous', saying that their ideas are but 'dreames and plaine dotage'. He refuses to tell his readers anything more about such neg-ative images of menstrual blood, concluding his chapter with reference to the foolish authors of such images, saying 'To reherse there fon[d] wurdes here were but losse of inke and paper'.[65]

Raynalde's positive valuation of menstrual blood was part of his larger emphasis on the importance of the mother. In his discussions of reproductive

[61] Raynalde, *Byrth* (1545), fo. 35[r-v]. [62] Ibid. fo. 35[v].
[63] Felicity Heal, *Hospitality in Early Modern England* (Oxford: Clarendon Press, 1990).
[64] Martin, *The Woman in the Body*.
[65] Raynalde, *Byrth* (1545), fos. 44[v], 45[r]. More generally, see Patricia Crawford, 'Attitudes to Men-struation in 17th-c. England', *Past & Present*, 91 (1981), 47–73.

anatomy and of conception, he makes mothers more important than fathers. These sections of the book do not come from the German original. He inserted them into the 1545 text and they remained in all subsequent London editions of the book, making the English version of this work significantly different from its Continental cousins. Raynalde's new section included pictures taken from Vesalius's groundbreaking anatomical text published two years earlier. His text, however, is a much more detailed discussion of female reproductive anatomy than that provided by Vesalius. He appears to have adapted parts of Berengario da Carpi's lengthy commentary on Mundino to construct his discussion of female anatomy.[66]

Raynalde's anatomical borrowings made his book much more positive about the roles of mothers than was the work's German original. As he says at the beginning of his anatomy section,

and allthough that man, be as principall moovar and cause of the generation: yet (no displeasure to men) the woman dothe confer and contribute much more, what to the encreasement of the child in her wombe and what to the nourisshement thereof after the birth, then doth the man.[67]

He continues by rhetorically showing the male reader how to assent. He says that if a man would ask to whom the child owes most in his generation, 'ye may wuurthely make answere that, to the mother'. Again, all this positive valuation of the maternal contribution to a child is new in the English version of this book—these sections are not in the German or Latin editions, and the German edition presents negative views of midwives and mothers.

The abilities of the maternal body are nothing short of amazing in Raynalde's account. It is as if the wonder and mystery of Jesus' Incarnation is dimly echoed in every conception. The womb is a marvellous structure, for in a non-pregnant woman it is tiny, but grows huge to contain the fetus. As Raynalde puts it, the womb

which in wemen being not with child is but very litel, contract and drawen together, so that the amplitude or largenesse therof, passith not the amplitude and largenes of the privy passage, the which thing to sum may seme uncredible, yet by annathomy ye may se it to be true.[68]

The non-pregnant womb was so tiny because it was carefully pleated or folded, 'full of rivelles or wrinkles', but it was so marvellously made that a body may

---

[66] Jacopo Berengario da Carpi, *Carpi Commentaria cum amplissimis additionibus super Anatomia Mundini una cum textu ejusdem in pristinum & verum nitorem redacto* (Bononiae, Impressum per Hieronymum de Benedictis, 1521). I cannot be certain that this is the source for Raynalde's anatomy, but it is the closest match. Many thanks to Pamela Long and Christine Ruggere for help on this point.

[67] Raynalde, *Byrth* (1545), fo. 1ʳ.   [68] Ibid. fo. 10ᵛ.

'scarce perceive in this innerside any wrinkle (all be it there be infinite) they be so finely and nere drawen together'. The non-pregnant womb was tiny not just for reasons of space or economy. Men's seed was very small in quantity, and the small size of the womb 'embracid' and 'contained' the tiny amount of seed so that it could be 'vivified'.[69] The wonders of the womb have a purpose, which is making seed into life.

Raynalde's text was composed in a variety of contexts and read in yet others. I am not arguing that we should understand Raynalde as 'Catholic' or 'Protestant' per se; after all, his text was made up of two nominally 'Catholic' predecessors, Mundino and the 1513 German text. Rather, I wish to call attention to the ways in which writings about the mechanics of conception and pregnancy had religious connotations in England in the 1540s. Raynalde's work looks back as well as forward. In its valorization of the miraculous qualities of women's bodies (drawn from Mundino) it fits well with the late medieval popular religious practices that made connections between Mary's miraculous motherhood and ordinary women's experiences of pregnancy and childbirth. In its refusal to adopt its German predecessor's misogynist views of midwives— indeed, of all women—Raynalde's text creates an alternative to some of the hardening of gender roles characteristic of the Continental Reformations.[70] Nonetheless, his prologue (like that of Richard Jonas) suggests that he was no stranger to reformed religion.

Two years after Raynalde's book was published, Henry VIII died and his 9-year-old son Edward succeeded him. The realm lurched forward into further religious reforms. English clerics like John Hooper returned from their Continental exile, and the tide turned the other way as European reformers no longer welcome in their own lands fled to a safe haven in England. Others were recruited by Thomas Cranmer, the Archbishop of Canterbury. Martin Bucer, the renowned Strasburg reformer, was named Regius Professor of Theology at Cambridge while the Italian Peter Martyr Vermigli occupied the equivalent chair at Oxford. By 1550 the pendulum had swung too far, and even reformers like Hooper were worried by the array of diverse beliefs flourishing in London. Hooper wrote to his Zurich mentor Heinrich Bullinger complaining about the 'Anabaptists' who came to his sermons, and a specific church for foreigners was set up in London, as a way of containing and regulating some of the wilder fringes of the exile community.

It is difficult to identify exactly to whom Hooper was referring when he complained about 'Anabaptists'. The term was often used to denote a range of

---

[69] Raynalde, *Byrth* (1545), fos. 11^r, 11^v.
[70] Lyndal Roper, *The Holy Household: Women and Morals in Reformation Augsburg* (Oxford: Clarendon Press, 1989).

unacceptable religious beliefs and social practices. However, he told Bullinger what worried him about these Anabaptists, saying that they 'give me much trouble with their opinions respecting the incarnation of the Lord; for they deny altogether that Christ was born of the virgin Mary according to the flesh'.[71] He was so troubled by this belief that he wrote a sermon on the topic, published by none other than Thomas Raynalde.

Historians have often understood Hooper's sermon as prompted by these unnamed Anabaptists.[72] Trouble lay a good deal closer to home, however. It was not just foreign-born Anabaptism that made the Incarnation a politically contentious topic. Hooper dated his sermon 20 June 1549. A few months earlier, a woman named Joan Bocher had been tried before Archbishop Cranmer and condemned to death on a single item of heresy:

that you beleve that the worde was made flesshe in the virgins Belly But that Christ toke flesshe of the Virgin you beleve not because the flesshe of the Virgin being the owtwarde man was sinfully gotton, and born in Sinne. But the worde by the consent of the inwarde man of the virgin was made flesshe.[73]

By the time that Joan Bocher found herself in front of Cranmer in 1549, she had a long history of unorthodox belief and trouble with the authorities. In the 1520s, she had been living in Steeple Bumpstead, a village well known for its long history of Lollard beliefs. Lollards supposedly gathered for meetings in her home.[74] Bocher also caused comment by conspicuously breaking the Easter fast by sharing a calf's head with two men on Holy Saturday, in 1540 or 1541. In 1541, evidently she was called up by a church court in Canterbury, suspected of heretical beliefs about the nature of the Eucharist. Given her Lollard connections, and her acquaintance with reformers such as the parson of Hothfield (who called the Virgin Mary an empty saffron bag), she had had ample opportunity to develop such views. It was rumoured that she had already been forced to abjure heretical beliefs in Colchester some years earlier. In 1542 she was up before the court again, but, brandishing a pardon, she was set free. In the following year Thomas Cranmer, Archbishop of Canterbury, himself commented on her deposition, taken in another sweep against heretics in Kent,

---

[71] Hooper to Bullinger, 25 June 1549, in *Original Letters Relative to the English Reformation*, trans. and ed. Hastings Robinson, for the Parker Society (Cambridge: Cambridge University Press, 1846), i. 65. Hooper complained that the Anabaptists also did not believe in Original Sin.

[72] E. W. Hunt, *The Life and Times of John Hooper (c.1500–1555), Bishop of Gloucester* (Lewiston, NY: Edward Mellen Press, 1992), 99–100.

[73] Davis, 'Joan of Kent', 232, quoting Cranmer's register, fo. 75ʳ, at Lambeth Palace Library.

[74] *Letters and Papers*, iv, pt. 3, 4242(3), 4850. The most detailed account of Bocher is now C. J. Clement, *Religious Radicalism in England, 1535–1565* (Carlisle: Published for Rutherford House by Paternoster Press, 1997). Unfortunately, I only became acquainted with Clement's work after completing this chapter.

writing 'offensive' in the margin. She had said that matins and evensong were no better than the 'rumbling of tubs', echoing a common complaint of reformers that preaching, not just services, was needed.[75] In the next few years, Joan Bocher risked danger repeatedly, becoming an agent for distributing William Tyndale's forbidden New Testament in English. Perhaps later hagiographers made up this detail, but supposedly Bocher tied forbidden books with strings and hid them under her skirts, even carrying them to the royal court, where she met Ann Askew, soon to be condemned as a heretic herself.

Joan Bocher's beliefs about the nature of the Incarnation have come down to us because she was a cause célèbre. Cranmer's recent biographer suggests that the moving of heresy trials behind closed doors may have been due to the sensation caused by her public trial, held in the Lady Chapel at St Pauls.[76] In addition to John Hooper, the reformers Hugh Latimer and Roger Hutchinson preached about her. After her execution, a small pamphlet in verse attempted to persuade the masses of the error of her ways. Edmund Becke, author of the pamphlet, called her 'the devil's eldest doughter' and 'the wayward Virago', calling up the most negative stereotypes of womanhood to blacken her reputation.[77] After the trial she was kept in jail for over a year in the hopes that she would change her mind, and young Edward VI was supposed to have been loath to sign her death warrant. Cranmer and Nicholas Ridley, both reformers, had her brought to their houses a few days before her execution in hopes of persuading her to recant.

Bocher's beliefs, for which she was burnt at the stake on 2 May 1550, were powerful. While he was preaching at Grimsthorp Castle in Lincolnshire, the home of his patron the Dowager Duchess of Suffolk, Hugh Latimer said that Bocher believed that the son of God penetrated through the Virgin Mary, taking no substance of her, 'as a light passes through glass'. Latimer was careful to label Bocher as 'foolish', and told his hearers that 'she could shew no reason why she should believe so'. He was attacking a broad range of beliefs about Mary in these sermons, both radical ones like Bocher's, and traditional ones. For instance, he devoted a good portion of the previous sermon to denying a vernacular belief that the Virgin Mary went on to have more sons with Joseph after Christ was born.[78] Latimer's vehemence about Marian

---

[75] *Letters and Papers*, xviii, pt. 2, 312–14, 359.

[76] Diarmaid MacCulloch, *Thomas Cranmer: A Life* (New Haven: Yale University Press, 1996), 424. My understanding of Bocher owes much to MacCulloch's careful parsing of the layers of meanings attributed to her execution. On the publicity attending Bocher's trial and execution, see Clement, *Religious Radicalism*, 58–9.

[77] Edmund Becke, *A Brefe Confutation of this Most Destestable, and Anabaptistical Opinion* (Imprinted at London by John Day dwellynge over Aldersgate, and William seres dwellynge in Peter College, 1550), STC2 1709. Quotes, unnumbered 1.

[78] Hugh Latimer, *Sermons and Remains of Hugh Latimer*, ed. George Elwes Corrie, for the Parker Society (Cambridge: Cambridge University Press, 1845), ii. 114. Latimer clearly says that he has

beliefs is all the more striking when we recall that he was preaching to a female patron.

Despite Latimer's attempts to paint them so, Bocher's beliefs were not foolish. Roger Hutchinson, another Protestant reformer, records a conversation that he and Thomas Lever and others had with Bocher about the Incarnation. He spends a page and a half specifically disputing her views, and the better part of the chapter on the larger topic of the Incarnation. According to Hutchinson, Bocher had a sophisticated view of the conception of Christ. She did not deny that he was Mary's seed, but averred that Mary had two kinds of seed, one natural or corporeal, the other spiritual or heavenly. It is from this second, non-bodily seed that Bocher said Mary conceived Christ. Christ was born from Mary's 'faith and belief', not from her sinful human flesh. Hutchinson went on to condemn Bocher as 'the eldest and firstborn daughter of the antichrist'.[79] We cannot know how Bocher developed her complex views about the Incarnation. Perhaps she read Continental Anabaptists who espoused similar views, perhaps she was recounting some older Lollard view not often seen, or perhaps she developed these ideas from her own intense and careful reading of the Bible. Her last words were 'Go, read the Scriptures'.

Bocher did not hesitate to tell the Archbishop of Canterbury that he would come around to her way of seeing things if he read Scripture carefully. After she was condemned, she said to Cranmer:

It was not long ago since you burned Anne Ascue for a piece of bread, and yet came yourselves soon after to believe and profess the same doctrine for which you burned her. And now forsooth you will needs to burn me for a piece of flesh, and in the end you will come to believe this also, when you have read the scriptures and understood them.[80]

Bocher was an astute observer. One of the troubling aspects of her ideas about the Incarnation was the way that doubts about the nature of Christ's body at conception seemed to resound with problems about the nature of his body in the sacrament of the Eucharist. In 1546 Ann Askew had been executed for denying that the Eucharist was literally Christ's body and blood. A year or so later, Cranmer too came to believe that Christ's literal body was not in the bread and wine. His path to this change of heart was complex, but it seems that

preached about Joan before, saying 'I told you, the last time, of Joan of Kent'. The previous Grimsthorp sermon does address the issue of the Incarnation, but in its printed version does not mention Joan of Kent.

[79] *The Works of Roger Hutchinson*, ed. John Brice, for the Parker Society (Cambridge: Cambridge University Press, 1847), 146–7.

[80] Strype, *Ecclesiastical Memorials*, ii, pt. 1, 335; Robert Parsons, *The VVarn-vvord to Sir Francis Hastinges Wast-vvord* ([Antwerp: Printed by A. Conincx] Permissu superiorum, Anno 1602), STC2 19418, 496–7.

his ally Nicholas Ridley, soon to be Bishop of London, was crucial to this shift. Ridley had been reading Ratramnus of Corbie, a ninth-century monk, in whose writings he had found support for a less literal reading of the words of the consecration, 'this is my body'.[81] Ratramnus was published in English translation in London in 1548 by none other than Thomas Raynalde, the printer of *The Byrth of Mankind*.

The various glimpses of Joan Bocher afforded to us in the historical sources, usually hostile or sometimes hagiographical, suggest a tough-minded and independent woman who did not avoid trouble. Eating a calf's head on Holy Saturday was a provocative act, one she must have known would not remain a private or personal matter. Smuggling English testaments under her skirts was courting danger. From the scraps of debate preserved in Latimer's and Hutchinson's accounts of her, we can see someone reasoning carefully, and articulating her positions with precision. Even after her death, she remained in the memory of Londoners.[82]

Critics of Bocher's beliefs used the same images and metaphors about conception that Raynalde did, although sometimes to different ends. In his sermon on her, John Hooper carefully refuted her understanding of the Incarnation, using citations from the Old and New Testaments, and then countering several specific objections. The care with which he refutes these detailed objections suggests that he had had several arguments with so-called 'anabaptists'. Hooper's primary method of argument is textual: he repeatedly exhorts his readers to look in the Bible themselves, and check the meanings of specific key words or phrases, such as 'fruit of the belly' or 'seed'.[83] His instructions to read the Bible resonate with historical irony, for the Lollard tradition from which Bocher came emphasized reading the Bible in the vernacular, and Bocher's last words were an injunction to go and read the Scriptures. English men and women had only been able to read the Bible in English legally since the accession of Edward, with a brief earlier period under Henry VIII. Lollards had treasured their illegal manuscript copies of parts of the Bible, and memorized large portions of the New Testament. Hooper's instructions to perform an analysis of biblical language were themselves the result of a historical process that produced Bocher as well.

Becke's verse pamphlet reads like a cheap knock-off of Hooper's sermon: it follows the same order and uses some of the same examples, albeit in greatly

---

[81] Peter Brooks, *Thomas Cranmer's Doctrine of the Eucharist*, 2nd edn. (London: Macmillan, 1992); MacCulloch, *Cranmer*, 354–5; 378–93.

[82] Clement notes that Bocher was considered a martyr by the English Familists. Clement, *Religious Radicalism*, 331, 335.

[83] John Hooper, *A Lesson of thee Incarnation of Christe* ([Imprinted at Londo[n]: In Paules Church yearde, at the signe of the Starre. By Thomas Raynalde, M. D. L.] [1550]), STC 13762, sig. Aiiiiᵛ.

abbreviated form. One of the images of conception that he, Hooper, and others shared was that of a lead pipe carrying water. Hooper advises:

> Where so ever ye finde this word, thee sede of a woman in thee holye scripture, ye shall see alwayes it is taken for thee childe, and birthe that hathe of thee substaunce of his mother: and not for anye thinge that passethe thoroughe thee mother, as thee water passethe thoroughe a pipe.[84]

Becke used the same image, 'and not as water which runnes to a Condit, And passes thorowe a pipe', adding 'as the Divell nowe hath found it'.[85] He often invokes the Devil, making a livelier and less intellectual picture of the reasons for Bocher's heresy, and denying her position any legitimacy. Roger Hutchinson, in his popular book published in the same year, also described Bocher's error in plumbing terms, 'as water gusheth through a pipe or conduit'.[86] In all likelihood, Hutchinson and Hooper were drawing on a common source, perhaps a much older work, in their refutation of Bocher. This image of the pipe meant something very different to Raynalde. For him, water did not pass through a pipe untouched. He uses this image to describe how women's seed was made, a part of his larger valorization of women's roles in reproduction: 'For every thing that is liquid, as the seede is, receavith always a nature of the place, mine, or conduit by which it runneth and passeth.' He continues with a lesson on fluid dynamics, talking about how narrow lead pipes infuse much more lead into the water than do large ones. Then he uses the homely example of a little wine left overnight in a pewter or brass pot, which picks up the flavour of the pot.[87] For Raynalde, the way in which the tiny pipes or conduits inside a woman's body transform blood into seed are amazing: 'what greater wonder or miracle is there?' he asks.[88]

The other primary image of reproduction that Bocher's critics employed was that of a tree. In part, Hooper, Becke, and Hutchinson used the tree image because of the biblical referent of the tree or branch of Jesse foretold by the prophet Isaiah. As Hooper explained, the Bible did not say that Christ was grafted onto the root, but was of the same root. Every flower, he alleged, took its substance from the root of its tree, and he challenged his listeners: 'Shewe us the floure of an Orange to springe of an Oke.'[89] Becke used the same image of an orange springing from an oak, similarly as an expression of disbelief, just after explicating Isaiah's prophecy (Isaiah 11: 1):

[84] Hooper, *Lesson*, sig. Aiiii^v.
[85] Becke, *Confutation*, unnumbered 3.   [86] Hutchinson, *Works*, 145.
[87] Raynalde, *Byrth* (1545), fo. 22^{r-v}.
[88] Ibid. fo. 23^v. Here Raynalde is tracing the entire process by which food is made into blood, and then blood is made into seed, so he may be referring to male as well as female bodies, although the discussion is of female anatomy.   [89] Hooper, *Lesson*, sigs. Aviii^r (Jesse), Bii^{r-v}.

> From the rote of Jesse procede shall a bud
> And a flower of this rote, for so the prophet saies.
> This bud was Marye, of whose fleshe and bloud,
> Came Christe the flowre, my faith shalbe alwayes.[90]

As we shall see in Chapter 7, the idea that like produced like, or that a fruit always owed its parentage to the tree on which it was found, was not always a self-evident fact, and examples could be drawn from the Bible itself to suggest that inheritance was not always a simple transfer from generation to generation. For Bocher's critics, however, the tree and fruit analogy seemed to play on both biblical reference and common-sense understandings of reproduction. As Roger Hutchinson put it, 'are grapes gathered of thorns, or figs of apple trees?'[91]

The controversy over the Incarnation suggests one of the ways that conception, pregnancy, and childbirth were sites of contest before and during the early years of the Reformation. Whether we look at Lollard critiques of Marian birth practices, or at Bishop Shaxton's indictment of them, or the sensation caused by Joan Bocher's beliefs, we see how women's reproductive bodies were the material with which people fought battles of belief. In the context of the controversies about the Incarnation sketched above, Raynalde's text, like Hooper's, could be read as holding the line against the wilder shores of Anabaptist or other claims that Mary contributed nothing to the body of Jesus. In his borrowings from Mundino, Raynalde created a book that emphasized the materiality of the maternal body and its contributions to the fetus, an emphasis that came to have religious connotations in the later 1540s. John Hooper tried to make just such arguments about the nature of pregnancy in his sermon against Bocher, although he (not surprisingly) drew upon Scripture rather than medical writings.

Beliefs about the Incarnation and childbirth practices continued to be the target of reformers. In 1550, Nicholas Ridley, the Bishop of London, enquired whether anyone in his parishes 'teacheth and sayeth that Christ took no Flesh and Blood of the Blessed Virgin Mary?'[92] Many of Ridley's questions were drawn from the Royal Injunctions and Articles of 1547, but this question was not, prompted in part by the very public controversy over Joan Bocher.[93] In the following year, John Hooper, who had published the sermon on Bocher's beliefs, expounded on proper belief in his directions to the parishes in his new dioceses: 'Item, Christ in the substance of our nature took flesh of the

---

[90] Becke, *Confutation*, unnumbered 3.   [91] Hutchinson, *Works*, 145.
[92] *Visitation Articles*, ii. 233.
[93] The questions came from Cranmer's *sede vacante* visitors to the Diocese of Norwich in early 1550, and thus can be understood as responses to Kett's rebellion as well as to concerns about Anabaptist ideas about the Incarnation. See Diarmaid MacCulloch, *Tudor Church Militant: Edward VI and the Protestant Reformation* (London: Allen Lane, 1999), 96–9.

substance of the Virgin Mary without the seed of any man, like unto us in all things, except in sin.'[94] Hooper had just been made Bishop of Gloucester and Worcester, and, unlike most previous bishops, he had personal knowledge about childbed practices since he had married and had a daughter four years earlier.

Hooper continued to try to reform 'superstitious' childbed rituals. He enquired about 'beads, images, relics, or any other monuments of superstition', not only in parish churches, but also in private homes. He adapted Shaxton's query about midwives, asking:

Whether the midwives at the labor and birth of any child do use any prayers or invocations unto any saint, saving to God in Christ, for the deliverance of the woman; and whether they do use any salt, herbs, water, wax, cloths, girdles, or relics, or any other like thing or superstitious means, contrary to the word of God and the laws of the realm.[95]

He highlighted the importance of relying on God himself, not on the Virgin Mary or any other saints, and he created a virtual inventory of traditional helps in childbirth: 'salt, water, wax, cloths, girdles, or relics'. Fifteen years later, a midwife was asked to swear that she would use no 'sorcery or incantation' in childbirth, and that she would perform emergency baptisms properly, using 'pure and clean water, not any rose or damask water, or water made from any confection or mixture'.[96] The specificity with which she was required to swear about pure water suggests that Hooper may have been worried about more than just holy water. Perhaps newborns were honoured or welcomed using perfumed water, as would be an honoured guest.

Hooper's queries also suggest that birthing rooms were not insulated from religious conflict at the parish level. He specifically asked if any midwives refused to attend women whose religious beliefs they did not like, or refused to attend the wives of ministers. Again, this is a new question, not derived from earlier bishops' enquiries. It suggests that, if anything, bishops were increasingly worried about the religious politics of reproduction, and sought to ensure that reform happened in the home and in the birthing room. Hugh Latimer, who had preached about the errors of Joan Bocher, thought that midwives were the source of much trouble, preaching that they were 'the occasion of much superstition and dishonouring of God'. He specifically blamed midwives for

---

[94] *Visitation Articles*, ii. 272.

[95] Ibid. 285, 292. Hooper cannot be taken as typical, rather he represents the leading edge of reform. See D. G. Newcombe, 'John Hooper's Visitation and Examination of the Clergy in the Dioceses of Gloucester, 1551', in Beate A. Kümin (ed.), *Reformations Old and New: Essays on the Socioeconomic Impact of Religious Change ca. 1470–1630* (Brookfield, Vt.: Scolar Press, 1996), 57–70.

[96] John Strype, *Annals of the Reformation*, in *Strype's Works* (Oxford: Clarendon Press, 1822), ii. 242–3.

propagating Marian birth practices, 'when the women be travailing, and so in peril of their lives, they cause them to call upon our Lady, which no doubt is very idolatry'.[97] For Hooper and for Latimer, calling upon the Virgin Mary was wrong, since she could not intercede with God. Only prayers to God himself were appropriate.

This shift from Mary to Christ was also made in prayers intended for women's use. In 1548 Thomas Raynalde published a little book of prayers, including those for the sick, for women giving thanks after childbirth, and for a burial. The women's prayer was part of a shift in the ritual of churching, a transformation from a late medieval rite of purification to a Protestant one of thanksgiving.[98] Women were instructed to say that unless Christ had helped them in their labour, 'all womans helpe and al physick had been in vaine'.[99] This simple phrase represents a huge change. No longer were prayers to the Virgin, holy relics, the help of women friends, and the midwife of paramount importance. Even medicine itself—'physick'—was useless without Christ's intervention. Every traditional help was rendered secondary to prayers to Christ. Raynalde's prayer book emphasized a second strand of Protestant thinking about pregnancy. Women were to connect their suffering in child-birth, not with the Virgin Mary, but rather with Eve. In this prayer, the speaker tells the Lord that she acknowledges that He has 'justly' increased the pain and sorrow with which women bring forth children because of Eve's 'original trans-gression'.[100] As we shall see, this double replacement of Mary by Christ and by Eve becomes central to the prayers offered to women later in the century.

Worrying about what was happening in the birthing room was not the sole prerogative of reformers. When Henry VIII's daughter Mary succeeded

---

[97] *Visitation Articles*, ii. 292–3. Latimer, *Sermons and Remains*, 114. Latimer urged bishops to control midwives more closely.

[98] Edward VI's prayerbook, published in 1552, created a new ceremony of churching. The litera-ture on the ceremony is growing, although its focus is mostly on events after 1552. See Jeffrey Johnson, 'Recovering the Curse of Eve: John Donne's Churching Sermons', *Renaissance and Reformation*, NS 23 (1999), 61–71; Will Coster, 'Purity, Profanity, and Puritanism: The Churching of Women, 1500–1700', in W. J. Sheils and Diana Wood (eds.), *Women in the Church: Studies in Church History*, 27 (1990), 377–87; Adrian Wilson, 'The Ceremony of Childbirth and its Interpretation', in Valerie Fildes (ed.), *Women as Mothers in Early Modern England: Essays in Memory of Dorothy McLaren* (London: Routledge, 1990), 68–107; Peter Rushton, 'Purification or Social Control: Ideologies of Reproduction and the Churching of Women after Childbirth', in Eva Gamarnikow (ed.), *The Public and the Private* (London: Heinemann, 1983), 118–31; David Cressy, 'Purifications, Thanksgiving and the Churching of Women in Post-Reformation England', *Past & Present*, 141 (1993), 106–46, further developed in his *Birth, Marriage and Death: Ritual, Religion, and the Life-Cycle in Tudor and Stuart England* (Oxford: Oxford University Press, 1997), 197–229.

[99] *A Newe Boke, Conteyninge an Exhortacio[n] to the Sycke. The Sycke Mans Prayer. A Prayer With Thankes, at the Purification of Women. A Consolacion at Buryall* ([London: T. Raynold?], M. D. XLVIII), STC2 3363, sig. C1ʳ.

[100] *New Boke* (1548), sig. B6ʳ. I doubt that the prayer is original to this text, but have not yet found it in an earlier source.

Edward in 1553, England was abruptly returned to Catholicism. The
reforms of the past decade were reversed: churches were told to rebuild
their rood screens, to repurchase their vestments and plate, and to return
to saying Mass. Bishop Bonner, restored to his London diocese, tried to
ensure that his flock was behaving appropriately in 1554. Even more
concerned than Hooper about midwives and childbirth, he devoted six
separate queries to the topic. Midwives were supposed to be examined by
the bishop, and so Bonner asked if there were any unexamined midwives
or women who functioned as such. Like Hooper, he was worried about
midwives who refused care, either because of religious difference or because of
money.

Bonner then enquired about superstitious practices, but he had to make
much finer distinctions than had his reforming predecessors. Many practices
that Hooper had found 'superstitious' were perfectly acceptable to Bonner.
So Bonner asked if any midwife or woman 'do use or exercise any witchcraft,
charms, sorcery, invocations or prayers, other than such as be allowable,
and may stand with the laws and ordinances of the Catholic church?'[101] He was
creating a dividing line between magical practices that were superstitious or
dangerous and those that were 'allowable'. The Catholic Church continued
to encourage women in labour to make connections between themselves
and the Virgin Mary, by means of prayer and relics, outlawing only practices
labelled sorcery or witchcraft. In the later sixteenth and early seventeenth
centuries, recusant women continued to employ girdles of the Virgin,
wax amulets of the *agnus dei*, and other sacred objects to ensure successful
childbirth.[102]

Bonner also wanted to regulate baptism and churching, the service of
thanksgiving that new mothers performed after their month of lying-in as a
kind of ritual that restored them to customary life. He seemed especially
worried about deviant practices concerning churching, asking if any women
'by themselves or by sinister counsel have purified themselves after their own
devices and fantasies, not coming to church according to laudable custom'?[103]
Churching was a ritual that the most radical reformers disliked. Some said it
was too reminiscent of the Old Testament (and thus Jewish) practice of ritual
purification. Many women, however, seem to have followed the practice, even
under circumstances where they might have evaded it.[104] Bonner's concerns
with churching seem to have been part of his larger attempts to control reproductive rituals and practices. He ends his list of queries with a kind of blanket
question:

---

[101] *Visitation Articles*, ii. 356–7.   [102] Thomas, *Decline of Magic*, 73.
[103] *Visitation Articles*, ii. 357.   [104] Cressy, *Birth, Marriage and Death*, 197–229.

Whether there be any other disorder or evil behaviour concerning the said midwives or the women brought abed, or lying in childbed, or any other woman coming to the labour, or visiting the woman that so lieth in childbed; and whether the nurse attempt to do anything unlawfully?[105]

Bonner and Hooper disagreed about many aspects of religious practice, but they were united in their concern to ensure that birthing rooms were not sanctuaries for forbidden religious practices—even though they had different ideas about what some of those practices might be. The intensity of their unlikely shared concerns suggests that the politics of women's reproductive bodies represented an important battleground for religious differences.

Bonner's ascendency was brief. In 1558 Mary died and Elizabeth ascended the throne. England experienced the see-saw of religious practices yet again. Reformers banished remnants of the older religious practices and re-established a Protestant church. Bishops' concerns about birthing rooms gradually evolved away from material things—relics, girdles, and the like—to a more generalized worry about witchcraft and a specific focus on the words used in childbirth. However, concern about childbirth practices did not completely vanish, and bishops continued to worry about what might be happening in birthing rooms.

Nor did women in childbirth instantly abandon the charms, relics, and prayers on which their mothers had relied. Instead, a gradual process of accommodation and appropriation occurred. References to the Virgin Mary and relics—the two aspects of childbirth practices that most distressed Protestants—were banished fairly quickly, while deeper structures of thought and feeling changed but slowly. We can see both how specific practices were eradicated and how deeper structures persisted in a book called *The Monument of Matrones*. Published in 1582, the *Monument* was a compendium of religious writings intended for the 'simpler sort of women . . . all godlie and devout women readers'.[106] Thomas Bentley, its author and compiler, was clearly an advocate of the Elizabethan reformation. He dedicated the book to Queen Elizabeth in glowing terms. Although the book as a whole would have been fairly expensive, it was divided into seven 'lamps' or sections, which may have been sold individually; each has its own title page, and some copies of individual lamps survive. Lamp 5, which survives as a separate book, includes a whole

[105] *Visitation Articles*, ii. 356–7.
[106] Thomas Bentley, *The Monument of Matrones conteining seuen seuerall Lamps of Virginitie, or distinct treatises* ([London]: Printed by H. Denham, [1582]), STC 1892, sig. B1ʳ. See Colin B. Atkinson and William Stoneman, '"These Griping Greefes and Pinching Pangs": Attitudes to Childbirth in Thomas Bentley's *The Monument of Matrones* (1582)', *16th-c. Journal*, 21 (1990), 193–205; Colin B. and Jo B. Atkinson, 'The Identity and Life of Thomas Bentley, Compiler of *The Monument of Matrones*', *16th-c. Journal*, 31 (2001), 323–47.

section of prayers to be used in connection with childbirth. There are prayers to be said by the midwife, for the midwife, by the labouring woman, and by and for her attendants. There are prayers to be said for a woman dying in childbirth, or, as this book puts it in homely terms, 'when she is departing, and yeeldeth up the ghost'.[107] Bentley was careful to make his prayers sternly Protestant; readers were not supposed to confuse them with superstitious papist invocations or charms.

Bentley revises childbirth traditions in a number of ways. First, he does away with the Virgin Mary's role as intercessor, enjoining women to pray directly to Christ. He reproduces the prayer printed by Raynalde in 1548, transforming it from a prayer for churching women to one said during labour. The labouring woman is to say 'I am right well assured, that onlesse thou prosper my travell, all womans helpe, and all physicke is in vaine.'[108] Another prayer makes a specific comparison of the pains of childbirth with the suffering of Christ on the Cross.[109] The Virgin Mary is mentioned in passing only twice.[110] No longer are labouring women invited to compare their sufferings with those of the Virgin Mary at the Crucifixion. Rather, they are to identify with Christ. This new focus on Christ inverted late medieval customs. It was an attempt to erase the habits of identification with the Virgin by pregnant women that had been fostered by the Catholic Church. More deeply, it denied the sanctity accorded to feminine roles. No longer was Christ imagined as a nurturing mother, whose body might even produce milk. Instead, women were to imagine themselves as suffering like Christ on the Cross, rather than drawing upon images that made Christ like a woman or that valorized Mary's role as a mother.[111]

The Virgin Mary was replaced in this text in another very powerful way. The role of Eve in causing all women to suffer in childbirth is emphasized repeatedly. Where pregnant women once identified themselves with the Virgin by going to Mass, praying specifically to her, and wearing relics or sanctified objects related to her, now women were to identify with Eve instead. One prayer has the woman in labour saying that her pains are 'just reward for my manifold sins', and highlights the dual heritage of Genesis: men must work for

[107] Bentley, *Monument*, 148. All page references to Bentley refer to Lamp 5, unless otherwise specified.

[108] Ibid. 98. For other prayers that highlight the labouring woman's relation with God, rather than the Virgin, see 99, 101, 104, 107, 112. 'Travell' or travail was one of the most commonly used terms for labour.

[109] Ibid. 121–2.

[110] Ibid. 121–2. Like many others in this collection, this prayer may be considerably older than the 1580s.

[111] The classic analyses of the feminization of Christ are Caroline Walker Bynum, *Holy Feast and Holy Fast* (Berkeley: University of California Press, 1987), and her *Jesus as Mother: Studies in the Spirituality of the High Middle Ages* (Berkeley: University of California Press, 1992). As Bynum argues, representations of Christ as feminine were already on the wane before the Reformation.

a living and women must labour in pain. Another, for a woman in difficult labour, says 'and lo, it seemeth that thou for my sins hast shut up the dores of my wombe, and causeth the babe to stand still like to be stifled'.[112] Here women deserve suffering and are to understand it in relation to their own sinfulness. Rather than a beneficent Virgin Mary alleviating the pains of another woman, we have a punitive God who inflicts the sins of Eve upon all women.[113] Many of these prayers make a point of stating that God was right to visit the pains of childbirth on women. One says 'I mislike not this thy decree, but I acknowledge it to be holie, irreprehensible and good.'[114]

It is difficult to know how such prayers were used by women. One of the most striking aspects of Bentley's work is its powerful and detailed descriptions of women's pain: 'Surelie, O God, thou knowest my strength is not the strength of stons, neither is my flesh or bones made of brasse, or iron.' 'How long Lord shall my bowels thus sound like a harpe, my bones and sinews be racked asunder, and mine inward parts be thus greevouslie tormented for my sins?'[115] Although such details seem to resound with a kind of authenticity of women's bodily experiences, we cannot know how they were read and heard by women of various religious beliefs.

Elizabethan bishops likewise turned their attention to the forms of words used in childbirth. In 1571 Edmund Grindal asked if any in his York diocese used 'any charms or unlawful prayers, or invocations in Latin, or otherwise?', specifically referring to midwives. York was thought to be a place where the old religion lingered. Interestingly, Robert Horne, Bishop of Winchester, enquired about midwives in his articles for the remote Channel Islands, all too close to Catholic France. He asked if midwives 'use any other prayers invocations and ceremonies than are to be allowed by God's Word according to the ecclesiastical laws of the Church of England'?[116] Concern about Latin prayers was not confined to the remote corners of the land. In 1575, Matthew Parker, Archbishop of Canterbury, asked about charms and Latin prayers, echoing Grindal. Parker also emphasized midwives' civic responsibilities. He enquired whether they were asking unwed women in labour about the fathers of their children, so that the parish could extract child support.[117] Here midwives teetered between two stereotypes: the superstitious crone, muttering in Latin, and the hard-nosed torturer, extracting truth from suffering women.

Although Elizabethan bishops and Thomas Bentley emphasized the correct form of words rather than the use of relics, Bentley was not entirely silent on

---

[112] Bentley, *Monument*, 100, 113; see also 96.
[113] The replacement of New Testament figures by Old Testament ones was typical of late 16th-c. Protestantism. See Watt, *Cheap Print and Popular Piety*, 201.
[114] Bentley, *Monument*, 99, see also 100, 126.   [115] Ibid. 117, 115.
[116] Grindal: *Visitation Articles*, iii. 270; Horne: ibid. 221.   [117] Ibid. 383.

the topic of material goods. Lamp 7 of his book is a series of biographies of bib-lical and other historical women. One nameless woman is discussed at length: the New Testament woman who suffered from 'bloody issue', or vaginal bleed-ing, for twelve years. In Matthew, Mark, and Luke, it is described how she humbly reached out to touch just the hem of Jesus' garment and was healed. Bentley wants to make it very clear that the garment did not possess magical qualities: 'So her faith that she had in Christ and not any superstitious opinion that she had to attribute any vertue to his garment' caused her cure.[118]

Thomas Bentley's *Monument of Matrones* suggests some of the ways in which religious change was a process of accommodation and appropriation.[119] While reformers targeted specific 'superstitious' childbirth practices, older habits of mind were not so easily eradicated. Bentley's rejection of such prac-tices and his allegiance to the Elizabethan settlement is clear, but we can also see older patterns retained in his text. For example, he includes a number of prayers on topics that were in the old Sarum Missal, such as prayers for women whose husbands are soldiers, or are merchants away at sea, or imprisoned or persecuted.[120] While the *Monument* purged childbirth practices of any associa-tions with the Virgin Mary, the Virgin lingers in his text in a number of ways. Bentley plays with the idea of a virgin queen in terms reminiscent of those applied to the Virgin Mary, virgin yet mother. He refers to the Queen as 'the most naturall mother and noble nursse' of the Church of England, but then in the next clause highlights her status as a virgin. Later on the same page he refers to Jesus Christ as Elizabeth's 'sweet spouse', evoking an image of nuns married to the Lord.[121]

Nor do Bentley's prayers dispense with the wondrous and magical female reproductive body. While women are no longer encouraged to identify with the Virgin Mary, they still imagine their bodies in terms deriving from her

---

[118] Bentley, *Monument*, Lamp 7, 262.

[119] In adopting this gradual and accommodationist view, I am indebted to Watt, *Cheap Print and Popular Piety*; Robert Scribner, 'The Impact of the Reformation on Daily Life', in *Mensch und Objekt im Mittelalter und in der frühen Neuzeit: Leben, Alltag, Kultur* (Vienna: Verlag der Österreichischen Akademie der Wissenschaften, 1990), 315–43 (I owe this reference to the kindness of Kathleen Crowther-Heyck); Ronald Hutton, 'The English Reformation and the Evidence of Folklore', *Past & Present*, 148 (1995), 89–116. The first formulations of the revisionist account that emphasize the slowness of England's reformation are J. J. Scarisbrook, *The Reformation and the English People* (Oxford: Blackwell, 1984); Christopher Haigh, *Reformation and Resistance in Tudor Lancashire* (Cambridge: Cambridge University Press, 1975). See more recently Nicholas Tyacke (ed.), *England's Long Reformation 1500–1800* (London: University College Press, 1998).

[120] See e.g. prayers such as those for a wife whose husband is travelling (p. 76), gone to war (p. 79), on a merchant voyage (p. 85) or returning home (p. 89), or comes home from a voyage on a ship (p. 90).

[121] Bentley, *Monument*, 2 of Epistle. On the issue of Elizabeth's use of the image of the Virgin, see Helen Hackett, *Virgin Mother, Maiden Queen: Elizabeth I and the Cult of the Virgin Mary* (Basingstoke: Macmillan, 1995).

miraculous conception of Christ. He describes marital relations in wondrous terms: 'And thou, O sonne of God, which hast ordained the love of married folks to be a mysterie of a Wonderfull and heavenlie thing.'[122] The conception and development of a child are described in similar terms: 'Thine almightie wisedome and power is manifest unto us in all thy works, but most chieflie in the wonderfull worke of the forming of man, who of a marvellous small and loathsome substance, is made a living creature.'[123] Here the older ideas about the miraculous qualities of a woman's body, which transforms a bit of semen into a baby, are readjusted, so that the miraculous qualities are God's rather than the mother's, but the tone of wonder and mystery remains.

The final part of the *Monument of Matrones* is devoted to biographies of notable women (both good and bad) from the Bible and other antique sources. Here too, Bentley echoes older beliefs. Although his prayers rarely mention the Virgin Mary, sternly refusing to admit of any intercessor, he includes a biography of the Virgin. All the elements common to older primers reappear: the Annunciation, Mary's visit to Elizabeth, Joseph's doubts about his pregnant bride, etc. The emphasis of the biography is on Mary's experiences of pregnancy, inviting women to identify with the Virgin when they are pregnant or the mothers of young children.[124]

So on the one hand, traditional childbirth practices that especially smacked of papistry were attacked. Catholic recusants continued to employ girdles of the Virgin, the *agnus dei*, and other traditional forms of childbirth protection, but ordinary English post-Reformation women seem to have gradually abandoned these papist practices.[125] However, women still suffered in childbirth and wanted all the help they could obtain, so other supernatural means came to the fore. Many of these practices were mentioned in books of secrets, compendia of all kinds of miscellaneous practical knowledge.[126] We cannot know if women learnt about them from such books, or if such books recorded women's

---

[122] Bentley, *Monument*, 51.

[123] Ibid. 101. In another version of this prayer, similar language stresses the miraculous qualities of conception and development: 'Of how small beginning dooest thou make so marvellous a living thing' (p. 104). See also a prayer in verse, 'and yet we find / No marvell nor no wonder such, as dailie forming of man-kinde' (p. 105).

[124] Bentley, *Monument*, Lamp 7, 197–200. There is considerable debate about the roles of women in the Reformation; some historians claim that women were among the most fervent Protestants; others that they were among the most devoted recusants. Perhaps both are true, given the ways in which men's and women's devotional lives were structured by gender roles and responsibilities. See Patricia Crawford, *Women and Religion in England, 1500–1720* (London: Routledge, 1993), for a very helpful overview, and Mendelson and Crawford, *Women in Early Modern England*, 225–31, for a thought-provoking discussion of the ways in which religion was gendered.

[125] Thomas, *Decline of Magic*, 73.

[126] William Eamon, *Science and the Secrets of Nature: Books of Secrets in Medieval and Early Modern Culture* (Princeton: Princeton University Press, 1994).

extant practices. Probably the process was two-way, with customs and practices circulating between books and birthing rooms. These practices were authorized very differently than earlier ones related to the Virgin. Belief in items in a book of secrets was not a matter of religious faith. Rather, the authenticity of such items was underwritten by many citations of ancient and medieval writers.

Thomas Lupton's 1579 *Book of a Thousand Things* includes many childbirth remedies and much else. It is a compendium of classical authorities, medieval writers, Renaissance books of secrets, and remedies told to Lupton personally, all arranged in individual bite-sized items. For a woman in labour, Lupton recommends ingesting the herbs vervain, dittany, or a complex mixture including the early modern cure-all theriac. He also suggests a number of things that can be tied to the outside of the body, in processes reminiscent of tying the girdle of the Virgin around the belly of a labouring woman. A woman could wear a snakeskin around her belly. Presumably this was a sympathetic remedy, and the woman would shed the baby as easily as a snake shed its skin. Gourd-root, oakfern, sage, or mugwort could be tied to the thigh or genitals of a woman in labour to speed the process.[127] However, these remedies had to be used very carefully. They were understood to work on the child by a sympathetic process, pulling the baby towards themselves. If the herb was not removed promptly after delivery, the woman risked losing her womb, as it too would be attracted downwards.

Lupton also recommends an eagle-stone for difficult labour. This was a small stone with another stone rattling around inside it. Dioscorides had described it as 'a stone with child'; such a stone mimicked a pregnant woman. It both protected pregnant women from miscarrying and hastened delivery for women in labour, because it had an attractive power for a fetus. If the stone was worn around the mother's neck, the fetus remained safely within her body protected from miscarriage. If tied to the mother's thigh, however, the stone exerted its sympathetic powers to draw the fetus downwards, thus hastening delivery. Like the herbal preparations Lupton recommended, the eagle-stone had to be removed promptly after labour lest the womb be pulled towards it. The eagle-stone was a powerful tool. Lupton said that it also promoted love between men and women, functioning as a sort of love magic, and that it could protect against poisoning.[128]

The eagle-stone seems to have grown in popularity in the seventeenth century. In 1633 the Countess of Newcastle was invited to wear one to ease the

[127] Thomas Lupton, *A Thousand Notable Things, of Sundry Sortes* (Imprinted at London: By Iohn Charlewood, for Hughe Spooner, dwelling in Lumbardstreete at the signe of the Cradle, [1579]), STC 16955: vervain, 62; dittany, 12; theriac, 146; snakeskin, 86; gourd, 93; oakfern, 193; sage, 168; mugwort, 181.   [128] Ibid. 38.

pains of labour.[129] John Bargrave bought an eagle-stone from an Armenian in Rome in the 1650s. When he returned to England at the Restoration and became a prebendary of Canterbury Cathedral, the stone was in the keeping of his wife Frances. She knitted a tiny bag for the walnut-sized eagle-stone and kept it in its own little box. Bargrave wrote: 'It is so useful that my wife can seldom keep it at home.'[130] He wanted to ensure that the stone remained the property of the Cathedral, recommending that in future the wife of the dean or the vice-dean keep the stone, and loan it out 'for the public good'. But she should take care to whom she loaned it; Bargrave wanted to be certain that everyone understood that 'it still be the Cathedral's stone'.[131] Although he may not have been aware of the historical ironies involved, his eagle-stone had taken the place of the relics and girdles of the Virgin loaned out by churches and monasteries before the Reformation.

By the 1650s, Nicholas Culpeper, author of best-selling popular health books, including one on midwifery, offered a veritable consumer's guide to eagle-stones. The best sort, he advised, came from Africa, and had been taken directly from an eagle's nest. Some thought that an eagle could not lay eggs without one. This type was female; there were also male eagle-stones that were red and hard and came from Arabia. Culpeper does not mention the sex of the third and fourth types, from Cyprus and Taphismus respectively. He explained that if a woman wore an eagle-stone around her neck, touching her skin, whilst she was pregnant, she would not miscarry. He instructed his readers that 'experience shal prove my words to be very true' and that the first thing a reader should do upon discovering his veracity was '1. Give glory and praise to God for it'. Next, 2. 'Admire his wonderful works in his Creatures'. The eagle-stone was not a saint's relic or an *agnus dei*, but Culpeper put it into a sacred context.[132] The detail with which he describes these stones suggests that they were relatively easily available, although he recognized that poor women would not have been able to afford one. He encouraged the rich to relieve the necessities of poor pregnant women, whatever they might be, warning that those who did not help others would have to account for their behaviour to 'the great God of Heaven'. When Jane Sharp borrowed these passages from Culpeper in her

[129] Thomas, *Decline of Magic*, 189.

[130] I am indebted to Trish Crawford for this rich story. Crawford, *Women and Religion*, 102. The original source is John Bargrave, *Pope Alexander the Seventh and the College of Cardinals, with a Catalog of Dr. Bargrave's Museum* (London: printed for the Camden Society, vol. 92, 1867), 125.

[131] Bargrave, *Pope Alexander*, 126.

[132] Nicholas Culpeper, *A Directory for Midvvives* (London: Printed by Peter Cole, at the sign of the Printing-Press in Cornhill, near the Royal Exchange, 1651), Thomason E.1340 [1], 151–3. His categorization of the four types of eagle-stone ultimately goes back to Pliny's *Natural History*. Pliny locates Taphismus between Ithaca and Cape Leucas. However, he does not describe the stones as sexed.

1671 midwifery guide, she emphasized community obligations between rich and poor more than religious duty.[133]

Culpeper's descriptions of eagle-stones derive from classical natural history texts but also represent a kind of blending of various traditions. The use of a material object tied to the body of a labouring woman to aid safe delivery derives its power both from late medieval customs involving amulets and relics and from the sixteenth- and seventeenth-century fascination with exotic curiosities and wonders.[134] Culpeper offered a large array of helps during child-birth in addition to the eagle-stone: the snakeskin Lupton mentioned, an ass's hoof or a piece of red coral hung near the labouring woman's genitals, a lode-stone in her left hand, etc.[135] The ancient remedies of the eagle-stone and the snakeskin thus came to function as replacements for the *agnus dei*, the girdles of the Virgin, and countless other sacred objects no longer countenanced by religious authorities.

I have argued that women's reproductive bodies were an important topic through which aspects of the Protestant Reformation were realized, however imperfectly. Because late medieval pregnancy and childbirth were understood in deeply religious terms, changes in one part of the equation—religion—meant changes in the other. The corporeal emphasis of late medieval Christianity, especially in terms of devotional practices, was very difficult to change. In particular, patterns of Marian devotion ran very deep, so deep that reformers like John Hooper and Hugh Latimer found themselves preaching on topics such as the details of conception or the question of how many children the Virgin Mary eventually bore. As always, practices changed more quickly than did ideas and beliefs. Reformers were able to alter the customs and rituals women used to protect themselves in childbirth within a generation or so. Deeper attitudes about the processes of reproduction, however, changed more slowly. As we shall see in the next chapter, eventually the female reproductive body itself was disenchanted, stripped of some of its mystery and wonder.

---

[133] Culpeper, *Directory*, 153. Jane Sharp, *The Midwives Book, or the Whole Art of Midwifery Discovered Directing Childbearing Women How to Behave Themselves* (London: Simon Miller, 1671), Wing2 S2969B, 183–4.

[134] Lorraine Daston and Katharine Park, *Wonders and the Order of Nature, 1150–1750* (New York: Zone Books, 1998).

[135] Culpeper, *Directory*, 170–1. Culpeper stated that his remedies come from Mizaldus, one of the best-known books of secrets in early modern Europe, although never to my knowledge published in English.

2

The Womb Goes Bad

Early in the seventeenth century, vernacular ideas about the uterus changed dramatically. Once the womb had been a wonderful body part, capable of transforming male and female seed into a new being, and marvellous in its ability to grow from the size of a walnut into a vessel containing a full-term baby. This positive view of the womb was challenged by a much darker vision, propounded in vernacular texts from 1603. No longer was the womb the bringer of life; instead, it was the source of many of women's maladies. Neither view, positive nor negative, was new. Instead, as we shall see, the writers of popular texts borrowed different pieces of classical learning to bolster their interpretations of the nature of the womb. Both positive and negative readings of the capacities of the uterus were resources available to the writers and compilers of popular manuals. Their choices among those resources were shaped by larger cultural concerns about the nature of women and the meanings of motherhood.

This transformation of the womb can be understood as the next step in the process of reform discussed in the previous chapter. The womb had been considered marvellous in a context in which women were taught to connect their own pregnancies with that of the Virgin Mary. When women were no longer encouraged to identify with the Virgin, some of the miraculous connotations of conception and pregnancy faded. At the same time, a new kind of story about motherhood was being printed in a new kind of small cheap pamphlet. In the later sixteenth century printers began to churn out sensational stories about murders, witchcraft, and monsters, framed by a religious discourse that emphasized God's providence. Within such narratives, all kinds of disorder ran riot—mothers murdered their babies, fathers their sons, witches attacked their social betters and lavished maternal care on rats and toads—disorder barely contained by a godly ending in which evil was punished and social order restored.[1] Many of these pamphlets describe terrible mothers, offering readers a profoundly troubling picture of maternity. Such stories provide a context for

[1] My reading of these pamphlets has been shaped by the work of four scholars: Frances E. Dolan, *Dangerous Familiars: Representations of Domestic Crime in England, 1550–1700* (Ithaca: Cornell University Press, 1994) and Lena Cowen Orlin, *Private Matters and Public Culture in Post-Reformation England* (Ithaca: Cornell University Press, 1994) both provide gendered interpretations of domestic

understanding how the womb went bad, and help to counter any assumptions
that the bad womb was more rational or scientific than the good womb.

As we saw in the previous chapter, Thomas Raynalde emphasized the marvellous qualities of the womb and made it a key player in conception. The
vivifying properties of the womb and its forming faculties transformed the tiny
quantity of male and female seed into a new person—if the womb were so
inclined. In Thomas Bentley's Protestant prayer book of 1582, some of the
miraculous qualities of the womb were repeated. However, in a subtle shift,
the womb became less active in the creation of the baby. At times, Bentley
sounds almost like Raynalde in his descriptions of how a baby is made in the
womb. Like Raynalde, he uses the metaphor of a workshop to describe the
womb. However, the artisan is now God himself, not the womb. One prayer
explains:

O eternall God, which of the seed of man framest the living infant in the mothers
wombe, and nourishest the same congealed in bloud, that the flesh within the time of
ten moneths may take shape, drawing nourishment from the mother; we are all the
workmanship of thine hand.[2]

Bentley continues with a striking image that makes God the author of all
human bodies: 'in thy booke were all of our members written'.[3] Both these
images—God as the master of a workshop and God as a writer—move attention away from a female womb towards a male maker as the key to the development of a fetus. In this compilation of prayers, Bentley takes a further step
away from the constellation of beliefs and practices that connected pregnancy
and childbirth to the Virgin Mary. Not only does he reconfigure childbirth so
that women are taught to identify with Eve rather than the Virgin. He also
subtly shifts away from a depiction of the womb as powerful and wondrous, the
source of new people.

In Bentley's account, the womb becomes a kind of container, the site within
which God works the wonders of fetal development. Two decades later, a sensational event in London remade the womb as a dangerous organ, capable of
destroying life rather than nurturing it. In 1602, Mary Glover, the 14-year-old
daughter of a London shopkeeper, fell ill. Her throat swelled shut and she
could not eat, she was stricken dumb and blind, and she suffered terrifying fits.

---

murder narratives, while Peter Lake with Michael Questier, *The Antichrist's Lewd Hat* (New Haven:
Yale University Press, 2002) offers a reading of the genre of murder pamphlets that emphasizes their
religious framing and the cultural roles of inversion. Tessa Watt, *Cheap Print and Popular Piety*, first
called attention to the richness of cheap print for students of religion.

   [2] Bentley, *Monument of Matrones*, 131. Since Bentley is a compilation of prayers from different
sources, his prayers offer a variety of interpretations of conception and pregnancy. This is one of the
most forceful depictions of the womb as a container; for another example, see 102.
   [3] Ibid.

The Glovers brought in a series of eminent physicians, but they were unable to heal the girl. As the doctors failed to cure her, or even agree about a diagnosis, suspicions grew that the girl was possessed, the victim of witchcraft. It is as if two parallel sets of diagnostic possibilities existed simultaneously. The doctors argued about whether or not Glover suffered from a disease called 'suffocation of the mother', while many Londoners debated whether she was bewitched or suffered from a natural but puzzling ailment.[4]

There was plentiful evidence for either case. The precipitating event for Glover's illness was an episode with an older woman that was, as we shall see, typical of the stories told in cheap pamphlets about witchcraft. According to the doctor Stephen Bradwell, in late April 1602 Mary Glover annoyed an older woman named Elizabeth Jackson by claiming that she had been begging fraudulently. When Glover was sent to Jackson's house on an errand, Jackson berated her for some incident in which Glover had meddled with Jackson's daughter's clothing. A few days later, Jackson stopped by the Glovers' house and told Mary, who was drinking some posset, that she wanted to see her mother. When Mary replied that her mother was not at home, Jackson got angry at her. After Jackson left, Glover's throat swelled shut, and she could not drink her posset. Eighteen days of illness and fits ensued, during which she was unable to eat or drink, although her body showed none of the customary signs of fasting. She was so ill that her parents thought death was imminent, and had the passing bell tolled for her at the parish church. Jackson, seemingly in an attempt to improve relations with the Glovers, sent Mary an orange, a very choice and expensive piece of fruit. Mary seemed to respond well to the gift, smelling it and keeping it in her hand, but later that same day, the hand and that side of her body became paralysed and insensate. After some weeks, Mary's health improved, but when she saw Jackson in church (they lived and

---

[4] Michael MacDonald has edited and republished the chief printed and manuscript works about this case with a helpful introduction in which he unpacks the complex religious politics at play in this episode. Michael MacDonald, *Witchcraft and Hysteria in Elizabethan London: Edward Jorden and the Mary Glover Case* (London: Tavistock/Routledge, 1991), pp. ix–xiii, drawing largely on the account of one of the doctors in the case, Stephen Bradwell. The works are: John Swan, *A True and Briefe Report, of Mary Glouers Vexation, and of Her Deliuerance by the Meanes of Fastinge and Prayer* ([London?: n.p.], Imprinted, 1603), STC2 23517; Edward Jorden, *A Briefe Discourse of a Disease Called the Suffocation of the Mother. Written Vppon Occasion Which Hath Beene of Late Taken Thereby, to Suspect Possession of an Euill Spirit, or Some Such like Supernaturall Power* (London: printed by Iohn Windet, dwelling at the signe of the Crosse Keyes at Powles Wharfe, 1603), STC2 14790. 'Suffocation of the mother' does not imply that doctors thought Glover was a mother; 'mother' is a word for womb. 'Suffocation of the mother' or 'fits of the mother' was one of the most common English translations of the ailment called *passio hysterica* or *hysteria* in classical sources.

On hysteria, the classic history is Ilza Veith, *Hysteria: The History of a Disease* (Chicago: University of Chicago Press, 1965), but see Helen King, 'Once Upon a Text: The Hippocratic Origins of Hysteria', in Sander L. Gilman, Helen King, Roy Porter, G. S. Rousseau, and Elaine Showalter (eds.), *Hysteria beyond Freud* (Berkeley: University of California Press, 1993), 3–90, for crucial revision.

worshiped in the same parish), she fell into a series of terrible fits that precipitated a series of daily convulsions.[5]

These interactions between Mary Glover and Elizabeth Jackson were just the sort of small social dramas that formed a kernel around which layers of interpretation and discussion grew, sometimes resulting in suspicions or accusations of witchcraft.[6] From the 1560s on, cheap pamphlets were published describing various witchcraft cases, and so those who heard about Mary Glover's troubles had a fund of stories about witchcraft with which to interpret the situation. In 1579, for example, one Mother Staunton went to Richard Saunder's house to beg some yeast. She was refused, and after she left, the Saunder baby was taken vehemently sick. When its mother picked it up to comfort it, the baby's cradle eerily rocked by itself.[7] When Mother Staunton was refused 'diverse things' by Robert Petie's wife, the Petie baby was strangely sick for a week, and was thought to be near death.[8] We can see two elements of a grammar of witchcraft in these examples. First there is some kind of minor social unpleasantness, often involving a older woman. Second, a person connected to the old woman's opponent in the social scuffle becomes sick. The illness is of a bizarre or 'vehement' nature, and often the family despairs of the person's life.

A third element that pointed to witchcraft involved the behaviour of the older woman. She was heard to say threatening things against the sick person, statements that shaded into curses. Elizabeth Jackson had threatened Mary Glover with the words 'my daughter shall have clothes when thou art dead and rotten'. When Jackson heard the passing bell tolled for Glover, she boasted to a

---

[5] Bradwell's account of the case remained in manuscript. Since it was not printed, I rely upon it here for some details of the Glover story, but not to analyse the ways in which it uses the story for its own ends. Bradwell, in MacDonald, *Witchcraft*, 3–6.

[6] The literature on witchcraft is vast. My interpretation of the witchcraft elements in the Glover case has been shaped by those historians who focus on the circumstances leading up to an accusation, such as Robin Briggs, *Witches and Neighbors: The Social and Cultural Context of European Witchcraft* (New York: Viking, 1996).

[7] *A Detection of Damnable Driftes, practized by three witches arraigned at Chelmissford in Essex* (Imprinted at London for Edward White, at the little North-dore of Paules, [1579]), STC2 5115, sig. A7ᵛ. The witchcraft story most closely related in theme to that of Mary Glover was that of the witches of Warboys, a case in Huntingdonshire in 1589 in which young girls were seemingly possessed. However, the printed narrative of the case is longer than the 'cheap print' stories analysed here. *The Most Strange and Admirable Discouerie of the Three Witches of Warboys, Arraigned, Conuicted, and Executed at the Last Assises at Huntington, for the Bewitching of the Fiue Daughters of Robert Throckmorton Esquire* (London: Printed by the Widdowe Orwin, for Thomas Man, and Iohn Winington, and are to be solde in Paternoster Rowe, at the signe of the Talbot, 1593), STC2 25019. Some of the procedures for testing witchcraft in the Glover case are strongly reminiscent of those described in the Warboys case. For an analysis of the meanings of community in the Warboys case, see Anne Reiber DeWindt, 'Witchcraft and Conflicting Visions of the Ideal Village Community', *Journal of British Studies*, 34 (1995), 427–63. As in the previous chapter, I have slightly modernized spelling in quotations, silently changing y and j to i where needed.   [8] *Damnable Driftes*, sig. A8ʳ.

neighbour that 'I thank my God he hath heard my prayer, and stopped the mouth and tied the tongue of one of mine enemies'.[9] Women charged with witchcraft were often described as uttering such threats. Mother Nokes, accused in the same wave of Essex accusations as Mother Staunton, insulted a tailor's wife by suggesting that she had committed adultery. When the woman protested, Mother Nokes said 'thou hast a Nurse childe but thou shalte not keepe it long', and the baby soon died.[10] When Mother Staunton was refused a small piece of leather by William Turnor's wife, Staunton asked Mrs Turnor an ominous question, 'how many children she had?' She answered one, and the young child was taken sick, 'and fell into suche shricking and staring, wringing and writhing of the bodie to and fro, that all that sawe it, were doubtfull of the life of it'.[11] In this period, utterances and written words might have magical powers, and a curse was understood as a kind of assault. Words could kill.[12] We will never know what Mother Staunton, Mother Nokes, or Elizabeth Jackson really said, or what they meant by their utterances. However, we can understand that the kind of threatening remarks allegedly made by these women might be interpreted within the frame of witchcraft, and that people who repeated these kinds of details saw them as evidence of maleficence.

Mary Glover's fits became more dramatic and intense, and rumours of witchcraft spread. Meanwhile, the doctors could not come to agreement or treat the illness successfully. So people began to test whether or not she was bewitched. They forced Elizabeth Jackson to come to her bedside and touch the girl. It sounds as though Glover's bedside was crowded with onlookers, curious to see if the girl was faking or if her derangement was truly supernatural. Michael MacDonald has unearthed a joke that circulated in London about this case, in which a gentlewoman had her pocket picked while praying at Glover's bedside. A wit replied, well, you forgot half your lesson: Christ bade us watch and pray, and you prayed only. Had you watched as well you would not have lost your purse! The currency of this joke suggests that the case had become a spectacle. London's authorities began to intervene. The bishop of London, Richard Bancroft, directed the city's chief legal officer, John Croke, to perform an extraordinary series of experiments to determine the true cause of Glover's illness. For example, he had another woman disguised as Jackson approach Glover's bedside. Glover did not respond. Next, Croke tested the genuineness of the fits by assessing whether or not Glover felt pain. Croke put

---

[9] Bradwell, in MacDonald, *Witchcraft*, 3, 4.   [10] *Damnable Drifies*, sig. B2^r.

[11] Ibid. sig. A8^r.

[12] On 'witch-speak' see Kirila Stavreva, 'Fighting Words: Witch-Speak in Late Elizabethan Docu-Fiction', *Journal of Medieval and Early Modern Studies*, 30 (2000), 309–38, esp. 312–17. On the powers of cursing, see Thomas, *Decline of Magic*, 502–12.

a hot pin to her cheek, and burned her hand, but she remained impassive, seemingly insensible of pain.[13] These tests were similar to those applied to witches, who were thought to have insensible spots on their bodies. In both cases, insensibility was abnormal and showed that the supernatural was involved. However, these tests also made Glover into a kind of odd double to a witch, a kind of mirror image. Indeed, her insensibility was highlighted by an unusual test for Jackson, whose hand was burned in the same manner as was Glover's. When Jackson could not abide the pain, Croke scolded her for accusing Glover of imposture.

After these dramatic tests, Jackson was formally accused of witchcraft and remanded for trial. At the trial, two doctors, Edward Jorden and John Argent, argued that Glover's illness was natural, although they were unable to make a specific diagnosis. The jury heard testimony about the tests that Croke had done, saw Glover confront Jackson, and heard Jackson repeat the Lord's Prayer and the Creed incorrectly. The judge, Sir Edmund Anderson, was not impressed by the medical evidence, and instructed the jury about the evils of witchcraft and the many points of evidence against Jackson. The jury found her guilty and she was sentenced to the maximum penalty, namely to stand in the pillory several times and be imprisoned for a year.[14] However, powerful officials were not persuaded, and it seems that Jackson was not punished and may have received a royal pardon.[15]

Mary Glover's fits continued unabated. About two weeks after the trial, a group of Puritans gathered around her and attempted to exorcize the evil spirit they thought was bewitching her. They prayed and fasted, and the girl's fits grew more and more intense; evidently the devil who possessed her put up a good fight. After hours of struggle, Glover was cured. As Michael MacDonald has reconstructed, the ritual of exorcism was highly contested at the turn of the seventeenth century. The Anglican church had condemned the ceremony, deeming it idolatrous and extra-biblical. However, there was plenty of demand for exorcism as people continued to suffer from bizarre or intractable illnesses, and Catholic priests performed a number of spectacular and well-publicized exorcisms. In response, Protestants combed their Bibles and devised an acceptable form of exorcism, which became increasingly associated with Puritans. Two very well-known Puritan exorcists were tried in London in 1599, accused of fraudulent practices. Supporters and accusers published a series of pamphlets about the case, the final one appearing in 1602. So Glover's fits and the conflict over the correct interpretation of them occurred in a context in which these issues were already the subject of considerable heated debate.[16]

[13] MacDonald, *Witchcraft*, pp. xiii–xiv.   [14] Bradwell, in MacDonald, *Witchcraft*, 22–30.
[15] MacDonald, *Witchcraft*, pp. xviii–xix.   [16] Ibid. pp. xix–xxvi.

Edward Jorden, one of the two physicians whose testimony at Jackson's trial was not believed, tried to have the last word by publishing a pamphlet in 1603 about the ailment known as 'fits of the mother'. Jorden's pamphlet is only twenty-seven pages long, and on the title page he makes it clear to the reader that this is no ordinary medical text, but 'written uppon occasion which hath beene late taken thereby, to suspect possession of an evill spirit'.[17] Although he does not name Glover explicitly, it would have been clear to anyone who had heard about the case that he was arguing that she had suffered from fits of the mother.

Jorden's account of the womb is profoundly negative. The opening lines of his text make women the sicker sex: 'The passive condition of womankind is subject unto more diseases and other sortes and natures then men are: and especially in regarde of that part from whence this disease which we speake of doth arise.'[18] Right at the beginning, he links the social status of women—their 'passive condition'—with their imperfect bodies and their troublesome wombs. The womb is subject to more ailments than other parts of the body because it suffers both from illnesses pertaining to it and from those in other parts of the body that communicate with the womb.[19] Jorden cites Hippocrates for these negative views. Hippocrates had been cited for positive views by Raynalde, such as his wonder at the way the womb closes itself after conception. These opposite uses of classical authority are typical of vernacular medical writing. Both positive and negative views of women's bodies could be found in ancient learning, and an individual writer's choice was shaped by the particular circumstances of writing.

The womb was a dangerous organ for at least two reasons, according to Jorden. First, it was intimately connected with other important organs of the body, by direct and by sympathetic links. Second, it was an active organ that could cause trouble in other parts of the body. If the womb found itself 'anoyed by some unkind humor' it 'endevoreth to expell that which is offensive'. If for any reason the womb was not functioning properly, 'the offense is communicated from thence to the rest of the body'. He went on to describe the function of the three principal organs of the body, the liver, heart, and brain, and showed how problems in the womb disrupted their usual actions.[20]

Jorden's description of the function of the womb is startling. The first function is to excrete. The preservation of the entire body is accomplished only by

[17] Jorden, *Briefe Discourse*. MacDonald suggested that Jorden's pamphlet was little read in its own day, although subsequent historians have seen it as significant. Given the substantial interest in the case, and the brevity of Jorden's text, the readership may have been broader than MacDonald believes. Although Jorden cites many scholarly authorities, he writes in clear prose and gives colourful examples of other cases. John Windet published a number of short devotional or advice manuals intended for broad audiences.
[18] Ibid. fo. 1r.　　[19] Ibid.　　[20] Ibid. fo. 6r.

the womb's ability to rid the body of the 'superfluities which abound in that sex'. Jorden puts the womb's reproductive functions second, acknowledging that it is the place where a baby is conceived and nourished 'untill it be able to appear in the world'.[21] Here, the womb is merely the space within which a baby matures, a space usually given over to excretion. The capacity of the womb to nourish a baby was also problematic. Jorden explains that the veins and arteries of the womb are large, in order to nourish the baby, 'But this provision of nature is oftentimes defective.' The womb's ability to feed a fetus is potentially dangerous to the mother. Jorden retells the story of a woman who accidentally cut a vein in her leg, whereupon the loss of blood provoked fits of the mother because the womb struggled to retain or acquire sufficient blood to nourish any possible fetus. A moist and nourishing diet restored her to health, but the underlying message of the tale was that the womb's reproductive faculties might endanger a woman's life.[22] Female seed and retained menstrual blood were the sources of other dire problems. As Jorden explains, seed is a perfect substance—but when that perfection decays, 'it passeth all the humors of our bodie, in venom and malignitie'. Just in case any reader failed to understand, Jorden then compares the decayed seed to the venom of a snake or a mad dog.[23] Compared with the vision of the womb described in the last chapter, Jorden's depiction was dire. No longer was the womb wonderful, capable of making a new person. Now it was a kind of sink, draining the superfluities of the body in menstrual blood. Its only wondrous qualities lay in the havoc it could wreak upon the female body. As we shall see, Jorden's text can be understood in a larger context where motherhood itself came to be portrayed in negative and dangerous terms.

Jorden's pamphlet was not a dry exposition of physiological facts. It was enlivened by a series of scary and dramatic stories about wombs gone wrong. For example, he recounts a story from the Dutch writer Peter van Forrest, in which a 22-year-old woman suffered from fits of the mother:

which held her many houres together with such violent horrible accidents, as he never sawe the like: her whole body being pulled to and fro with convulsive motions, her belly sometimes lifted up, and sometimes depressed, a roaring noise heard within her, with crying and howling a distortion of her armes and handes; insomuch as those about her thought her to be possessed with a divell.[24]

[21] Jorden, *Briefe Discourse*, fo. 7[r].

[22] Ibid. fo. 19[r]. This folio is marked 17, but it is really 19.   [23] Ibid. fo. 20[r].

[24] Ibid. fo. 4[v]. Jorden probably took the story from Pieter van Forrest, *Observationum et Curationum Medicinalium Liber Vigesimusoctavus, De Mulierum Morbis. Una cum scholiis* ([Lugduni Batavorum] Ex Officina Plantiniana, apud Christophorum Raphelengium, 1599).

Jorden made a cunning choice in telling this story. Not only was it scary and dramatic, but it also echoed many of the key symptoms of the Glover case. However, the precipitating cause of the young Dutchwoman's affliction was her own will: she had fallen in love with a young man. Perhaps, Jorden hinted, Glover's will was implicated in her case as well. Forrest was more fortunate than Jorden: he cured his young patient in a short time.

Even more frightening than these depictions of young women seemingly tortured by their faulty wombs are the tales Jorden told about the threat of being buried alive. Because of the womb's connection to the heart, the pulse might slow down, and the woman become 'the very image of death'. Jorden warns that the body could lie like a dead corpse for hours or days, devoid of sense, motion, breath, heat, 'or any signe of life at all'.[25] He cites a number of authorities about the length of time that families should wait before burying an apparently dead woman, noting that three days was usual. However, he adds, there was a case where a woman lay for seven days as if dead and was then restored to life, and then mentions a six-day case, rendering his three-day advice troubling.[26] Jorden concludes a whole litany of these cases with what he tells the reader is 'the most pitifull example of all other in this kinde', taken from the French surgeon Ambroise Paré. The sixteenth-century anatomist Vesalius began to dissect the body of a Spanish gentle-woman. At the second cut, 'she cried out, and stirred her limbs', and came back to life.[27]

Jorden's profoundly pessimistic view of the womb, and thus of female physiology in general, became a much more general perspective when it was incorporated into popular midwifery and gynecological manuals. Although Raynalde was reprinted up to 1654, two works of the 1630s provided readers with a very different view of female reproductive physiology that incorporated Jorden's more pessimistic perspective. In 1636 John Sadler, a Norwich physician, published a small book called *The Sicke Woman's Private Looking-Glasse*. This book does not discuss childbearing, but focuses on the many ills to which women's reproductive systems were prone. Sadler hoped that women, who, he claimed, were often too ignorant or too modest to tell their physicians about their ailments, would read his book and be better able to recount their troubles to a medical man.[28] The following year, a German work, *The Expert Midwife*

---

[25] Jorden, *Briefe Discourse*, fo. 9^{r-v}.   [26] Ibid. fo. 9^v.

[27] Ibid. fo. 11^r. This was also a cautionary tale for doctors. Jorden says that the young woman's physician was so remorseful that he went on a pilgrimage and died.

[28] John Sadler, *The Sicke-VVoman's Private Looking-Glasse* (London: Printed by Anne Griffin, for Philemon Stephens, and Christopher Merideth, at the Golden Lion in S. Pauls Church-yard, 1636), STC2 21544. In his dedicatory epistle, Sadler writes: 'Considering therefore the manifold distempers of the body, which yee Women are subject unto through your ignorance & modestie, I could not but do my best, to informe and advise you in the conservation of your own health.' Sig. A4^{r-v}.

by Jacob Rueff, was translated into English.[29] Sadler's work had drawn heavily on this text: Rueff, a Lutheran physician in Zurich, had published his book in both German and Latin back in 1554.[30] The identity of its English translator remains a mystery, but its publication was clearly linked to Sadler's book, since Rueff was published by Edward Griffin, the husband of Anne Griffin, who had published Sadler. Rueff had been available for translation into English for decades, but his negative vision of the womb seems to have resonated in England only after the turn of the century. Both Rueff's and Sadler's books are important not just in their own right, but because parts of these books were incorporated into many subsequent popular medical works.

Rueff and Sadler created a very different female body than that envisioned in Raynalde. Although traces of older ideas about wonder and mystery remain, the female body became a dangerous and unstable entity. In particular, the womb, formerly wondrous, was now a threat. Both texts introduced two themes into English popular medical manuals: the idea that the womb can threaten a woman's health and even her life, and a fascination with what happens when reproduction goes awry and monsters are produced. Both Sadler and Rueff drew on Hippocratic models of the female body, models that were newly available to Latin readers after the 1525 publication of the most important works of Hippocrates on the diseases of women.[31] In particular, both propounded a very negative view of the ways in which women's reproductive systems affected their entire bodies, and both offered a plethora of remedies for such ailments. Again, none of these themes were novel, but their appearance in how-to books intended for lay readers was new.

A female reader of Sadler's book might well be alarmed by the many troubles she could expect. As Sadler tells her in his introduction to the book,

When I had spent some meditations, and consulted with Galen and Hippocrates for my proceeding; amongst all diseases incident to the body, I found none more frequent, none more perilous then those which arise from the ill affected wombe: for through the evill quality thereof, the heart, the liver, and the braine are affected.[32]

---

[29] Jacob Rueff, *The Expert Midwife, or An Excellent and Most Necessary Treatise of the Generation and Birth of Man* (London: Printed by E. G[riffin] for S. B[urton] and are to be sold by Thomas Alchorn at the signe of the Greene Dragon in Saint Pauls church-yard, 1637), STC2 21442. Like similar texts, although the title suggests that the work is intended for women who work as midwives, the introduction makes clear that the book is intended for 'all grave and modest Matrons'.

[30] Jakob Rüff, *De Conceptu et Generatione Hominis, et iis quae circa hec potissimum* ([Zurich]: Christophorus Froschoverus excudebat Tiguri, anno M.D.LIIII. [1554]). On Rueff, see M. Dunn, 'Jacob Rueff (1550–1558) of Zurich and *The Expert Midwife*', *Archives of Disease in Childhood*, 85 (2001), 222–24; H. L. Houtzager, 'Jacob Rueff', *European Journal of Obstetrics, Gynecology, and Reproductive Biology*, 13 (1982), 105–7.

[31] Helen King, 'The Power of Paternity: The Father of Medicine Meets the Prince of Physicians', in David Cantor (ed.), *Reinventing Hippocrates* (Aldershot: Ashgate, 2002), 21–36, esp. 28–9.

[32] Sadler, *Looking-Glasse*, sig. A4ᵛ.

Just like Jorden, Sadler drew on classical authorities to link the womb with the three most important organs of the body—the brain, liver, and heart—with dire results for women's health. He went on to list the ailments that derived from the womb: 'from the wombe comes convulsions, epilepsies, apoplexies, palseyes, hecticke fevers, dropsies, malignant ulcers, and to bee short, there is no disease so ill but may procede from the evill quality of it'.[33] Sadler alluded to Hippocrates' aphorism that the womb was the source of all diseases that happen to women.

In particular, both Sadler and Rueff describe how fits of the mother were caused by the retention of the menses or of female seed, and detailing its dire consequences. The womb moved up towards the diaphragm, pressing upon it in a way that led to the cessation of breathing. As Sadler describes, 'whereby the body, being refrigerated, and the actions depraved, she falls to the ground as one being dead'.[34] Rueff puts it even more simply: 'there is no motion of the body, and indeed nothing else but a similitude of present death'.[35] Sadler cites a number of authorities, including Rueff, each more frightening that the last, and repeats the story about the Spanish woman coming to life on the dissecting table.[36] Sadler and Rueff detail the ways in which apparent death could be distinguished from the real thing, employing tests such as holding a mirror to the mouth and looking for moisture, or placing a feather on the lips and watching for movement.

These negative attitudes about the womb were incorporated into subsequent books about childbearing. For example, *The Compleat Midwifes Practice Enlarged*, first published in 1656, was a compilation of older texts about childbearing, including Rueff.[37] In its discussion of reproduction, the attitude

[33] Sadler, *Looking-Glasse*, sig. A5ʳ.   [34] Ibid. 62.
[35] Rueff, *Expert Midwife*, Bk. 6, ch. 8, p. 63. Pagination starts anew with book 6; unless specified, page references are to the first five books.
[36] Sadler, *Looking-Glasse*, 62–3. It is interesting that this story comes from Spain. I have seen very few examples of such willingness to dissect in England. Katharine Park has suggested that there were profound differences in attitudes to the dead body and autopsy in southern and northern Europe in the Middle Ages; stories such as these suggest that such a divide may have continued well into the early modern period. Katharine Park, 'The Life of the Corpse: Division and Dissection in Late Medieval Europe', *Journal of the History of Medicine and Allied Sciences*, 50 (1995), 111–32.
[37] *The Compleat Midwifes Practice, in the most weighty and high Concernments of the Birth of Man* (London: Printed for Nathaniel Brooke at the Angell in Cornhill, 1656), Wing2 C1817C; Thomason E.1588[3]. This text, whose authors are listed as 'T.C. I.D. M.S. T.B. Practitioners', is a compilation of works by Jacob Rueff and Louise Bourgeois, among others; libraries often catalogue it as being by Thomas Chamberlayne, but its authorship is disputed. See Doreen Evenden, *The Midwives of 17th-c. London* (Cambridge: Cambridge University Press, 1999). It was subsequently republished a number of times as *The Compleat Midwife's Practice Enlarged*. See also Nicholas Fontanus, *The Womans Doctour, Or, an Exact and Distinct Explanation of All Such Diseases as Are Peculiar to That Sex* (London: Printed for John Blague and Samuel Howes, and are to be sold at their shop in Popes Head-Alley, 1652), Wing2 F1418A, 51–60; Alessandro Massaria, *De Morbis Foemineis, the Womans Counsellour: Or, the Feminine Physitian* (London: printed for John Streater, and are to be sold by the booksellers in London, 1657), Wing2 M1028; Thomason E.1650[3], 72–9.

towards the womb was neutral or positive, with a few echoes of the wonderful qualities mentioned in earlier texts. For instance, one of the functions of the womb is 'to cherish the Seed thus attracted, to alter it, and change it into the Birth, by raising up that power which before lay sleeping in the Seed'.[38] This image of the womb is reminiscent of older ideas about the mother's body as hospitable, cherishing the fetus like a guest, as well as the idea that the womb has the power to transform seed into a new being. However, the same book includes an extensive section on the diseases of the womb, including tentigo, narrowness of the neck of the womb, condyloma, ulcers, four different kinds of 'intemperancy', puffing up of the womb, inflammation, scirrhus, dropsy, and many others, echoing Sadler and other writers who emphasized women's diseases. This new emphasis on the dangers of the womb undercut the more positive connotations in this text's discussion of reproduction.

Other 1650s discussions of the womb also lack the wondrous qualities emphasized by earlier books. In Raynalde's 1545 book, the substance of the womb was described as minutely pleated so that it could expand greatly when a woman was pregnant. The intricacy of this pleating was a cause for admiration. However, in books of the 1650s, these properties of the womb are no longer highlighted as admirable. In *The Compleat Midwifes Practice Enlarged*, the pleats of the womb are mentioned in passing: 'In this concavity there are certain folds, or orbicular pleights [*sic*]; these are made by a certain Tunicle so wrinkled, as if a man should fold the skin with his fingers.'[39] This image calls to mind a man assessing the quality of a fabric he might purchase, folding it between his fingers to feel its weight and texture, rather than minute pleats whose intricacy testified to God's amazing workmanship in the human body.

Rueff and Sadler portrayed women's bodies as dangerous in a second way: each discusses the production of monsters. The arrival of a profoundly deformed baby is always a deeply unsettling event that stretches a community's interpretive resources. As is well known, in the sixteenth century Martin Luther used two animal monsters, the 'monk-calf' and the 'Pope-ass', to represent the evils of the monastic life and the papacy. Other interpretative strategies focused on collective or individual sins. The monstrous child was an emblem of sinfulness, either of the community as a whole or of the

[38] *Compleat Midwifes Practice*, 40–1.
[39] Ibid. 27–8. See p. 45 for a discussion of the way in which the womb closes itself after conception that lacks any of the sense of wonder generated in earlier texts. The figure of speech—that the mouth closes itself so tightly that not even the point of a needle may penetrate it—is originally taken from Hippocrates. However, as with so much else in these texts, early modern writers could choose to represent bits of classical wisdom in ways that made women's bodies praiseworthy or objects of derision, shame, or disgust.

parents.[40] Or the child had been conceived during the mother's menstrual period, implying that she and/or her partner had been overcome by lust.[41]

Jacob Rueff describes the production of moles, lumps of flesh similar to monstrous births, but lacking a human form. He runs through a variety of explanations before coming to his preferred one. Some authors, he says, claim that moles are produced from the normal seed of man and woman that corrupts, or from the 'weakness and debility' of both the seeds, or from excessive menstrual blood 'congealed and clotted together' by the excessive heat of the womb. But those who 'more narrowly pry and search into the Natures of things' have a better explanation, Rueff avers. It is:

especially in those women which are somewhat more lascivious than others are . . . by desire of the Matrix [the womb], doe stirre up copious seede of their owne, which augmented with the flowers [menstrual blood], by the heat of the Matrix, is congealed together . . .[42]

The womb, because it is lusty, stirs up seed, blends it with menstrual blood, and a monstrous being is made.[43] Where the womb was previously wonderful because it turned a little bit of semen into a new person, here it becomes a more ambiguous organ. It is as if the womb mimicked the woman herself. The woman lacked control, being too lascivious—and the womb lacked the careful direction of the male seed, that 'proper contriver'.

When Rueff moves on to discuss monstrous births, he invokes older ideas about the judgement of God, but he does not leave the discussion there. Instead, he describes a variety of ways in which the mother's body might produce monstrosity. Both male and female seed may be weak or become corrupted. Conjoint births, what Rueff called two infants growing together, are due to 'terrours and affrightments, and also other evill chances' in which the children already conceived 'are squashed together' in the womb.[44] Babies with harelips, or with spots and marks, are due to a mother's fright or to her unsatisfied longings. A mark like a bunch of grapes, for example, results from a pregnant woman's unfulfilled craving for grapes. In his discussion of these kinds of deformity, Rueff emphasizes the role of the maternal body: it is the womb squashing two conceptions together, or a mother's fright or longing that

[40] The secondary literature on monstrosity is now extensive. See in particular Katharine Park and Lorraine Daston, 'Unnatural Conceptions: The Study of Monsters in 16th and 17th-c. France and England', *Past & Present*, 92 (1981), 20–54, and Daston and Park, *Wonders and the Order of Nature*, 173–214. On the maternal imagination and its relation to monstrous births, see Marie-Hélène Huet, *The Monstrous Imagination* (Cambridge, Mass.: Harvard University Press, 1993).

[41] Ottavia Niccoli, ' "Menstruum quasi Monstruum": Monstrous Births and Menstrual Taboo in the 16th c.', trans. Mary M. Gallucci, in Edward Muir and Guido Ruggiero (eds.), *Sex and Gender in Historical Perspective* (Baltimore: Johns Hopkins University Press, 1990), 1–25.

[42] Rueff, *Expert Midwife*, 139.

[43] Ibid. Here Rueff is following a classic Aristotelian model of conception.   [44] Ibid. 153–4.

produce monstrosity. However, when he describes the woodcuts he included of classic monsters, such as that born in Ravenna in 1512 or in Cracow in 1547, he uses the older framework of divine displeasure: these 'wee ascribe to God alone'.[45] A reader of this text could choose amongst these interpretations of the cause of monstrosity, perhaps making Rueff's text less negative about maternity than it appears at first glance.

Like Rueff, Sadler attributes monstrous births either to God or to natural causes, although he defines the role of God somewhat more narrowly. Divine causation, he says, 'proceeds from the permissive will of God, suffering parents to bring forth such abominations, for their filthie and corrupte affections which are let loose unto wickednesse'.[46] Sadler divides the natural causes of monstrosity into faults in the matter or in the agent. Faults in the matter result in babies with extra or missing parts. However, he does not explain why such faults might occur. He focuses instead on faults in the agent, by which he means the womb. As he says, 'The agent, or wombe may be at fault in three ways.'[47] The formative faculty of the womb may be too strong or too weak, creating deformity. Second, there may be an 'evill conformation' of the womb, resulting in a monstrous birth.[48] Third, a mother's imagination may mark the fetus. Sadler devotes most of his discussion of monsters to this third cause, retelling a number of classic tales, such as that of the white woman who gave birth to a black child due to the painting of a black person hanging in her bedroom.[49] As Marie-Hélène Huet has shown, the topic of the maternal imagination is rich and complex, and I discuss its further ramifications in Chapter 7. Here I merely wish to point out that Sadler places the blame for monstrosity on the mother. In the context of his book, which depicts the many ways in which the female body is dangerous and unstable, the attribution of monstrosity to the female becomes another instance of the transformation of the female body from the wondrous to the terrible.

Both Rueff and Sadler offer English readers a new way to think about the production of horribly deformed infants. Cheap-print pamphlets about monstrosity emphasize God's will rather than defects of the womb. For example, the minister John Hilliard includes a brief mention of a monstrous child in his pamphlet detailing a mysterious fire that consumed John Hitchell without any visible flames, and the burning of the godless town of Dorchester. Although he refuses to describe the form of the infant, he notes that it was born without lips, 'to teach us (as I suppose) that we want sanctified lippes to glorifie the powerfull name of our gratious God', and without an anus, to teach that 'the filth of

[45] Rueff, *Expert Midwife*, 157.   [46] Sadler, *Looking-Glasse*, 135.   [47] Ibid. 137.
[48] Ibid.   [49] Ibid. 138.

sin remaineth still within us because there wanteth true Repentance in us'. Nowhere does he mention the infant's mother; its birth resulted from collective, not individual, sin.[50]

A pamphlet about a monstrous birth in Kent strives to make a dubious mother blameless in the production of her deformed infant. It opens by setting the scene: the old and virtuous Mother Watts kindly took in a very pregnant young woman, who begged for help for God's sake and 'for womanhood sake'. The young woman went into labour, and could not be delivered by the group of women who come to help until the skilled midwife Goodwife Hatch arrived. The infant was 'strange & dreadful to behold', and indeed, the pamphlet includes two copies of a horrifying woodcut image of the baby (see Fig. 2.1).[51] Under these circumstances, it would have been very easy to blame the infant's shape on the sins of its mother. No decent woman would have been wandering around homeless, begging charity at such a time. Even if poor, a married woman would have had a circle of neighbours and acquaintances who could have offered assistance—or at least that is what the advice literature would have us believe.

Equally suspicious, the new mother vanished. She asked Mother Watts to go into town to get her the things necessary for a lying-in woman, giving her money for the purchases. Then she disappeared, leaving eight shillings beside the body of her now dead infant, for its burial. As the pamphlet emphasizes, 'it could not be knowne by any meanes what she was, from whence she came, nor whither she was going'.[52] The women who gathered to help this unfortunate, however, and the writer of the pamphlet, strove to avoid any easy moralizing about the mother's lack of virtue, saying of the birth, 'whether it were for the sinnes of the Parents, or that God would have his Justice, in the estranging of nature for our sinnes here shewen, let the wiser sort imagine'.[53] The pamphlet frames the story of the monster birth as a warning to all, rather than a condemnation of this mysterious mother.

The role of the supernatural, and thus the idea that the baby was the expression of God's direct will, is highlighted in the detail that the unfortunate mother offered before she fled, namely that 'this monster a little time before her delivery, moved in her belly, not like unto other naturall children, but as if shee had been possessed with an evill spirit'.[54] This detail, like so much else in this

[50] John Hilliard, *Fire from Heauen. Burning the body of one Iohn Hittchell* (Printed at London: [By E. Allde] for Iohn Trundle, and are to be sold at his shop in Barby can [*sic*] at the signe of Nobody, 1613), STC2 13507.3, sig. B8ᵛ.
[51] *Strange Nevves out of Kent, of a Monstrous and Misshapen Child, Borne in Olde Sandwitch, Vpon the 10. Of Iulie, Last, the like (For Strangenes) Hath Neuer Beene Seene* (Imprinted at London: By T. C[reede] for W. Barley, and are to be sold at his shop in Gratious-street, 1609), STC2 14934, sig. B1ʳ, B1ᵛ.   [52] Ibid. sig. B4ʳ.   [53] Ibid. sig. B1ᵛ.   [54] Ibid. sig. B3ʳ.

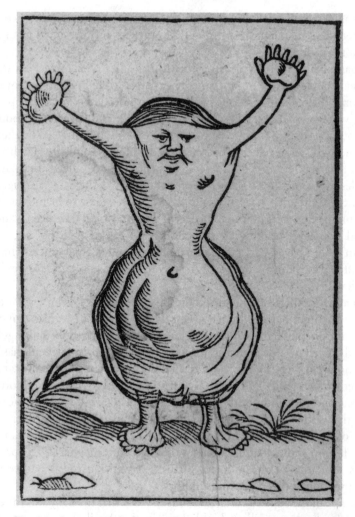

Fig. 2.1. A monster baby born in Kent. *Stranges Nevves out of Kent, of a Monstrous and Misshapen Child* (1609). Courtesy of the British Library, shelf mark C.31.b.16

weird story, makes the mother blameless and the infant the result of a super-natural or divine intervention. Again, it would have been very easy to make this into a story of a sinful mother, but instead the story suggests that the baby was emblematic of everyone's sin.[55] And in none of these tales was there any sug-gestion that the mother's womb might be at fault. It was only with Rueff and

[55] For other examples that make monster births signs of God's displeasure with a community or nation, see *Strange Newes of a Prodigious Monster, Borne in the Towneship of Adlington in the parish of*

Sadler that the womb became an agent in the production of monstrosity in cheap print.

In Jacob Rueff's midwifery manual, monstrosity was just one of the ways in which women's bodies were troubling. He also tells stories about abortion and witchcraft. He warns that the 'wicked Arts and policies of old Witches and Harlots' should be forbidden by magistrates, and then he tells a long story of a woman, 'deflowered' and 'robbed of her best Jewell', who discovers some alteration in her body. She feels sick with her accustomed meat and drink, vomits, swoons, and feels pains of the heart and teeth. At first, she tries to remedy the alteration by lacing her bodice tighter, so that she may 'extinguish and destroy' the fetus. When tight lacing does not restore her health, she proceeds to consult 'some old Witch', who prescribes a series of herbal remedies to restore menstrual regularity, and sends the woman to an apothecary for further medicaments. When these remedies do not work, the woman seeks to have blood let from her foot, 'which being done', says Rueff, 'that perisheth by and by which was conceived in the womb'.[56] This intervention, bloodletting from the saphenous vein in the foot, made logical sense in the seventeenth century, when men and women understood the human body in humoral terms. Bleeding from the foot encouraged the downward movement of blood throughout the body, thus provoking menstruation.[57]

Rueff worries that women such as these were profoundly deceitful. He continues by retelling his story from the point of view of the household, making the protagonist a domestic servant, the commonest occupation for a young woman in England. The master and mistress of the household begin to suspect pregnancy. But the now plural young women 'pretend and make a shew that they are troubled with wringings and gripings in the belly, with paines of the brest and head, and do shadow and dissemble the truth of the matter'. Once

---

Standish in the Countie of Lancaster, the 17. day of Aprill last, 1613 ([London]: Printed by I. P[indley] for S. M[an] and are to be sold at his shop in Pauls Church-yard at the signe of the Ball, 1613), STC2 15428; *Gods Handy-vvorke in VVonders. Miraculously Shewen Vpon Two Women Lately Deliuered of Two Monsters: with a Most Strange and Terrible Earth-quake, by Which, Fields and Other Grounds, Were Quite Remoued to Other Places* (London: Printed [by George Purslowe] for I. W[right], 1615), STC2 11926. Even a story about the incestuous relationship between cousins that produced a monster birth is couched in terms of the extent of sexual sins nationwide: I. R., *A Most Straunge, and True Discourse, of the Wonderfull Iudgement of God. Of a Monstrous, Deformed Infant, Begotten by Incestuous Copulation, Betweene the Brothers Sonne and the Sisters Daughter, Being Both Vnmarried Persons* (Imprinted at London: [By E. Allde] for Richard Iones, 1600), STC2 20575.

[56] Rueff, *Expert Midwife*, 59–61.

[57] See Angus McLaren, *Reproductive Rituals: The Perception of Fertility in England from the Sixteenth to the 19th c.* (London: Methuen, 1984), and Cressy, *Birth, Marriage and Death*, 48 for the argument that the knowledge of abortion was widespread in the female subculture of early modern England. John Riddle has argued more generally that effective knowledge of herbal remedies for contraceptive and abortifacient purposes was widespread in medieval and early modern Europe: John M. Riddle, *Contraception and Abortion from the Ancient World to the Renaissance* (Cambridge, Mass.: Harvard University Press, 1992).

such women get their periods again, 'when they know they are free', they compound their wickedness by sharing their knowledge with other women. As Rueff warns, 'they impart and communicate likewise those murthering arts and cruell practices to others' so that many infants are aborted. Rueff spends three full pages of his book worrying about such practices, and at the end of the discussion he seems to realize that he had been led astray, for he writes, 'Now let us returne to the matter', in other words, let us get back to the proper subject of the book.[58] Rueff's twice-told tale of abortion suggests how anxiety-provoking the secret nature of women's reproductive bodies might be. Men simply could not know if their potential child might be destroyed, nor was sexual immorality made apparent in unwanted pregnancies. His use of emotive words like 'witch' and 'harlot' to describe the women in his story points to the ways in which female sexuality might threaten social order, represented in his tale by the household, headed by master and mistress.

In Rueff's story, the woman consults other women, who advise her about a range of practices. None of these, however, is written down. All the discussions are oral, between women—and all of Rueff's tale, therefore, is imagined. His book, in which the tale is written, exemplifies the differences between women's and men's access to understandings of the female body. Women talked with other women—but men were no part of those conversations. The social practices surrounding childbirth emphasized the exclusion of men from women's knowledge. Well before a woman went into labour, she extended invitations to her closest female relatives, friends, and neighbours to support her through the birth. As many as a dozen women stayed with the labouring woman, trying to keep up her spirits by talking, telling jokes, and drinking a special kind of wine thickened with grain.[59] These hours of labour were dangerous and frightening, but the men excluded from the birthing room imagined the women telling jokes about sex, belittling men's performances and reputations. The women invited to the birth were called 'gossips', from which our modern use of the word to mean scandalous and intimate personal details is derived. By extension, the word 'gossips' was also used to describe the visitors to the new mother, who expected to be feasted to celebrate the new arrival.[60]

Popular books about women's bodies proclaim themselves to be written, at least in part, for women readers. However, few women in England in the first half of the seventeenth century could read—perhaps only one of every six, although such estimates are very crude. In their introductions, the books them-

---

[58] Rueff, *Expert Midwife*, 59–61.

[59] Wilson, 'The Ceremony of Childbirth and its Interpretation'; Cressy, *Birth, Marriage and Death*, 55–79.

[60] On gossips, see Cressy, *Birth, Marriage and Death*, 55–9, 84–7; Caroline Bicks, *Midwiving Subjects in Shakespeare's England* (Aldershot: Ashgate, 2003), esp. 27–9.

selves reveal the tensions implicit between male and female knowledge of the body. Although the books assert that they are written for women, they fret about potential male readers of the text.

For example, Thomas Raynalde worried about communicating the knowledge of women's bodies to men. He starts his preface to women readers by comparing the prologue to a menu, spoken aloud at the beginning of a banquet, to invite guests to partake of it. However, he explains the metaphor by referring to a male reader, saying: 'Likewise it is a great prick or allurement, entising and moving a man to reade any Book, when he is somewhat first admonished of the matters comprehended and contained therein.'[61] Here he alludes to the potential for male readers to be attracted to the book for the wrong reasons by using a metaphor 'prick or allurement' with sexual overtones. He switches back to a female implied reader a few pages later, telling her that the book will be the means 'to better understand how every thing cometh to passe within your bodies, in the time of conception, bearing, and birth'.[62] Later in the introduction, he worries that some of his critics will consider his book a dishonour to women. Men who read the book or heard it read aloud 'shalbe mooved thereby the moore to abhorre and loothe the company of Woomen' or 'to jeste and bourde of Wymens privitees'.[63] Raynalde hastens to defend his book, by noting that the wonders of the body can promote godly devotion, and adds that any item can be used for good or evil. He goes on to warn his reader than anyone who uses his book to speak irreverently of women's bodies does 'great injury, dishonor, and contumely to nature' herself, and is guilty of 'mortall and dedly sin'.[64] Almost half of his introduction is taken up with concerns about his book being read by lascivious or misguided men.

Jacques Guillemeau, whose French midwifery text was intended in part for young male surgeons, was translated into English in 1612 by a writer concerned with the potential impropriety of writing about women's bodies. The translator worries:

if I have been offensive to Women, in prostituting and divulging that, which they would not have come to open light, and which beside cannot be exprest in such modest termes, as are fit for the virginitie of pen & paper, and the white sheetes of their Child-bed.[65]

---

[61] Raynalde, *Byrth* (1545), sig. B1ʳ. Of course, this kind of framing device, in which an author attempts to discipline his/her reader in the introductory matter, also characterizes the cheap print pamphlets analysed below, and derives from medieval manuscript traditions.

[62] Ibid. sig. B2ʳ.

[63] Ibid. sig. C2ʳ. 'Bourd' is an archaic usage; it means to accost or make advances towards.

[64] Ibid. sig. C5ᵛ–6ʳ.

[65] Jacques Guillemeau, *Child-birth Or, the Happy Deliuerie of VVomen. VVherein Is Set Downe the Gouernment of Women. In the Time of Their Breeding Childe* (London: Printed by A. Hatfield, 1612), STC2 12496, sig. ¶¶2ᵛ.

This image, in which ink on white paper is metaphorically transposed into virginal blood on white sheets, suggests some of the multiple anxieties men had in talking about women's private parts in print. The translator defends himself by saying that he has tried to be 'private and retired' in the way he writes about women's bodies.[66]

Books about women's bodies, therefore, were often written in part for men. Women might learn from books, but more often learned from each other. These differences in male and female cultures only amplified men's concerns about the powerful and mysterious qualities of women's reproductive bodies. On the one hand, the generative qualities of women's bodies excited wonder and amazement. On the other, those same qualities provoked anxiety and concern, leading men to mutter about witches and harlots. When men imagined the hidden interiors of women's bodies, this same dichotomy of wonder and anxiety created powerful and bizarre images.

One of the underlying reasons for these male concerns about women's reproductive bodies was the widespread idea that women were much more desirous of sex than men. From joke-books to medical works, writers reiterated that women were lascivious, driven by physiological needs for sex that led to all kinds of immorality and disorder. In 1602 a small pamphlet was published in London called 'Well met Gossip: or, Tis Merry when Gossips meet'. It is a dialogue among a widow, a wife, and a maid or an unmarried woman. These three sit drinking in a tavern and discussing which of them has the best life (Fig. 2.2). The pamphlet reveals how men, who wrote and published it, imagined women's talk, and portrayed them as the lustier sex. The maid declares: 'I'le have a handsome Man, or none at all', and then goes on to describe what she wants:

> I'le have a comely Man from head to foot,
> In whose neat Limbs no blemish can be spied
> Whose Leg shall grace his Stocking or his Boot,
> And wear his Rapier Manly by his side.
> With such a one my humor doth agree
> He shall be welcome to my Bed and me.[67]

The knowing laughs from her companions make it clear just what sort of 'Manly Rapier' this young woman seeks. The widow urges the maid not to stay

---

[66] Guillemeau, *Child-birth*, sig. ¶¶3ʳ. The translator also defends himself by pointing out that Guillemeau himself wrote in the vernacular.

[67] Samuel Rowlands, *Tis Merrie VVhen Gossips Meete* (At London: Printed by W. W[hite] and are to be sold by George Loftus at the Golden Ball in Popeshead [*sic*] Alley, 1602), STC2 21409, sig. D4ᵛ. This work went through a number of editions up to 1675 under a variety of titles. Fig. 2.2. is taken from a later edition; Samuel Rowlands, *Well Met Gossip: Or, Tis Merrie When Gossips Meete*, (London: I. W. for I. Deane, 1619), STC2 21411.

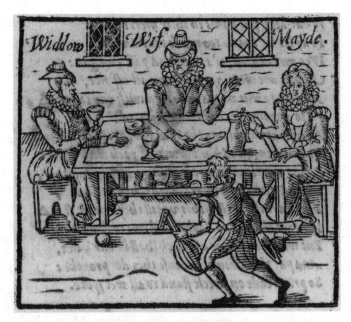

Fig. 2.2. Well-met Gossips: Samuel Rowlands' idea of women talking with other women about men. Samuel Rowlands, *Tis Merrie VVhen Gossips Meete* (1613). Courtesy of the Bodleian Library

single too long, saying 'I could not for a World have liv'd a Nun: Oh flesh is frail, we are a sinful sort.'[68] The consequences of women's sexual desires are made plain. The gossips laugh at men who are cuckolded by their wives. Often, cuckolds were depicted as growing horns on their foreheads, and these gossips joke about the men who, unknowingly, 'every night sleep in Horn work caps'.[69] Rowlands's description of gossips meeting in a tavern can be understood as a kind of lighter version of the scene in Rueff when the women servants confer with a witch about procuring abortions. Both stories reveal to us the ways in which men imagined women's reproductive knowledge as secret and powerful.

The remaking of the womb as a problematic or troubling body part is, as I have suggested, a part of the longer reform of the body. As most Englishmen and women came to think of themselves as Protestant, and no longer remembered their grandmothers and great-grandmothers' devotional practices that linked pregnancy with the Virgin Mary, eventually they came to adopt a new view of the female reproductive body that did not echo the divine. However, the gradual transformation of normative English religious practices is only part of the reason that the womb became dangerous. It might have become merely

---

[68] Rowlands, *Tis Merrie*, sig. C2ᵛ.   [69] Ibid. sig. C4ᵛ.

a container, just a kind of nourishing but largely inert space within the female body.

Instead, almost like the seed that Jorden described, the womb moved from being very good to very bad. Although Jorden may have tried to depict his view of the womb as scientific or rational, in contradiction to the supernatural beliefs held by Glover's prosecutors, a broader understanding of the meanings of the womb does not follow this trajectory of a move completely away from the supernatural. The new emphasis on the womb's bad qualities comes in part from a larger cultural shift in the meanings of motherhood. From the 1560s onwards, cheap print began depicting bad mothers in dramatic and sensational ways.[70] Stories of witches and infanticidal mothers depicted women, and mothers in particular, as dangerous figures. These narratives were the stuff of cheap print, tales of bad mothers written in simple language in small pamphlets accessible to readers and listeners alike. Many of these cases have been analysed by social historians interested in the dynamics of village life. Here I am not concerned with the truth of these sad stories or with the complex patterns of witchcraft accusations and confessions or with the relationship of witchcraft pamphlets to actual accusations and trials. Real witches, in other words, matter less to my analysis than the stories told about witches. My emphasis is on the repeated patterns in these stories, patterns that tell us something about ideas on motherhood that were available to a large proportion of the population.[71] These stories of terrible mothers are inversions of the commonly accepted models of good mothers emblematized in religious tracts and the like, and as we shall see, their transgressions are managed textually by encasing their gory

[70] For other studies that suggest a turn towards portrayals of mothers as dangerous, see Janet Adelman, *Suffocating Mothers: Fantasies of Maternal Origin in Shakespeare's Plays, 'Hamlet' to 'The Tempest'* (London: Routledge, 1992); Mary Beth Rose, 'Where Are the Mothers in Shakespeare? Options for Gender Representation in the English Renaissance', *Shakespeare Quarterly*, 42 (1991), 291–314; Diane Willis, *Malevolent Nurture: Witch-Hunting and Maternal Power in Early Modern England* (Ithaca: Cornell University Press, 1995). These studies employ a broad range of genres, usually including Shakespeare's plays. My focus is on the texts that circulated very widely, more widely than most canonical literature, although as Peter Lake points out, theatre performances in London might be considered akin to cheap print in the breadth of audience they reached, albeit a breadth limited to London. Lake, *Antichrist's Lewd Hat*, pp. xix–xxii.

[71] On witchcraft as narrative, see Jonathan Barry, 'Introduction: Keith Thomas and the Problem of Witchcraft', in Jonathan Barry, Marianne Hester, and Gareth Roberts (eds.), *Witchcraft in Early Modern Europe* (Cambridge: Cambridge University Press, 1996), 1–45. Both Diane Purkiss and Lyndal Roper have explored a different aspect of witchcraft as narrative, looking at the ways that the stories witches tell are important fictions whose concerns tell us much about the social and cultural worlds these women inhabited. Diane Purkiss, 'Women's Stories of Witchcraft in Early Modern England: The House, the Body, the Child', *Gender and History*, 7 (1995), 408–32, which is incorporated into her larger study, *The Witch in History* (London: Routledge, 1996); Lyndal Roper, *Oedipus and the Devil* (London: Routledge, 1994). For the evolution of generic types of witchcraft pamphlets, see Marion Gibson, *Reading Witchcraft: Stories of Early English Witches* (London: Routledge, 1999). On infanticide narratives, see Dolan, *Dangerous Familiars*, 121–70.

acts within a religious frame.[72] Usually, these errant women repent and accept their fates on the last page before they are executed.

For us, the crimes of infanticide and witchcraft are different. Infanticide is a real crime, that is, we still understand it as a criminal act and prosecute it today, while witchcraft is not a crime but instead a marker of an 'unenlightened' past. However, as we shall see, these two kinds of deviance were not understood as categorically different in early modern England. The cheap pamphlets that describe these sensational crimes share crucial sets of references.[73] At times, the crimes blur into each other; a witch and a murdering mother are each tempted by the devil into their wicked ways. At others, these two kinds of dangerous women function as opposites, either end of a spectrum in which a good mother might occupy the centre. Witches can be understood as excessively maternal towards their familiars, the small magical animals that supposedly did their bidding, while murdering mothers were insufficiently maternal towards their offspring. In both kinds of pamphlets, motherhood in all its depraved varieties is described in intensely bodily terms, with a near obsession with blood and milk.[74]

Murdering mothers and witches intersected in the harm they caused to children. They also resembled each other in their links to the supernatural. Witches, of course, were defined by their ability to tap into the powers of

[72] These stories of bad mothers are the dark twins of another emerging genre about maternity, namely, the mother's posthumous blessing to her children. See e.g. Dorothy Leigh, *The Mothers Blessing. Or the Godly Counsaile of a Gentle-woman Not Long since Deceased* (Printed at London: For Iohn Budge, and are to be sold at the great South-dore of Paules, and at Brittaines Burse, 1616), STC2 15402. (This work went into at least fifteen editions to 1729.) Elizabeth Joceline, *The Mother's Legacie to her Vnborne Childe* (London: Printed by Iohn Hauiland, for William Barret, 1624), STC2 14624. (This work went into at least eight editions to 1724.)

[73] What follows is based on a reading of all the shorter pamphlets about witchcraft and infanticide from the 1550s to 1637. Although a number of scholarly works on demonology and witchcraft were published in this period, they were large and expensive books. Most witchcraft pamphlets are fifty pages or fewer, while infanticide ones are even shorter, usually about twenty pages. Although I highlight certain cases in what follows, I allude to other examples in the footnotes. Not all infanticides were women (just as not all accused of witchcraft were female), although stories told about killing babies or very young children usually focus on mothers as killers. In cheap print, men who killed their children tended to kill older children or adults, as in *Newes from Perin in Cornwall* (London: Printed by E.A[llde] and are to be solde at Christ-Church gate, 1618), STC2 19614. Exceptions include *Sundrye strange and inhumaine murthers* (Printed at London: By Thomas Scarlet, 1591), STC2 18286.5, although here the killing is done by a hired hit-man; and *Two Most Vnnaturall and Bloodie Murthers* (Printed at London: By V. S[immes] for Nathanael Butter dwelling in Paules churchyard neere Saint Austens gate, 1605), STC2 18288.

[74] Stuart Clark has analysed how the 'inversionary thinking' central to witchcraft contained a contradiction, namely, that as each good or worthy aspect of culture was defined by its opposite, it was also constantly under threat of being destabilized by that opposite. While Clark focuses on a much broader range of discourses about the nature of witchcraft than I do, his insights into the instabilities produced in these patterns of thought is very relevant to this analysis of cheap print. Stuart Clark, *Thinking with Demons: The Idea of Witchcraft in Early Modern Europe* (Oxford: Clarendon Press, 1997), esp. pt. 1, pp. 1–147.

darkness. Many of the witches in cheap print had familiars. Ursley Kempe, for example, confessed to having four familiars in 1582. She specified that it was Pigen, a black toad, who harmed Annis Leatherdell's baby.[75] Joan Prentice was accused of witchcraft in Chelmsford in 1589. One night when she was in bed in the almshouse where she lived, the devil appeared to her in the shape of a dun-coloured ferret with fiery eyes. The ferret said that he would do her bidding. Some while later, Prentice went begging to the home of the Glascocks. Master and mistress being out, the maidservant refused to give her any alms. Later that night, Prentice told her ferret to nip one of Glascock's children. When the ferret returned from its errand, it informed Prentice that young Sara Glascock would die. Prentice told her examiners that she scolded the ferret, reminding it that she had only asked it to nip a child, not kill it. The ferret went off in a huff, never to be seen again.[76]

Murdering mothers were also connected to the supernatural. Margaret Vincent, for example, was described as bewitched by the devil. She killed her two children because she and her husband had feuded over her conversion to Catholicism, which he refused to emulate, and she thought that her children were damned because they were being reared as Protestants. The reader is warned to consider 'how strangely the Divell here set in his foote, and what cunning instruments hee used in his assaylements'. Vincent was 'converted to a blinde beliefe of bewitching heresie' by some 'close Papists'. Both the devil and the papists seem to be agents of the supernatural here. Vincent is portrayed as nearly blameless: 'hardly the female kinde can escape their inticements'.[77] The picture of Vincent on the title page shows a large devil offering her the cords with which she strangles her children, and perhaps even the executioner's rope that will kill her (see Fig. 2.3). Vincent's story ends with her remorse and execution, and again she is shown as nearly blameless. The reader is told: 'Forgive and forget her good Gentlewomen. Shee is the not first that hath beene blemished with blood, nor the last that will make a husband wifelesse, her offense was begot by a strange occasion.' Were it not for 'Popish perswa-

---

[75] W. W., *A True and Iust Recorde, of the Information, Examination and Confession of All the Witches, Taken at S. Ofes in the Countie of Essex: Whereof Some Were Executed, and Other Some Entreated According to the Determination of Lawe* (Imprinted in London: At the three Cranes in the Vinetree by Thomas Dawson, 1582), STC2 24922, sig. A8ʳ. On the larger topic of familiars, see James Serpell, 'Guardian Spirits or Demonic Pets: The Concept of the Witch's Familiar in Early Modern England, 1530–1712', in Angela Creager and William Chester Jordan (eds.), *The Animal/Human Boundary: Historical Perspectives* (Rochester: University of Rochester Press, 2002), 157–90.

[76] *The Apprehension and Confession of Three Notorious Witches. Arreigned and by iustice condemned and executed at Chelmes-forde, in the Countye of Essex, the 5. day of Iulye, last past. 1589.* ([London]: E. Allde, 1589]), STC2 5114, sig. B1ʳ–2ᵛ.

[77] *A Pittilesse Mother. That Most Vnnaturally at One Time, Murthered Two of Her Owne Children at Acton Within Six Miles from London Vppon Holy Thursday Last 1616.* ([London]: Printed [by G. Eld] for J. Trundle, and sold by J. Wright, [1616]]), STC2 24757, sig. A2ʳ. See also sig. B1ᵛ, where Vincent is described as the victim of 'a witchcraft begot by hell'.

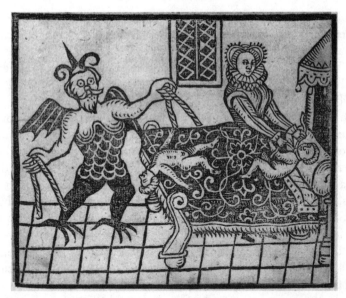

Fig. 2.3. An infanticidal mother tempted by the devil. *A Pittilesse Mother.
That Most Vnnaturally at One Time, Murthered Two of her Owne Children*
(1616). Courtesy of the British Library, shelf mark 1077.i.20

sions' and the work of the devil, the writer assures his readers, Vincent would
have carried the name of virtue even to her grave.[78]

Elizabeth Barnes, a poor woman who murdered her 8-year-old daughter,
was similarly described as a victim of 'diabolicall seduction'. After the murder,
the devil tempted her to throw herself into a pond and drown herself, but she
resisted. The minister who spoke with her in jail told his readers that she
thought her crime was due solely to the devil's temptation.[79]

Vincent and Barnes were not typical of the women tried for infanticide in
this period. Most who were prosecuted were single women whose newborn
children had been found dead, perhaps stillborn, perhaps killed at birth by
intention or neglect. Married women were given the benefit of the doubt if a
newborn died, or if a young baby died under almost any circumstances short of
spectacular marks of violence on its body.[80] Perhaps the pamphlet writers
needed the plot device of the devil in order to make their subject's crimes

---

[78] *Pittilesse Mother*, sig. B2ʳ.

[79] Henry Goodcole, *Natures Cruell Step-dames: or, Matchlesse monsters of the female sex; Elizabeth
Barnes, and Anne Willis* (Printed at London: [By E. Purslowe] for Francis Coules, dwelling in the
Old-Baily, 1637), STC2 12012, 2, 3, 5.

[80] On the history of infanticide in England, see Laura Gowing, 'Secret Births and Infanticide in
17th-c. England', *Past & Present*, 156 (1997), 87–115; Peter C. Hoffer and N. E. H. Hull, *Murdering*

explicable, or perhaps the women themselves found diabolical intervention a way to explain or understand their murderous impulses.[81] In either case, the result was a vision of infanticide tied closely to witchcraft.

Like infanticide stories, witchcraft pamphlets dwelt on harm to children. In one of the earliest English witchcraft pamphlets, the witch Elizabeth Frauncis is described as a murdering mother. She wanted to bewitch one Andrew Byles so that he would marry her. Although he had sex with her, he would not marry her. Frauncis found herself pregnant, and Byles died, so she asked her familiar to destroy the fetus. The familiar, a white cat named Sathan, 'bad her take a certaine herbe and drinke it which she did, and destroyed the childe forthwith', just as a witch in the Rueff account provided a herbal abortifacient to the servants. Subsequently Frauncis married another man and had a baby three months after the wedding. She and her husband lived unquietly, and 'she willed sathan her Cat to kill the childe, beinge about the age of half a yere olde and he did so'.[82] More commonly, witches were portrayed as killing other women's children. In a 1579 pamphlet, Mother Staunton was accused of making four babies violently ill, although none died, while Mother Nokes was supposed to have caused the death of a tailor's child.[83]

A 1582 pamphlet about witches in St Osyth is replete with stories of witches harming children. Ursley Kempe fell out with Grace Thurlowe over the care of Thurlowe's babies. Although Kempe had stopped by to see how the baby was doing a number of times, when Thurlowe asked her to stay the night to take care of the baby, Kempe refused, saying that 'the child would do well enough'. The text does not comment directly on the outcome of this disagreement but just notes in a chilling aside that the baby was fine but its hands were turned backwards, a detail denoting witchcraft in other pamphlets.[84] When Thurlowe

---

Mothers: Infanticide in England and New England, 1558–1803 (New York: New York University Press, 1981); McLaren, *Reproductive Rituals*, 129–35; Keith Wrightson, 'Infanticide in Earlier 17th-c. England', *Local Population Studies*, 15 (1975), 10–22. Frances Dolan's work on the meanings of infanticide has shaped my reading of the pamphlets; Dolan, *Dangerous Familiars*, 170. For a cross-border perspective, see Deborah Symonds, *Weep Not for Me: Women, Ballads, and Infanticide in Early Modern Scotland* (University Park, Pa.: Penn State Press, 1997).

[81] Michael MacDonald suggests that mothers might interpret their murderous feelings as resulting from diabolic intervention. Michael MacDonald, *Mystical Bedlam: Madness, Anxiety, and Healing in 17th-c. England* (Cambridge: Cambridge University Press, 1983), 83; Dolan, *Dangerous Familiars*, 140. Peter Lake has called attention to the way in which the plot device of the devil was used in many murder pamphlets and often featured in the title page woodcut; Lake, *Antichrist's Lewd Hat*, 40–53.

[82] *The Examination and Confession of Certaine Wytches at Chensforde in the countie of Essex: before the Quenes Maiesties judges, the xxvi daye of July, anno 1566* (Imprynted at London: By Wyllyam Powell for Wyllyam Pickeringe dwelling at Sainte Magnus corner and are there for to be soulde, anno 1566.the.23.August), STC2 19869.5, sig. A7ᵛ, sig. A7ᵛ–8ʳ.

[83] *Damnable Driftes*, sig. A7ᵛ, A8ʳ, A8ʳ, B1ʳ, B2ʳ.

[84] W. W., *A True and Iust Recorde*, sig. A1ᵛ. For another example of a child's hands turned backwards, see *A Rehearsall Both Straung and True, of Hainous and Horrible Actes Committed by Elizabeth Stile, alias Rockingham, Mother Dutten, Mother Deuell, Mother Margaret, fower notorious witches,*

had another baby, she and Kempe quarrelled because she did not hire her to be the baby's nurse. At three months of age, the baby fell out of the cradle, broke its neck, and died.[85] After Annis Leatherdell refused to give Kempe some scouring sand, Leatherdell's baby got sick, with strange swellings in its belly and privy parts. After Leatherdell confronted Kempe, the baby got worse.[86] Cisley Selles, another woman accused of witchcraft in the same pamphlet, had the same kind of problematic relationships with other women's children. Selles was nursing George Battelle's child, and Battelle took the child away from her and gave it to Thomas Death's wife instead. Cisley threatened Death's wife, saying she should lose more than she would gain by it. Death's 4-year-old son went out into the yard to play in fine health, but then dropped down dead. Although he was revived, he was but a 'pitious case, and so died presently'.[87]

Wet-nursing was one of the most lucrative employments available to a poor woman, and it is easy to understand how hostilities broke out when Selles lost her job to the unfortunately named Mrs Death.[88] In these examples, as in some of the ones involving Kempe, the accused witch was acting as a kind of substitute mother, as a nurse or a wet-nurse. However, like infanticidal mothers, these women caused harm to children rather than providing nurturance. The implicit assumption in both cases is that women are maternal by nature, and that their nurturing qualities can extend from their own children to those of others. Witches and murdering mothers highlight the centrality of these norms by the very violence with which they deviate from them.

Of course, these intersections between murdering mothers and witchcraft also speak to the social facts of early modern women's lives.[89] There must have been countless conflicts about who would wet-nurse a child, and many a

---

apprehended at Winsore in the countie of Barks (Imprinted at London: [By J. Kingston] for Edward White at the little north-doore of Paules, at the signe of the Gun, and are there to be sold, [1579]), STC2 23267, sig. B1r.

[85] Ibid. sig. A1v.   [86] Ibid. sig. A3r.

[87] Ibid. sig. D8v. See also the interesting moment when Selles's husband accuses her of harming their children (or perhaps her step-children?). He yells at her: 'Ye stinking whore, what mean yee? Can ye not keepe your imps from my children?' Henry Selles's comment, as reported by their 6-year-old son, positions Cisley as yet again harming someone else's children—even when, as in this case, they are hers; sig. D2r.

[88] Most of the social history of wet-nursing is on a slightly later period: Dorothy McLaren, 'Nature's Contraceptive: Wet-nursing and Prolonged Lactation, the Case of Chesham, Buckinghamshire, 1578–1601', *Medical History*, 23 (1979), 426–41; ead., 'Fertility, Infant Mortality, and Breast Feeding in the 17th c.', *Medical History*, 22 (1978), 378–96; David Harley, 'From Providence to Nature: The Moral Theology and Godly Practice of Maternal Breast-Feeding in Stuart England', *Bulletin of the History of Medicine*, 69 (1995), 198–223; Marylynn Salmon, 'The Cultural Significance of Breastfeeding and Infant Care in Early Modern England and America', *Journal of Social History*, 28 (1994), 247–69.

[89] On this point, see especially Purkiss, 'Women's Stories of Witchcraft in Early Modern England', and James Sharpe, *Instruments of Darkness: Witchcraft in Early Modern England* (Philadelphia: University of Pennsylvania Press, 1997), 173–86, as well as the many fine social histories of witchcraft and

pregnant unwed woman took herbal remedies in an attempt to cause an abortion. Since married women's work was centred on household and child-rearing, those are the very spaces within which conflicts between women were most likely to occur. Given the importance of the role of motherhood, an angry woman who had been refused some household necessity like scouring sand might well find it easy to curse another woman's child. In cheap pamphlets, these social facts come to have cultural meanings, serving as cautionary tales and as suggestions that not all mothers were beneficent.

Witches' relationships with their familiars are portrayed as depraved versions of motherhood while infanticidal mothers are described as savage or unnatural because they lack what is presumed to be the natural tenderness of a mother towards her children. In each case we see a kind of dark version of assumptions about motherhood expressed through images of animality. Margaret Vincent was called a tiger, and compared to cannibals and other inhuman creatures. Elizabeth Barnes was labelled a savage and a wolf, while Anne Willis, another murdering mother, was described as an unnatural beast.[90] The rich descriptions of witches' relationships with their familiars provided readers with images of anti-mothers, a kind of double perversion of the maternal relationship. First, as described, these women killed babies and children rather than cherishing them. Second, they lavished maternal attentions on spirits in the shape of small animals. This focus of devotion seemed a lot more problematic to sixteenth- or early seventeenth-century readers than it does to us. Domestic pets were not yet common, and, as we shall see, these women's animals were often not pet-like: they might be toads or rats. Joan Cunny, for example, was supposed to have had a series of toads, and in the woodcut that accompanies her confession, two of the toads are given human names, but the other two are not (see Fig. 2.4).

These small animals made a mockery of motherhood. They lived on blood or milk. The blood they sucked from their witch, just as a baby nursed from its mother. Mother Dutten fed her toad with blood that issued from her flank. Elizabeth Stile fed her rat with blood from her wrist.[91] Every time her familiar, the cat Sathan, did her bidding, Elizabeth Frauncis was obliged to feed him with a drop of her blood, pricking herself in order to provide for him.[92] Other witches fed their familiars on milk as well as blood. The curiously named

of infanticide. See e.g. Annabel Gregory, 'Witchcraft, Politics and Good Neighborhood in Early 17th c. Rye', *Past & Present*, 133 (1991), 31–66; J. A. Sharpe, 'Witchcraft and Women in 17th-c. England: Some Northern Evidence', *Continuity and Change*, 6 (1991), 179–99; Clive Holmes, 'Women: Witnesses and Witches', *Past & Present*, 140 (1993), 45–78; Gowing, 'Secret Births and Infanticide'.

[90] *Pittilesse Mother*, sigs. A3ʳ, B1ʳ⁻ᵛ; *Natures Cruell Step-dames*, 2, 17.
[91] *Rehearsall Both Straung and True*, sig. A5ʳ⁻ᵛ, A6ʳ.   [92] *Examination and Confession*, sig. A7ʳ.

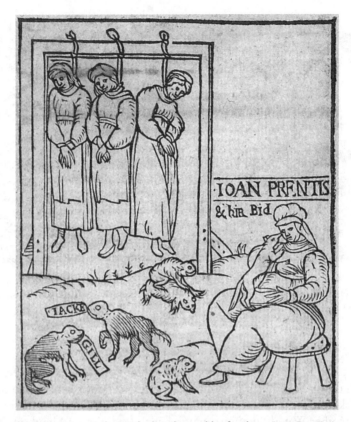

Fig. 2.4. Four witches with their humanlike familiars. Joan Prentis is pictured holding her ferret Bid as a mother might hold her baby. *The apprehension and confession of three notorious witches* (1589). Courtesy of the Lambeth Palace Library

Mother Devell, a poor young woman, had a black cat named Gille, whom she fed 'with Milke, mingled with her owne bloud'. Mother Margaret, who lived in the almshouse in Windsor, had a kitten named Ginnie, whom she fed with crumbs of bread and her own blood.[93] Margery Sammon's mother passed on to her two familiars who were shaped like toads. Her mother instructed Margery: 'if thou doest not give them milke, they will sucke of thy blood'.[94] Other famil-iars, like toddlers, were fed spoonful by spoonful, as in the illustration to the 1579 Windsor pamphlet (Fig. 2.5).

Animal familiars resembled babies, not only in their need to be fed, but also in the care that their 'mothers' gave them. These women were described as

[93] *Rehearsall Both Straung and True,* sig. A5ᵛ, A6ʳ.   [94] W. W., *A True and Iust Recorde,* sig. C4ᵛ.

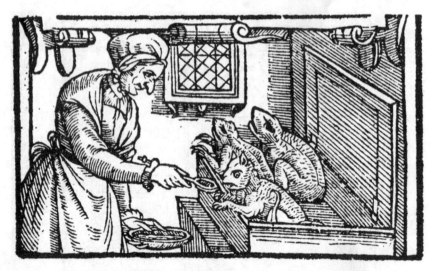

Fig. 2.5. A witch's familiars fed like young children. *A rehearsall both straung and true, of hainous and horrible actes committed by Elizabeth Stile* (1579). Courtesy of the British Library, shelf mark C.27.a.11

taking pains to provide a comfortable place for their familiars to sleep even though they lacked material resources. Elizabeth Frauncis kept the cat Sathan in a basket, as her grandmother had instructed her.[95] Frauncis handed Sathan on to Mother Waterhouse, instructing her to feed him on blood, milk, and bread. Waterhouse kept Sathan in a bowl lined with wool to make a soft bed. When 'being moved by povertie' she had to use the wool, she cleverly transformed Sathan into a toad so that he could be kept in the bowl without wool.[96] These women are described as keeping their little animals with care and tenderness, underlining the curious way in which this relationship was seen as an inversion of motherhood.

Finally, familiars were given names that granted them individuality and a kind of semblance of personhood. Some familiars had non-human names, such as Suckin, a name perhaps emblematic of this black dog's infantile needs. Others, however, had human names, such as Mother Devell's Gille, or Mother Margaret's Ginnie. Joan Cunny's toads were called Jack and Gill, and were identified as such in the woodcut illustration (see Fig. 2.4). Elizabeth Stile's rat

---

[95] *Examination and Confession*, sig. A6^{r-v}.

[96] Ibid. sigs. A8^r, B2^{r-v}. For other familiars kept in a bowl of wool, see Elizabeth Bennet's Lierd and Suckin, small dogs. W. W., *A True and Iust Recorde*, sig. C1^v.

was named Philip.[97] Ales Manfielde had four imps, like black cats, called Robin, Jack, William, and Puppet, alias Mamet, whom she kept in a box with wool. Robin, Jack, and William were all common men's names. 'Puppet' referred to a small doll or poppet, and 'mamet' also meant a small doll or other figure. Both words might also mean an idol, that is, a figure who took someone away from a true God. Manfielde's familiars were called 'imps', a word that meant young children. Her imps formed a set of siblings. The older ones, Jack, Robin, and William, were fed on beer, just as children were given small beer to drink. The baby Puppet was still fed with milk/blood from Manfielde's shoulder.[98]

Milk, blood, bread. Witchcraft pamphlets and those describing infanticidal mothers are full of references to these three substances. Each of these is related to the other by a transformative property. Breast milk was understood to be purified, whitened blood. The blood of Christ, shed for mankind, was transformed into communion bread—or, in the Anglican service, consubstantiated in the Eucharist. In the cheap print pamphlets I discuss here, there is no one simple set of meanings associated with these three substances. Instead, they refer to each other and to the material facts of women's lives in complex networks of meaning. Here I trace a few of these associations, highlighting the ways in which references to these substances suggest a context for the making of the bad womb. For, as I have suggested, the womb was a synecdoche for motherhood itself. In cheap print, there is a burst of stories about bad mothers, women who are the dark side of the good mothers held up as exemplars in conduct manuals and the like. The womb is the bodily analogue of this double image of motherhood, shaped both by these representations of witches and infanticidal mothers, and by the long consequences of the Protestant Reformation's turning away from the Virgin Mary as an exemplar for all women. In cheap pamphlets' fascination with blood, milk, and bread we can see these themes come together in an intensely corporeal way.

The narrative of Margaret Vincent inverts the usual blood and milk equation. The text constantly uses the term 'bloody' to describe her actions in killing her children. She used a ploy to get the maidservant out of the house. All of the wives of Acton were going to a riot over a conflict with the neighbouring town of Willesden about grazing rights on a local common. When the women asked Vincent to join them, she offered her maidservant instead, 'having a minde as then more setled on bloudy purposes then countrey occasions'. As the narrative moves towards the actual moments of killing, it draws an elaborate

---

[97] *Rehearsall Both Straung and True*, sig. A5ᵛ, A6ʳ, A6ʳ (Gill, Ginnie, Philip); *Apprehension and Confession*, sig. A3ʳ (Jack and Gill). On the names of familiars, see Serpell, 'Guardian Spirits or Demonic Pets'.   [98] *True and Iuste Recorde*, sig. D5ᵛ–7ᵛ.

metaphor of blood and milk. It describes a 'mother who by nature should have cherisht them [her children] with her own body, as the Pellican that pecks her owne brest to feed her yong ones with her blood'. A human mother fed her young with milk from the breast, but common lore had it that the mother pelican fed her chicks with blood pecked from her own breast, a metaphor for all kinds of maternal and sacred sacrifice. After Vincent killed the younger of the two children, the text describes in hyperbolic terms how

This Creature not deserving Mothers name, as I said before, not yet glutted, nor sufficed with these few drops of Innocent blood, nay her owne deare blood bred in her owne body, cherished in her own wombe with much dearenes full forty weekes.[99]

Rather than feeding on her children's blood, this mother should have been feeding them with her own milk/blood. The eater and eaten are reversed, and the relation of blood to milk is inverted. In the midst of this unnatural scene, the writer of the story strives to remind the reader of what a good mother should be like by emphasizing that this woman does not deserve even the name of mother.

In these narratives of infanticide, writers return to images of blood repeatedly, as when Vincent is described as not the first to be 'blemished with blood'.[100] Elizabeth Barnes's crime is described with the adjective 'bloody': 'bloody fact', 'bloody hand', and 'bloody crying-fact'.[101] In part, this emphasis on blood is due to the early modern belief that a murdered person's body would literally bleed afresh in the presence of a murderer, but it also underlines the perversion of motherhood that these women are made to represent in cheap print.

As suggested, the first network of meanings of blood, milk, and bread connects good motherhood with the appropriate feeding of infants. In witchcraft stories, this network links the care of familiars to the care of babies to provide one kind of inversion. In the womb, the infant was nourished with maternal blood, which was transformed after the birth into milk.[102] When babies were weaned, one of their first foods was bread that had been chewed by the mother or nurse in order to soften it. Familiars' diet of blood, milk, and bread thus highlighted their similarity to babies. In the infanticide pamphlets, the connection between blood and milk also echoes infant feeding practices as a way of demonstrating the perverse nature of these mothers who kill. Instead of spending their own blood in the form of breast milk, they shed the blood of their children. These descriptions of witches and infanticidal mothers emphasize the

---

[99] *Pittilesse Mother*, sig. A3ᵛ–4ʳ. The trope of Vincent feeding on the blood of her young continues. The text describes how she still desires more blood, but fortunately her third child was a baby being cared for by a wet-nurse, here a figure of appropriate maternity.   [100] Ibid. sig. B2ʳ.
[101] *Natures Cruell Step-dames*, 3, 4.   [102] Rueff, *Expert Midwife*, 39.

importance of mothers' roles in literal physical nurturance by depicting those roles gone horribly wrong.

A second set of meanings of milk was highlighted in the St Osyth witchcraft case. Women were in charge of dairying. They made butter, cheese, and other milk products.[103] Robert Sanneret testified that the summer after he'd had some trouble with his servant Elizabeth Ewstace, he tended seven milk cows, 'and very often times, his saide beasts did give downe blood in steede of milke'.[104] Margaret Grevill and Annis Herd were each accused of witchcraft in making milk go bad. Grevill had asked the butcher Nicholas Strickland for some mutton, which he refused, telling her to come back later. His wife then had trouble preparing milk. She was seething some milk for their workers, and it went bitter and stank. A few days later, she was churning butter, but the butter would not come, though she churned from morning until night. Her husband advised her to heat the milk and try again, but it would not heat properly, so she poured half of it into the fire, whereupon it stank so much that everyone had to leave the house. The next time she went to make butter, it wouldn't churn either, so she put the milk in the cow swill, but the cow sickened so much that Strickland had it killed before it died. Bennet Lane had similar troubles in making butter after she had refused Annis Herd the loan of tuppence. She described to the magistrate how she scrubbed out her vessels carefully, but the only remedy that worked was a magical one—putting a red-hot horseshoe into the cream.[105]

To us these incidents might speak of the chanciness of material life in the early modern period, or to the profound concerns women had in providing food for their families and servants under uncertain circumstances.[106] Here I suggest another layer of meaning. Just as witches' familiars seem to be an inversion of the usual pattern of motherhood, so these disruptions in dairying point towards a perversion of maternity. Instead of providing milk—either breast milk for babies or cow's milk, butter, and cheese for adults—these witches transformed milk into blood or into nasty stinking substances that would not churn into butter or be boiled into a pudding. They made the normal tasks of motherhood impossible for the woman against whom the witch held a grudge.

---

[103] Deborah Valenze, ' "The Art of Women, the Business of Men": Women's Work and the Dairy Industry c. 1740–1840', *Past & Present*, 130 (1991), 142–69.

[104] *True and Iuste Recorde*, sig. C7ʳ. For a similar case, see *Damnable Drifies*, sig. B1ʳ.

[105] *True and Iuste Recorde*, sigs. E3ʳ⁻ᵛ, E8ʳ⁻ᵛ.

[106] Barbara Rosen speculated about modern explanations for the causes of these incidents; *Witchcraft in England, 1558–1618*, (ed.) Barbara Rosen (Amherst: University of Massachusetts Press, 1991). See e.g. p. 99, where she mentions glanders (an animal ailment) and hysteria as possible causes for the events described in a witchcraft pamphlet. Diane Purkiss interprets these and other such moments as reflective of women's own fears about domestic processes and domestic integrity. Purkiss, 'Women's Stories of Witchcraft in Early Modern England'.

The third set of meanings of blood, milk, and bread has to do with religious belief. The nature of Christ's body and blood in the bread and wine of the Eucharist was a central issue in the Protestant Reformation, with the Anglican church denying the Catholic doctrine of transubstantiation that bread and wine were literally transformed into Christ's body and blood. Many of the older women in the witchcraft pamphlets discussed here had lived through this period of upheaval, and would have been familiar with the kinds of religious and magical beliefs associated with the consecrated host that persisted long after the Reformation. There are various pointers to religious controversy in witchcraft pamphlets. For example, Mother Waterhouse was asked by her interrogators if she went to church. She said yes, and then was asked what she did in church. She answered cautiously that she did what other women did, and prayed 'right hartely' there. Her examiner pressed on, asking what prayers she said, and whether she said them in English or in Latin. This last question was Waterhouse's undoing, for she replied that she said the Lord's Prayer, the Ave Maria, and the 'belefe' (the Creed) in Latin. The questioner asked why 'she saide it not in englishe but in laten, seing that it was set out by publike auc-thoritie and according to goddes worde that all men should pray in the englishe & mother toung that they best understande'.[107] Mother Waterhouse was 64 years old, and had thus had spent most of her life in a church in which prayer in Latin had been the rule. She replied that the cat Sathan, her familiar, would never let her say her prayers in English.

The pamphlet closes here, noting that for this and many other offences she was condemned to die, 'trusting to be in joye with Christe her savior, whiche dearely had bought her with his most precious bloudde'.[108] Mother Water-house and the other witches in this pamphlet were described as buying a very different soul, for they gave their familiars drops of their blood for the harm that the familiars caused their enemies. It is as if the writer of the pamphlet sought to restore an appropriate relationship mediated by purchases of blood after spending pages describing how women 'rewarded' their familiars with drops of blood, reminding the reader that Christ redeemed their souls with his blood. The pamphlet is framed by religious discourse, for it opens with an epistle to the reader, a preface, and an exhortation to the reader, setting the sensational stories to follow in a godly paradigm. Even the illustration on the title page refers to a godly subject: it is a woodcut of Christ washing the feet of the Apostles, a scene with no obvious reference in the text (see Fig. 2.6).

The story of Joan Prentice and her ferret is cast within a religious framework that also emphasizes Christ's blood, shed for the sins of mankind. Her story was framed in sacred time. It opened 'about six yeeres last past, betweene the

---

[107] *Examination and Confession*, Pt. 3, sig. B5ʳ.   [108] Ibid. Pt. 2, sig. B5ᵛ–B6ʳ.

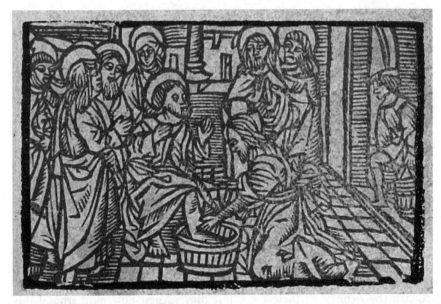

Fig. 2.6. Christ washing the feet of his apostles on Maundy Thursday. *The Examination and confession of certaine wytches at Chensforde in the countie of Essex* (1566). Courtesy of the Lambeth Palace Library

feastes of all Saintes, and the birth of our Lord God', setting the scene for Prentice's first encounter with the ferret within the liturgical year. Prentice was resting in her almshouse bed at 10 at night when the fiery-eyed animal arrived. The ferret sat in her lap and said to her: 'Joan Prentice give me thy soule.' Prentice, shocked, replied: 'In the name of god what art thou?' The ferret told her that he was Satan, that he had come to do her no harm, but that he must have her soul. Prentice told the ferret that he asked for something that was not hers to give, saying 'her soule appertained onely unto Jesus Christ, by whose precious blood shedding, it was bought and purchased'. The ferret immediately picked up on this reference to blood, saying 'I must then have some of thy blood'. Without any explanation for Prentice's sudden change of heart, the story continues 'which she willingly graunting', the ferret settling itself in her lap and sucking blood from her left forefinger.[109] The rapid shift from Prentice's staunch refusal, citing Christ's blood, to her acquiescence emphasizes for the reader the inversive qualities of witchcraft. Blood moves from a eucharistic to a demonic meaning in the space of a sentence. The extent of Prentice's sin was

[109] *Apprehension and Confession*, sig. B1ʳ⁻ᵛ.

also highlighted by the rapidity of her about-face, because she seemed to be clear about the religious stakes implicit in the ferret's request—only to subvert them a moment later. As in other examples, blood served here as a kind of marker that might be sacred or demonic or both.

As discussed above, the entire narrative of Margaret Vincent's killing of her children is a religious tale about the evils of papistry. Vincent is described as bewitched by clandestine Catholics, and/or tempted by the devil. In her story, blood is a marker, not of salvation, but of crime. Again and again, the writer uses the adjective 'bloody', and the metaphor of bloodstains, to describe her unnatural act. At the very end of her story, however, just as in the story of Mother Waterhouse, the writer attempts to restore an appropriate religious meaning to the substance of blood. He makes an allusion to the biblical phrase about being washed clean in the blood of the Lamb, saying 'the blood of her two innocent Children so wilfully shed (according to all charitable judgements) is washed away by the mercies of God'.[110] It is as if the seemingly indelible stain of her crime can be erased by the blood of Christ.

These three sets of meanings associated with blood, milk, and bread do not exhaust the richness of these texts, but they suggest how motherhood was represented in profoundly corporeal terms. In these stories of bad mothers, the substances of blood, milk, and bread, usually associated with nurturant mothering, signify the multiple inversions through which these texts define a good mother by means of her opposites. A good mother feeds her baby with breast milk, a witch feeds her familiar with blood. A good mother expends her own blood to make a new baby and then converts blood into milk to feed it. A bad mother sheds, not her own blood, but the blood of her child, or another's child.

I am suggesting that these extended stories of bad motherhood, expressed in deeply corporeal terms, provide some of the context in which the womb itself became understood in negative terms. All these examples—witches, infanticidal mothers, and wombs that threaten to suffocate women—are presented as abnormal, outside the usual life course of women. However, the sensational ways in which they are presented threaten all women with the possibility that the powers of maternity might go bad. Here I have suggested that the invention (or reinvention) of the bad womb was due in part both to the long shock-waves of the Protestant Reformation, the final disenchantment of reproduction, and to the cultural concern with stories about bad mothers. Perhaps 'disenchantment' is not quite the right word, because the terrible womb could be described in terms just as supernatural as was the miraculous womb, but in the same way that relics, pilgrimages, statues, and other religious items gradually lost their powers during and after the Reformation so too did the womb lose its associa-

---

[110] *Pittilesse Mother*, sig. B2^r.

tions with the miracle of Christ's conception. As I have argued in this chapter, that interpretative space was not filled by only one story or only one way of explaining the womb's power, but nor was the womb transmuted into just another body part.

At the same time, however, Raynalde's 1545 midwifery manual continued to be reprinted and so readers had multiple versions of the female body available to them. In any individual case, a woman's exposure to one midwifery text or another was shaped by factors we can rarely recover—the handing down of a book within a family, or chance encounter with a particular book on a second-hand stall in a market. Whatever stories a woman read or heard about the womb, however, by the early seventeenth century she had access to new kinds of sensational stories about bad mothers.

I can only speculate about the deeper causes for the production of these stories of bad mothers. Part of any explanation is the overall increase in sensational pamphlets about murders, disasters, and the like, perhaps amplified by a tendency to depict calamity as divine Providence.[111] Another strand of explanation lies in the social circumstances of the 1590s, a decade of bad harvests, social dislocation, and famine. Perhaps stories in which the most elemental form of nourishment—a baby's nursing—was presented in grossly perverted ways resonated with peoples' experiences of hunger and want, expressing a kind of deep and inarticulate anger and frustration about dearth and famine. Whatever the local circumstances that produced these images of bad mothers, the power of these representations outlived the moment that created them. The bad womb persisted long after the possession controversy that launched it into popular print, and the stories of bad mothers that made it plausible and compelling.

[111] On providence, see Alexandra Walsham, *Providence in Early Modern England* (Oxford: Oxford University Press, 1999); on the role of providence in murder pamphlets, see Lake, *Antichrist's Lewd Hat*, esp. 3–54.

3

Protesting and Preaching

In the 1640s England was torn apart by civil war. For the first time since the Wars of the Roses two centuries earlier, Englishmen faced their brothers, cousins, and neighbours on the field of war. Traumatic as those battles were, they pale in comparison with the larger social upheavals of the decade. 'The world turned upside down' is the way a contemporary commentator tried to describe how all kinds of social truths were questioned, inverted, or discarded. In 1649 the very pinnacle of the social hierarchy tumbled: King Charles I was executed after a trial for treason. England became a republic, governed by Parliament and a Lord Protector, Oliver Cromwell. By 1660 the political experiment had failed, and the King's son was crowned as Charles II. Restoring a king was easy, but restoring the past was not possible. As we shall see, too many radical ideas had been unleashed in the 1640s to ever put the genie back in the bottle. No sooner had war stopped than historians began to try to understand what had happened. Each generation has reinterpreted the Civil War, casting its own heroes and villains according to its own needs.

In this chapter, I tell the story of the 1640s as a tale of gender trouble. All kinds of authority were questioned in this decade, and none more profoundly than that of man over woman. First, because of the ways in which early modern English people thought about relations of power, the authority of a husband and father over his household was considered analogous to that of other governors, such as the King. Today we think of these kinds of human interaction differently. By and large, domestic relations are private, and governmental ones are public. In the seventeenth century, however, these relations were very similar, the one a kind of miniature of the other. So when the authority of the King or the authority of bishops was called into question, those debates echoed in the household. Second, and more directly, gender relations were contentious in the 1640s because large numbers of women acted in new ways: they preached, prophesied, and protested in public. Their actions contravened widely held norms of female behaviour and those actions were broadcast in cheap print as never before. As descriptions of these women's actions evolved over the course of the 1640s, debate became increasingly polarized, with women insisting that they had the right to speak as women, and their critics resorting to ever more sexualized slanders in attempts to contain them.[1]

In the last chapter, we saw how cheap-print pamphlets about murdering mothers and witches offered readers and listeners chilling stories of women gone wrong, women who dramatically contravened gender norms about maternal behaviours. Such murdering mothers had been treated as exceptional, and the disorder they wreaked was carefully resolved at the end of the story by repentance and execution. Cheap print of the 1640s offered no such consolations. Stories about women preachers or protesters were not framed in godly narrative, and order was not restored on the last page. Instead, as newsbooks (the ancestors of our newspapers) came to be issued twice weekly, they developed their own satirical and ongoing forms of narrative that had no closure. As I discuss further in Chapter 6, politics itself became sexualized as parliamentary matters were constantly satirized in sexual terms—even politics that were not 'about' gender relations were described in terms that were about women and men.[2]

These tensions in relations between men and women were not resolved easily. One of the ways in which people tackled these issues was in thinking about the body. In the 1650s, a spate of new popular books about conception and pregnancy offered readers ways to imagine gender relations through the medium of the body. If the macrocosm—the larger social world—no longer provided a steady model for gender relations, perhaps the microcosm—the human body itself—might provide an image of stability and hierarchy. This shift, in which bodies came to serve as sites for imagining the correct relations between men and women, did not depend on new scientific knowledge. As always, vernacular texts purveyed earlier learning, compiled and rearranged by popularizers. What was new was the attitude of male writers. As we shall see in

[1] In casting 'the world turned upside down' as gender trouble, I draw on Sharon Achinstein, 'Women on Top in the Pamphlet Literature of the English Revolution', *Women's Studies*, 24 (1994), 131–63; Crawford, 'The Challenges to Patriarchalism'; Hilary Hinds, *God's Englishwomen: 17th-c. Radical Sectarian Writing and Feminist Criticism* (Manchester: Manchester University Press, 1996); Phyllis Mack, *Visionary Women: Ecstatic Prophecy in 17th-c. England* (Berkeley: University of California Press, 1992).

[2] On the larger topic of women and the formation of public opinion at this moment, see Dagmar Freist, *Governed by Opinion: Politics, Religion, and the Dynamics of Communication in Stuart London, 1637–1645* (London: Tauris Academic Studies, 1997). On politics and sexual satire, see David Underdown, *A Freeborn People: Politics and the Nation in 17th-c. England* (Oxford: Clarendon Press, 1996), ch. 5, '*The Man in the Moon*: Loyalty and Libel in Popular Politics, 1640–1650', 90–111; Lois Potter, 'The *Mistress Parliament* Dialogues', ed., with an introduction, *Analytical and Enumerative Bibliography*, 1 (1987), 101–70; Tamsyn Williams, ' "Magnetic Figures": Polemical Prints of the English Revolution', in Lucy Gent and Nigel Llewellyn (eds.), *Renaissance Bodies: The Human Figure in English Culture c.1540–1660* (London: Reaktion Books, 1990), 86–110; Susan Wiseman, ' "Adam, the Father of All Flesh": Porno-Political Rhetoric and Political Theory in and After the English Civil War', in James Holstun (ed.), *Pamphlet Wars: Prose in the English Revolution* (London: Frank Cass, 1992), 134–57.

the next chapter, about a female prophet and the man who wrote her story down, it was not easy for men to write about women's bodies or to make those changeable bodies into stable producers of truths. Nor had men been comfortable describing women's 'secrets'. In 1651, however, Nicholas Culpeper wrote a revolutionary book on midwifery that changed these conventions and made women's reproductive bodies the stuff of social debate. His work is the subject of Chapter 5, but it must be understood in relation to the gender troubles described here.

In order to grasp the tensions that grew into civil war in the 1640s, we need to go back to the previous decade, if not much earlier, when Charles I ruled without calling a Parliament for eleven years, the so-called 'Personal Rule'. In that time, three interrelated issues simmered, reaching boiling point in 1641. First was Charles's troubled relationship with his Parliaments. After some years of tension, in 1629 he dissolved Parliament and arrested five members who resisted its closure. The second grew from the first. Without a Parliament to grant him revenues, Charles revived and expanded ancient taxes that were resented bitterly. He also used the courts aggressively to repress criticism of his regime, and the combination of taxation and prosecution made him seem far too authoritarian to many of his subjects. Third, and perhaps most explosive, Charles seemed to many to be far too popish. With the help of William Laud, Archbishop of Canterbury, he revised church practices, downplaying the importance of preaching, emphasizing the role of the sacraments, restoring the altar to a Catholic configuration, and encouraging the use of devotional images and statues. To English Protestants, these actions suggested that Charles wanted to restore Catholicism or at least many Catholic practices. These issues were not restricted to Charles's English kingdom. Scotland rebelled when Charles attempted to make its religious practices conform more closely with those in England, and tensions between Catholics and Protestants in Ireland intensified. The Scots invaded England in August 1640, and in the autumn of 1641 rebellion broke out in Ireland.

Two circumstances made this unstable situation even more volatile. In July 1641 Charles abolished the Court of Star Chamber and the Court of High Commission, courts he had used to silence criticism in the previous decade. An unexpected by-product of this attempt at reconciliation was the freedom of the press. Star Chamber had been the court where all kinds of violations of censorship had been prosecuted, and with it gone, cheap print exploded. In the late 1630s about 600 titles were produced in England per year. In 1641 that number tripled to almost 2,000, and in 1642 more than 4,000 titles were published. For the rest of the decade, anywhere from 1,200 to 2,000 items were produced every year, a pattern that continued into the

1650s.[3] It is not just that there were many more items printed. English men and women craved information about the political and religious upheavals in which they found themselves, and unfettered printers obliged with a mountain of cheap pamphlets and news-sheets. Prior to 1641, it was illegal to print domestic news, and the first newsbook was published in November 1641. As conflict ripened into war, a host of partisan newsbooks flourished, continuing into the 1650s.[4] Their commentary was bold and satirical, unlike anything seen before, taunting the King and Members of Parliament with sarcastic nicknames and sexually loaded jokes. Events such as the rebellion in Ireland were described to readers in sensational and vivid prose, creating a string of atrocity tales. Politics became a form of public conversation in cheap print as never before.[5] Women's preaching, prophesying, and protesting was amplified by this rush of cheap print. All of a sudden, people all over the land could read about a woman preacher or a petition presented to Parliament by a group of women.

The second circumstance that made the 1640s particularly volatile was the extent to which London crowds took political action. Riots had long been a part of London life. Apprentices, for example, customarily rioted on Shrove Tuesday, often attacking brothels and/or foreigners, a kind of collective action often treated leniently by those in authority. Or mobs might take direct action, such as the moment in 1628 when a crowd attacked and killed John Lambe, the magician associated with the King's despised favourite, the Duke of Buckingham. These sorts of riots were episodic, moments of unrest that crossed the political heavens like shooting stars, dramatic but very short-lived. By late 1640, however, the mob was there to stay. Its actions, and fears about its future actions, began to shape the political process.

From 1641 onwards, cheap print was full of accounts of women preaching and prophesying. Women, of course, had spoken in public about religion before. Some of the best-known English martyrs of the previous century, Protestant and Catholic, had been women. Female parishioners had been

---

[3] These numbers were generated from a search of the online ESTC on 30 Jan. 2001, including all books published in England. As the ESTC adds new entries, the totals will change, but the overall picture has long been known. See e.g. Nigel Smith, *Literature and Revolution* (New Haven: Yale University Press, 1994), 23–31; F. S. Siebert, *Freedom of the Press in England 1476–1776* (Urbana: University of Illinois Press, 1952), 165–263; John Barnard, 'London Publishing, 1640–1660: Crisis, Continuity, and Innovation', *Book History*, 4 (2001), 1–16. Many thanks to Yvonne Noble for this last reference.

[4] On newsbooks, see *Making the News: An Anthology of the Newsbooks of Revolutionary England, 1641–1660*, ed. Joad Raymond (New York: St. Martin's Press, 1993); id. (ed.), *News, Newspapers, and Society in Early Modern Britain* (London: Frank Cass, 1999). On the pre-history of newsbooks, see the very illuminating essay by Richard Cust, 'News and Politics in Early-17th c. England', *Past & Present*, 112 (1986), 60–90.

[5] On the creation of a kind of public sphere, see David Zaret, *Origins of Democratic Culture: Printing, Petitions, and the Public Sphere in Early Modern England* (Princeton: Princeton University Press, 2000).

rowdy protesters, as a Bishop of London discovered when he preached at
St Margarets, Old Fish Street, London in 1567. The women hooted at him,
loudly comparing his cap to a cuckold's horn.[6] Women had preached in public,
albeit rarely, before the 1640s. For example, Arthur Lake, Bishop of Bath and
Wells, preached a sermon at a service of penance for those men and women
who had frequented a conventicle where a woman preached sometime in the
1610s or early 1620s.[7] In Salisbury in the 1620s and 1630s, Joan Slowe was
repeatedly in trouble with the authorities for preaching and for teaching school
without a licence.[8]

   However, in the 1640s a rare occurrence became a common one: women
were talking about religious matters in public as never before. A 1641 pamphlet about six women preachers tells us about Anne Hempstall, in the parish
of St Andrewes, Holborn, who preached about a dream that she understood as
a prophecy.[9] It also describes Mary Bilbrow, the wife of a bricklayer in the
parish of St Giles in the Fields, as well as women in Gravesend, Ashford, Ely,
and Salisbury, who preached in their homes or in public places.[10]

   Ironically, the best known-accounts of women preachers come from one of
their bitterest enemies, the minister Thomas Edwards. In 1646 he published
Gangraena, a book detailing the religious excesses he saw around him. For
instance, there were the two women who preached in London every Tuesday at
four o'clock in the afternoon, namely, Mrs Attaway, a lace-woman who sold her
wares in Cheapside and lived in Bell Alley in Coleman Street, and a major's wife
living in the Old Bailey.[11] Edwards records another woman's explanation of
how she had come to preach. First she gave biblical justification for speaking to
women, such as in Titus, 'that the elder women ought to teach the younger'.

---

   [6] John Stowe, *Three 15th-c. Chronicles*, ed. James Gairdner, The Camden Society, 28 (London,
1880), 140. I owe this reference and many others to Dorothy Ludlow's Ph.D. dissertation, ' "Arise and
Be Doing": English "Preaching" Women, 1640–1660' (Ph.D. diss., Indiana University, 1978); see
esp. 49.
   [7] Arthur Lake, 'A Sermon Preached at St. Cutberts in Welles When certaine persons did Penance
for being at Conventicles where a Woman Preached', in *Sermons with Some Religious and Divine
Meditations* (London: W. Stansby for Nathanial Butter, 1629), STC2 15134, pt. 4, 67–73.
   [8] Martin Ingram, 'Puritans and the Church Courts, 1560–1640', in Jacqueline Eales and
Christopher Durston (eds.), *The Culture of English Puritanism, 1560–1700* (New York: St. Martin's
Press, 1996), 84.
   [9] *A Discovery of Six Women-Preachers* ([London?]: Printed, 1641), Thomason E.166[1], sig. A2ʳ⁻ᵛ.
The Thomason Tracts are a huge collection of pamphlets assembled by the London bookseller George
Thomason in the 1640s and 1650s, now held by the British Library. On women's dreams, see Patricia
Crawford, 'Women's Dreams in Early Modern England', *History Workshop Journal*, 49 (2000),
129–41.
   [10] *Discovery of Six Women-Preachers*, sig. A3ʳ, A3ᵛ.
   [11] Thomas Edwards, *Gangraena: Or a Catalog and Discovery of many of the Errours, Heresies,
Blasphemies and Pernicious Practices of the Sects* (London: Printed for Ralph Smith, at the Signe of the
Bible in Corn hill near the Royall-Exchange, 1646), Thomason E.323[3], 84–5. All cites are to pt. 1
unless otherwise noted. On Edwards and *Gangraena*, see Ann Hughes's forthcoming work.

Then she began speaking to men also 'when she considered the glory of God was manifested in Babes and Sucklings, and that she was desired by some to admit all those that pleased to come, she could not deny to impart those things which the Spirit had communicated to her'.[12] The impact of these women preachers was greatly magnified by Edwards's work, as well as by the cheap pamphlets that decried all kinds of religious deviance or excess. In some measure, it did not matter which of such items was literally 'true' and which imagined or satirical—the world was turned upside down in the imagination of cheap print before armies took to the field and civil war and regicide shattered patterns of governance.[13]

Other women eschewed the role of preacher per se, publishing books or prophesying instead. Mary Cary, for example, claimed the kinds of learned authority usually accorded to ministers, but, as far as we know, she did not speak in public, publishing her writings instead. Women also prophesied, claiming direct inspiration from God.[14] Again, their impact was greatly amplified by printing.

One of the best-known women preachers was Katherine Chidley, who was alleged to have set up a conventicle with her son at Bury, in Suffolk, in addition to very public preaching in London. Chidley and her husband Daniel had long been involved in religious controversy.[15] They were married and had children in Shrewsbury, where Daniel was a tailor. The Chidleys came into conflict with their minister, Peter Studley, who presented them in a church court for absenteeism in 1626; presumably the Chidleys were attending services in other parish churches or some form of separate congregation. Katherine Chidley was also presented for refusing to be churched after childbirth, a practice that, as we shall see, she despised.[16] In her later writings, Katherine describes being 'driven out' of Shrewsbury. Although details are lacking, it is certain that the Chidleys moved to London shortly after the birth of their eighth child in 1629. Once in London, they joined with John Duppa and others to form a separate congregation in 1630.[17] Such independent gatherings were the object of harassment and persecution by church authorities. Some congregations emigrated, first to the Netherlands, and then to New England, while others continued to meet clandestinely.

[12] Edwards, *Gangraena*, 88.
[13] Cressy, 'The Protestation Protested', characterizes the opening up of the political nation by the Protestation as 'the revolution that preceded the civil war' (p. 279); I suggest that the early 1640s explosion of cheap print about politics had a similar effect to that he discusses for the Protestation.
[14] Mack, *Visionary Women*, 1.
[15] Ludlow, 'Arise and Be Doing', 82–143; Ian Gentles, 'London Levellers in the English Revolution: The Chidleys and their Circle', *Journal of Ecclesiastical History*, 29 (1978), 281–309; Rachel Trubowitz, 'Female Preachers and Male Wives: Gender and Authority in Civil War England', in Holstun (ed.), *Pamphlet Wars*, 112–33.
[16] Ludlow, 'Arise and Be Doing', 84–5.   [17] Ibid. 86.

Chidley burst into print in 1641, replying to Thomas Edwards's *Reasons against the Independent Government of Particular Congregations* with her first book, *The Justification of the Independent Churches of Christ*.[18] Chidley used an inflammatory biblical citation on her title page: 'Then Jael, Hebers wife tooke a naile of the tent, and tooke an hammer in her hand, and went softly to him, and smote the naile into his temples and fastened in unto the ground, (for he was fast asleepe and weary) and so he died (Judges 4: 21).' Just as Jael killed Sisera, we might infer, Chidley will demolish Edwards. Her citation may also be an allusion to the first part of the same chapter, in which the prophetess Deborah calls together the Israelites to fight their enemies.

Indeed, Chidley is especially fond of military metaphors in her disputes with Edwards. As we shall see, she often reminds the reader that she is a woman, but she also casts herself in a male military role. Having demolished two of Edwards's arguments about the function of authority within a church, she gloats:

So that these two first Reasons being (as I conceive) the greatest Champions, which you have sent out in this skirmage, are now both slaine . . . Now, these two being thus turned aside, by one of the meanest of all the Army of Jesus Christ, you may justly feare, that all the rest of your souldiers will run away wounded.[19]

At the close of her text she challenges Edwards to intellectual combat:

Then chuse you sixe men (or more, if you please) and I will chuse as many, and if you will we will agree upon a Moderator: and trie it out in a faire discourse & peradventure save you a labour from publishing your large Tractates, which you say you intend to put out in print.[20]

Chidley's challenge to Edwards becomes more military and less humorous three years later: 'But (*Mr Edwards*) now I will counsell you, to *muster up all your army you bragge of*, and *come forth, set up your colours*, and pitch a field with the *Separation*.'[21] In 1644, in the midst of Civil War (the King

---

[18] Thomas Edwards, *Reasons against the Independent Government of Particular Congregations* (London: printed by Richard Cotes for Jo. Bellamie, & Ralph Smith, dwelling at the signe of the three Golden Lions, in Corne-hill neere the Royall Exchange, 1641), Thomason E.167[16]; Katherine Chidley, *The Justification of the Independent Churches of Christ* (London: Printed for William Larnar, and are to be sold at his Shop, at the Signe of the Golden Anchor, neere Pauls-Chaine, 1641), Thomason E.174[7]. Edwards's book was an attack on Henry Burton's *The Protestation Protested*. Edwards was mortified that Chidley was his only respondent to *Reasons against the Independent Government*. Thanks to Ann Hughes for this and many other points.

[19] Chidley, *Justification*, 9. See also 20: 'and yet neither this Scout, nor the joyned, nor the sub-joyned forces, shall be able to discover what strength is on my side, although they be formed by you in battle array'. William Larner, Chidley's publisher, was later associated with the Levellers, as was Chidley.   [20] Ibid. 80.

[21] Katherine Chidley, *A New-Yeares-Gift, or a brief exhortation to Mr. Thomas Edwards* (S.l.: s.n., printed in the year, 1645), Thomason E.23[13], sig. A3ᵛ.

had first raised his colours in the summer of 1642), such an image was very powerful.

Women like Chidley were not only causing trouble in the realm of religion. They were also taking unprecedented political action, marching on Parliament to present their petitions. My separation of 'religion' and 'politics' is purely analytical; no such division would have been understood by English men and women of the 1640s, plunged into a civil war triggered in part by religious differences.[22] The first evidence we have of a women's petition concerns itself with religious issues. There is a pamphlet dated 1641 called *The Petition of the Weamen of Middlesex* in the Thomason Tracts. Its title page disparages its supposed actors, claiming that the women, who had collected 12,000 signatures, withheld the petition 'untill it should please God to endue them with more wit, and lesse Non-sence'.[23] The rest of the pamphlet is typical of the many petitions presented in late 1641 and early 1642, and may well have been presented to Parliament. It is as if the disclaimer title page and the text are the products of two very different writers, one belittling women, the other asserting women's political views.

At this moment, long-running tensions about the role of bishops in the English church had come to a head, as well as deeply held enmity to William Laud, the Archbishop of Canterbury. Many thought that there was no biblical grounding for bishops and that they were a remnant of a popish past that needed to be extinguished. Worse yet, bishops sat in the House of Lords, giving them temporal as well as spiritual authority. In late 1640 a number of petitions were presented to Parliament to do away with Laudian innovations. Some went further, including the so-called 'Root and Branch' petitions, which suggested abolishing the entire church hierarchy, 'root and branch', archdeacons, bishops, and archbishops.[24] The pamphlet by the Women of Middlesex voices concerns typical of this movement. For example, it proclaims 'Let not Bishops tryumph, nor corrupted Judges goe too long . . . We desire, that Altars may be altered'.[25] The pamphlet continues with concerns about the survival of stained-glass church windows with superstitious images, the use of the surplice by ministers, the persistence of hymn-singing, and the Laudian insistence on the prayer book rather than extempore preaching.

---

[22] David Cressy, 'Conflict, Consensus, and the Willingness to Wink: The Erosion of Community in Charles I's England', *Huntington Library Quarterly*, 61 (1998), 131–49; Kenneth Fincham, 'The Restoration of Altars in the 1630s', *Historical Journal*, 44 (2001), 919–40.

[23] *The Petition of the Weamen of Middlesex* (London: Printed for William Bowden, 1641), Thomason E.180[17], title page.

[24] On Root and Branch see, among others, Anthony Fletcher, *The Outbreak of the English Civil War* (New York: New York University Press, 1981), 91–124; Keith Lindley, *Popular Politics and Religion in Civil War London* (Aldershot: Scolar Press, 1997), 4–19.

[25] *Petition of the Weamen of Middlesex*, sig. A2ʳ.

A newsbook describes how a group of more than 400 women went to the House of Lords on 1 February 1642 to deliver a petition. Evidently this was not the first one, since the account refers to a prior petition. The women were waiting for a response from the Lords when the Duke of Lenox came to attend the House. The women tried to present him with their petition, but he sneered 'Away with these women'. Some women tried to block his way, and in the confusion the Duke's staff was broken, so that he had to send for another. Despite what might seem like unacceptably unruly behaviour—breaking the phallic badge of the Duke's office—when the women were able to present their petition to Lord Savage, they were well received. The Lords evidently read the petition, and asked that twelve of the women be called into the House to declare their grievances, 'which was done accordingly'.[26]

Three days later, an even larger group of women petitioned the House of Commons. They declared themselves to be gentlewomen and tradesmen's wives 'in and about the city of London'. There is some evidence to suggest that they too had already tried to present a petition, even threatening the Sergeant-Major that 'where there is one woman now here, there would be five hundred tomorrow'.[27] The petition was presented on the fourth of February by Mrs Anne Stagg, who is described as 'a gentlewoman and a brewers wife'.[28] The pamphlet of the petition includes not just the text of the petition, but a justification for its production and presentation and a description of its reception at the House of Commons.

The petition is in one way utterly typical of its moment—it centres on the issue of bishops and invokes sensationalist descriptions of the likely fate of the English should proper religion not be upheld. The gentlewomen's petition warns 'great danger and feare do still attend us, & will, so long as Popish Lords & superstitious Bishops are suffered to have their voice in the House of Peers'.[29] These concerns can be found in many other contemporary petitions. Five days earlier, for example, a petition from 'many thousand poore people' made very similar references.[30]

---

[26] *The True Diurnall Occurances*, 31 Jan.–7 Feb. 1642, Thomason E.201[13].

[27] Ellen McArthur, 'Women Petitioners and the Long Parliament', *English Historical Review*, 24 (1909), 698–703, quote at 698. Unfortunately, McArthur does not specifically footnote this quote and I have not been able to trace its origin.

[28] *A True Copie of the Petition of the Gentlewomen, and Tradesmens-wives* (London: Printed by R.O. and G.D. for John Bull, 1641), Thomason E.134[17], 6 (really p. 7). The pamphlet uses Lady-day dating, i.e., 1642 does not begin until 25 March under this system. The pamphlet is reprinted in the *Harleian Miscellany* (London: printed for White and Cochrane, 1811), vii. 605–8.

[29] *True Copie*, 2.

[30] *To the Honourable House of Commons Assembled in Parliament. The Humble Petition of Many Thousand Poore People, in and Around the City of London* (London: Printed for Will. Larner and T.B. This 31 of January 1642), Thomason 669.f.4[54].

While the issues raised by these women were familiar, another aspect of their petition is novel: women's claims to a form of equality with their husbands. In the body of the petition, the women play with their subordinate gender role, referring to 'our frail condition' and using sensationalist language about the fate of women in the recent Irish rebellion, describing 'savage usage and unheard of rapes', which had been reported extensively in the unfettered English press. The petition then conjures up a threat of similar barbarities to happen in England, 'to see our Children dashed against the stones, and the Mothers milk mingled with the Infants blood, running down the streets'.[31] Here women invoke their customary roles as chaste wives and devoted mothers as justification for their speech, albeit in highly sensationalist ways. However, at the end of the pamphlet there is a list of the reasons why these women speak in public that does not rest on traditional gender roles. As the writer notes, 'It may be thought strange, and unbeseeming our sex to shew ourselves by way of Petition to this Honourable Assembly.' Here women claim equivalent rights and status with men:

First, because Christ hath purchased us at as deare a rate as he hath done Men . . . Secondly, because in the free enjoying of Christ in his own Laws, and a flourishing estate of the Church and Common-wealth, consisteth the happinesse of Women as well as Men. Thirdly, because Women are sharers in the common Calamities that accompany both Church and Common-wealth when oppression is exercised.[32]

The women then remind Members that women as well as men have suffered in Newgate (the London prison), Smithfield (where martyrs were burnt at the stake in London), and other places of persecution. Then the women cite biblical precedent in Queen Esther, who risked her life to petition King Ahasuerus. Finally, the pamphlet steps back from its claims for a moment, saying 'We doe it not out of any selfe conceit, or pride of heart, as seeking to equall our selves with Men, either in Authority or wisdome.'[33] Perhaps they do not claim equality of authority or wisdom, but they do claim equality in rights to petition and speak in public.

Two themes are particularly important in these claims. The women who petitioned Parliament in early 1642 articulated new arguments about their rights as women. They point out that they are equal to men in God's eyes and that they have suffered for their religious beliefs in the same ways that men have, making a kind of translation from the realm of the spirit to the temporal

[31] *True Copie* (NB. pagination of this pamphlet is idiosyncratic; quotes are sig. A2ʳ and A2ᵛ). On the larger topic of women and the formation of public opinion at this moment, see Freist, *Governed by Opinion*, and Achinstein, 'Women on Top'. On women and politics in the Civil War, see Hughes, 'Women, Men and Politics in the English Civil War'.   [32] *True Copie*, sig. A4ʳ.
[33] Ibid. sig. A4ᵛ.

world of Newgate and Smithfield. Second, these women are claiming the right
to speak in public. They made those claims in a kind of nascent public sphere
created by cheap print.[34] Female rioters had often engaged in acts, sometimes
deeply symbolic acts, such as reselling grain at a fair price, or pulling down the
fences that marked enclosures. In 1629, for example, Ann Carter had led
rioters in Maldon, Kent, who were angry about grain prices and scarcity. She
titled herself 'Captain', like a man, and she supposedly explained her actions as
motivated by 'the Crie of the Country and Hir owne want'.[35] The women petitioners of the 1640s, however, justified their actions in terms of their own
gender, and those justifications circulated widely in print.

It is difficult for us to recover just how shocking these women's public
actions were to their contemporaries. Silence was a virtue closely associated
with the female sex in early modern England. For example, a pamphlet critical
of women's preaching was quick to invoke biblical injunctions, 'To learne in
silence what all subjection' and 'But I suffer not a Woman to teach, nor usurp
authoritie over the man; but to be in silence.'[36] Prescriptive and recreational literature for women abounded in advice about silence. Historian Suzanne Hull
took her book's title, *Chaste, Silent and Obedient,* from a late sixteenth-century
moralizing tale listing these as the three special virtues for women.[37] Laura
Gowing characterizes the domestic advice literature as construing women's
virtue in terms of 'silence, obedience, submissiveness, restraint, and above all
chastity'.[38] In his 1631 book of needlework patterns John Taylor also enjoined
women

> To use their tongues lesse, and their Needles more.
> The Needles sharpenesse, profit yeelds, and pleasure,
> But sharpenesse of the tongue, bites out of measure.[39]

[34] Zaret, *Origins of Democratic Culture*; Achinstein, 'Women on Top'.

[35] John Walter, 'Grain Riots and Popular Attitudes to the Law: Maldon and the Crisis of 1629', in
John Brewer and John Styles (eds.), *An Ungovernable People: the English and their Law in the Seventeenth and Eighteenth Centuries* (New Brunswick, NJ: Rutgers University Press, 1980), 47–84. More
generally, see the helpful discussion in Mendelson and Crawford, *Women in Early Modern England*
380–94.

[36] *A Spirit Moving in the VVomen-preachers* (London: Printed for Henry Sheppard, at the Bible in
Tower-Street, William Lay, at Pauls Chaine neere the Doctors Commons, 1646), Thomason
E.324[10], 6. The citations are 1 Timothy 2: 11–12.

[37] Suzanne Hull, *Chaste, Silent and Obedient: English Books for Women 1475–1640* (San Marino,
Calif.: Huntington Library, 1982), 81; citing Robert Greene, *Penelopes VVeb: VVherein a Christall
Myrror of Fæminine Perfection Represents to the Viewe of Euery One Those Vertues and Graces* (Imprinted
at London: [by Thomas Orwin?] for T[homas]. C[adman] and E[dward] A[ggas], [1587]), STC2
12293, title page. The work was reprinted in 1601.   [38] Gowing, *Domestic Dangers*, 2.

[39] John Taylor, *The Needles Excellency* (London: Printed for James Boler and are to be sold at the
Signe of the Marigold in Paules Churchyard, 1631), STC2 23775.5, sig. A1ᵛ–2ʳ. This work was republished at least twice, in 1634 and 1640. Since the 1640 text claims to be the 12th edition, it is likely
that there were many more editions than are extant today.

From fiction to embroidery patterns, from sermons to household guides, women were everywhere reminded that silence was to be their adornment.

As Taylor's reference to the sharpness of women's tongues suggests, everyone knew that women were not as silent as advice manuals would wish. Proverbs point to women's tongues as troublesome: 'A woman's weapon is her tongue'; 'A woman's tongue is the last thing that dies'; 'Many women many words, many geese many turds'; 'Women must have their words' and many others.[40] William Gouge, author of *Domesticall Duties*, a best-selling 1622 compendium of sermons that functioned as a conduct manual, experienced a reality rather different from the precepts he preached. When he delivered a sermon to his London congregation that included a proscription of a wife disposing of common goods without her husband's prior consent, he was hissed and booed by the women in church. When he published the sermon, he was still so upset about this experience that he took special pains in the introduction to rejustify his position.[41] Many women worked in their husbands' shops or took goods to market to sell, and many others ran their own businesses. Had these women needed their husbands' consent to sell specific goods, their work would have ground to a halt.[42]

Two other locations remind us that women were far from silent in early modern England. First, they could be taken to court for being 'scolds', that is, for speaking out of turn and/or saying harsh things, and special punishments were devised for these unruly women. Often women were ducked in the local pond, immersed in water completely.[43] This punishment is reminiscent of the practice of 'swimming' suspected witches, and also plays on some kind of association with women's humoral physiology—women were thought to be colder and wetter than men. In a 1630 ballad, a young woman scolded a constable for pissing against the wall of her house. She not unreasonably complained that 'every Cuckold now against her wall must pisse', but the ballad writer repeatedly characterized her tongue and her speech as devilish. She already had a reputation as a scold, and the constable threw her into jail and then saw that she

---

[40] Morris Tilley, *A Dictionary of the Proverbs in England in the Sixteenth and Seventeenth Centuries* (Ann Arbor: University of Michigan Press, 1950), proverbs W675, W676, W687, W701. On women's tongues as sexual weapons, see Lisa Jardine, *Still Harping on Daughters* (Sussex: Harvester Press, 1983), 121–6, and Carla Mazzio, 'The Sins of the Tongue', in David Hillman and Carla Mazzio (eds.), *The Body in Parts* (London: Routledge, 1997), 53–81.

[41] William Gouge, *Of Domesticall Duties Eight Treatises* (London: Printed by John Haviland for William Bladen, and are to be sold at the signe of the Bible neere the great North doore of Pauls, 1622), STC 12119, sig. ¶3ᵛ.

[42] On women's work, see Lindsey Charles and Lorna Duffin (eds.), *Women's Work in Pre-Industrial England* (London: Routledge, 1985); Peter Earle, 'The Female Labour Market in London in the Late Seventeenth and Early Eighteenth Centuries', *Economic History Review*, 2nd ser. 42 (1989), 328–53; Mendelson and Crawford, *Women in Early Modern England*, 327–36.

[43] On scolds, see Underdown, 'The Taming of the Scold'. Underdown's findings are disputed in Ingram, ' "Scolding Women Cucked or Washed" '.

was paraded to the waterfront and ducked, wearing only her shift and a humil-
iating necklace of neats' tongues.[44]

Second, the work of scholars such as Laura Gowing on London church
courts makes it clear that women used sexual slander, went to court when slandered, and testified for each other with great frequency in the decades before
the Civil War. As Gowing shows, women and men were acutely aware of legal
boundaries, tiptoeing around the word 'whore', for example, if they wished to
avoid actionable speech.[45] Some women did not hesitate to speak in the streets
or in the court, using colourful and slanderous language, contravening any
ideas about women being chaste, silent, and obedient.

However, in the 1640s and 1650s, women were even less constrained than
before about speaking in public in a number of contexts. The Court of Star
Chamber, which heard riot cases, was abolished. The church courts, which
heard defamation cases, were closed. Men and women such as Katherine
Chidley enjoyed greater freedoms of worship once ecclesiastical authority had
been called into question. And women and men had the novel forum of an
unfettered press eager to publish contemporary dispute and polemic. Not only
were women speaking in public in new ways; that speech was greatly amplified
by the popular press.[46]

Initially, the responses to these women's actions were satirical. Religious and
political activists were caricatured as whores or as sexually voracious. This
translation of one kind of transgression into another points us back to the triad
chaste, silent, and obedient—if a woman was outspoken, surely she was
unchaste and disobedient too. The sexualizing of dissent also relies on a very
old trope, that of women as cuckold-makers. The persistence of the figure of
the cuckold in all kinds of literature suggests just how fragile men felt their
authority over women truly was.

The equation of women speaking out with women in sexual disarray was
invoked almost immediately in 1641. The first extant pamphlet that describes
women preachers characterizes them as creatures carried away by fleshly
desires. The women who came to hear Anne Hempstall, for example, were
'bent more upon the strong water bottle, then upon the uses or doctrines which
their sister entended to expound unto them'. Mary Bilbrow is depicted as

---

[44] *The Cucking of a Scould. To the Tune Of, the Merchant of Em[d]en* (Printed at London: by G.P.,
[*c*.1630]), STC2 6100.

[45] Gowing, *Domestic Dangers*; see also Martin Ingram, *Church Courts, Sex and Marriage in England,
1570–1640* (Cambridge: Cambridge University Press, 1987).

[46] Women also played a key role in the distribution of these novel forms of print. Women 'mer-
curies' hawked the news in the streets. For their role in a slightly later period, see Margaret Hunt,
'Hawkers, Bawlers, and Mercuries: Women and the London Press in the Early Enlightenment',
Women & History, 9 (1984), 41–68; more generally, see Paula McDowell, *The Women of Grub Street:
Press, Politics, and Gender in the London Literary Marketplace, 1678–1730* (Oxford: Clarendon Press,
1998).

leaving her preaching in a rush to go to a gentleman in Bloomsbury. Her gossips feasted on the roast pig she had promised them and we are left to presume Bilbrow satisfied other desires.[47]

Not long after this pamphlet was published, another writer attempted to build on its evident success by going one better: it describes not six women preachers but seven Catholic women confessors! Drawing on recent arrests of Jesuit priests in London, this writer says that seven women 'impudently resolved to supply their places, and privately proclaimed themselves Confessors, ordained by Father Ciprian'.[48] Six of the women are young and pretty, and the older seventh one takes the pieces of silver from the men who select one of the 'confessors' with whom he will meet privately. As the pamphlet concludes, 'By which way they stuffe their purses with gold, and their bellies with children'.[49] The writer of this pamphlet cleverly combined topics of sempiternal interest to early modern English readers—Catholics and sex—and spiced them with current events—the sudden appearance of preaching women, and the arrest and trial of Jesuit priests.

Katherine Chidley was also the subject of sexual slander in much the same way as other women preachers. Patricia Crawford has found a rhyming libel which runs

> Oh Kate, O Kate, thou are unclean I heare,
> A man doth lye betweene thy sheetes, I feare.[50]

This couplet neatly twins sexual licence with the idea that only a man could have written the sheets that made up her books.

Women's new political activities were greeted in a very similar way, with satirical remarks about their sexual desires. In the summer of 1642, just months after the women's petitions to Parliament, the bookseller William Watson produced a mock-petition. Entitled *The Resolution of the Women of London to the Parliament*, it details women's clever employment of political fortunes to achieve their desires for extramarital sexual adventures.[51] Even now, the

---

[47] *Discovery of Six Women-Preachers*, sigs. A2ᵛ, A3ʳ⁻ᵛ. Historians have usually treated this pamphlet as if it reported on real women who were preaching. The effect of facticity is produced by the details—the women's names, their locations, etc. I remain somewhat more agnostic about the relationship of this text to real events, but whatever that relationship, the pamphlet probably reached many more readers than those who went to hear these preachers, and is especially useful in terms of the fears and tropes it embodies.

[48] *The Seven Women Confessors* (London: Printed for John Smith, [1641]), Thomason E.134[15], sig. A3ʳ. On the meanings of 'Cyprian' see Gordon Williams, *A Dictionary of Sexual Language and Imagery in Shakespearian and Stuart Literature* (London: Athlone Press, 1994).

[49] *Seven Women Confessors*, sig. A3ᵛ, quote at sig. A4ʳ.

[50] Crawford, *Women and Religion*, 129, citing a MS collection in the British Library.

[51] *The Resolution of the Women of London to the Parliament* ([London]: for William Watson, 1642), Thomason E.114[140]. Thomason's copy is dated 26 Aug.

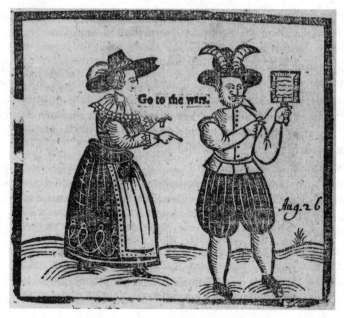

Fig. 3.1. Go to the Wars! Sexual satire and women's political action. *The Resolution of the Women of London to the Parliament* (1642). Courtesy of the British Library, shelf mark E.114[140]

pamphlet gives one a feeling of London in the buildup to war: 'if there should be warrs, as wee doe shrewdly suspect it by the daily noise of Drummes, the great preparations which are made, and the powder which is continually spent, together with the cracking of Guns in the streets'.[52] The oft-repeated trope of women's tongues as weapons is invoked next, the female narrators declaring that they plan 'to use our tongues in such a violent manner, that our continuall scolding shall make them [their husbands] goe to the warres'.[53] Just in case anyone was fooled by the title into thinking that this was a genuine petition, the picture on the title page makes plain the real theme of the work (see Fig. 3.1). It shows a woman telling her husband to go to the wars; the husband is depicted with a cuckold's horns. The pamphlet is not all spoof, however. It sounds a very common note about the true causes of the King's difficulties with Parliament, blaming it on his 'evill wicked counsellors'.[54] Like the seven con-

---

[52] *The Resolution of the Women of London to the Parliament*, sig. A2^r.   [53] Ibid.

[54] Ibid. sig. A3^r. The 'evil counsellors' was a very common trope in criticisms of the monarch, preserving the writer from accusations of treason, and maintaining hope that the monarch might return to his senses. It dates back at least to the reign of Elizabeth.

fessors pamphlet, the *Resolution* cleverly clothes an old theme—cuckoldry—in the contemporary dress of women's new political initiatives.[55]

The equation of verbal and sexual disorder was easy to make, and as we have seen, it appeared in print almost as soon as women began speaking in public in new ways. However, this quick equation did not neutralize the threat to gender relations inherent in women speaking in public, conspicuously not remaining silent. Women's protests and responses to them continued to evolve in the 1640s, playing off one another and becoming more sophisticated and complex in the process. One of the most important aspects of this process was the ways in which women activists and writers continued to call attention to the fact that they were women, even as the responses to them became ever clearer about the extent to which these women's actions appeared to threaten the entire gender hierarchy.

Responses to women preachers, for example, quickly moved beyond sexual slander to deeper arguments about the true nature of woman.[56] In 1642 a female religious visionary was the supposed trigger for a pamphlet subtitled *Wherein is Plainely Expressed the True Nature of Most Women.*[57] The pamphlet envisages a group of women getting together in a tavern, a kind of echo of the scene in *Well Met Gossips* described in Chapter 2. The first woman boasts: 'I thanke God I never cal'd my husband Knave nor Drunkard, I never strove to wear the Breeches.' The narrator points out that she has done just these on many occasions as well as cuckolding her husband. The second woman commends the first, saying that she's been a little too hasty with her tongue. The third woman parodies the advice literature by suggesting that women, being the weaker sex, are bound to fail much more often than men, 'Truely Goshopp [i.e. gossip] quoth she the Tounge is an unruly member, besides, you know that Woman are the weaker Vessels, & men ought to beare with our infermeties.'[58] The drunken women then lurch home, greeted by husbands asking them where they've been. Women's tongues cause trouble again: 'they look presently

[55] For additional sexual satires based on women's petitions to Parliament, see *The Virgins Complaint for the Losse of their Sweet-Hearts* (London: printed for Henry Wilson, 1642), Thomason E.86[38]; *The Widovves Lamentation* (Printed at London for John Robinson, 1643), Thomason E.88[26]; *The Mid-Wives Just Petition* (Printed at London, 1643), Thomason E.86[14]. Thomason dates this as 26 Jan. 1642; *The Humble Petition of Many Thousands of Wives and Matrons* (Printed at London for John Cookson, 1643), Thomason E.88[13]. Thomason dates this 4 Feb. 1643. For more on sexual slander, see Ch. 6.

[56] Debates about the nature of woman had, of course, been a staple of early modern print culture. The so-called *querelle des femmes*, originally a late medieval discussion, heated up in the 1620s with the publication of the famous misogynist pamphlets collected and reprinted in Katherine Usher Henderson and Barbara McManus, *Half Humankind: Contexts and Texts of the Controversy about Women in England, 1540–1640* (Urbana: University of Illinois Press, 1985). However, the Civil War period saw a shift in these kinds of rhetoric as women took on new roles.

[57] L. H., *A Strange Wonder or Wonder in A Woman* (London: Printed for I.T., 1642), Thomason E.144[5]. [58] Ibid. 3.

on their Apron Strings, which inspires them with a Lye with which they slapp their too credulous Husbands in the Mouth'. One has been to see an aunt, another to the childbed of a gentlewoman. Lying is equated with cuckoldry and then with religious dissent: 'there is no Whore to a holy Whore . . . she can cover her Lust with Religion'.[59] Here a single female visionary provokes an entire catalogue of women's failings: dishonesty, drunkenness, sexual infidelity.

Some of the same themes are invoked in a work with a very different tone, a critique of women preachers grounded in scriptural citations. Here too, however, women's new religious activities threaten all gender hierarchy. Just a few women preaching seem to undermine the entire construct of gender roles. Women preachers are decribed as 'wearing the breeches, and so draw and lead their husbands by the nose'.[60] The writer expands with a discussion of the fact that women are not equal to men:

1. By Creation, we find her equall unto the man, a helper meet for him, Gen. 2.18. 2. By Degeneration, we find her to be his inferiour, the weaker vessell, as the Apostle speaks, 1 Pet.3.7 made subject unto mans government, her will forever subjected unto his will, he to beare rule over her, Gen 3.16. she becoming therwith ignorant, shallow, proud, ambitious, fantastike, inconstant, passionate, and vaine-glorious, indiscreet, easily led into extreames.[61]

Just as a single woman visionary leads to the pamphlet describing women's drunkenness, lying, etc., here preaching women invoke a response designed to show the inherent instability of all women.

Responses to women's new religious activism were not limited to pamphlet-writers. The flowering of all kinds of new religious activities worried Parliament as early as 1641, when the House of Commons passed a resolution to reprove lay preachers.[62] But by the mid-1640s the sense of crisis was much more acute. In January 1646 the Lord Mayor of London and the aldermen presented a petition to the House of Lords to suppress all private meetings on Sundays, claiming that there were as many as eleven independent congregations in a single parish. All over London, groups of people were meeting, not just for religious discussion, but for worship. Voluntary gatherings were evolving into congregations.[63]

1646 saw increased policing of unorthodox religious expression, as well as the publication of Edwards's *Gangraena*. Women were not the only targets of

---

[59] L. H., *Strange*, 4. The remark about the apron strings plays upon a very well-known proverb that a woman need look no further than her apron string to find an excuse for herself. Tilley, *Dictionary*, W659.

[60] *Spirit Moving*, 3.   [61] Ibid. 4.

[62] This paragraph rests on the work of Ethyn Morgan Williams, 'Women Preachers in the Civil War', *Journal of Modern History*, 1 (1929), 561–9.

[63] Francis Bremer, *Congregational Communion: Clerical Friendship in the Anglo-American Puritan Community, 1610–1692* (Boston: Northeastern University Press, 1994).

repression, but they were among the most visibly outrageous examples of the proliferation of religious excess. There is tantalizing but incomplete evidence that in January 1646 women were hauled before the House of Commons' Committee of Examinations to testify about the female preachers already committed to custody.[64] Later in the year Parliament passed a number of acts designed to rein in a variety of religious offenders. For example, the Commons passed an act against blasphemy and heresy, and, after some discussion, decided that the punishment for the crime should be death.[65] A few weeks later, the Lords passed an act punishing anyone who interrupted or otherwise caused a disturbance in a religious service. The Lords further ordered that the act be read out in every church in the land.[66] Finally, on 30 December, the Commons passed a law that no person could preach or expound the Scriptures in any church, chapel, or other public place unless ordained in the Church of England or some other Reformed church. Nor was any minister or any other to preach or publish anything 'against or in derogation of' the form of church government instituted by Parliament.[67] Obviously, both men and women preachers were targeted by this act, but men might at least aspire to some form of ordination in some kind of church. Women could not.

Women responded to these strictures in a variety of ways, but interestingly, their responses often reminded their readers that they were women. As the dialogue between women and their critics continued, women writers became more insistent on their identities as women. For example, Mary Cary did not take kindly to the persecution of women preachers or the clamping down on religious diversity. In June 1647 she published a pamphlet urging Parliament to reconsider, exhorting them repeatedly, 'be wise ye rulers'. She told them: 'be sure you do not stop the mouths of the Prophets of Jesus Christ' and enjoined 'for though you do permit some to Preach Jesus Christ, yet if you do prohibit any from Preaching Jesus Christ, you do quench the spirit and oppose the freeness of the spirit, who is a free agent'. Just in case her readers missed the specificity of her argument, she continued: 'Do not you enact any law against any Saints exercising the gifts of the spirit.'[68] Cary places her own authority as a religious seeker above the authority of the Parliament.

Cary uses a metaphor about this pamphlet that might remind readers that she is a woman: she subtitles it 'A precious cordiall for a distempered Kingdom'.

[64] *A Diary, or an Exact Journall*, 22 Jan. to 29 Jan. 1645 [i.e. 1646], Thomason E. 319[19], 4. I have not found references to these events in other newsbooks.

[65] *A Perfect Diurnall*, 30 Nov. to 7 Dec. 1646, Thomason E.513[27], 1399.

[66] Ibid. 11 to 18 Dec. 1646, Thomason E.513[30], 1424.

[67] Ibid. 28 Dec. 1646 to 4 Jan. 1647, Thomason E.513[31], 1436.

[68] Mary Cary, *A Word in Season to the Kingdom of England* (London: Printed by R.W. for Giles Calvert, and are to be sold at the Black-spred Eagle at the West end of Pauls, 1647) Thomason E.393[26], 2, 4–5.

She extends the metaphor at the close of the pamphlet: 'If now this cordiall shall be received, it may allay the violence of (& expell) that distemper which is upon this kingdom, which may otherwise prove its death.' And to whom was this cordial to be administered? 'Now it must be first taken in by the head, by those that are in the highest Authority, and from thence the sweet and comfortable effects of it shall descend to all the members, the whole body.'[69] Women made cordials and other healing preparations as a part of their household duties. Both manuscript remedy books and printed works testify to the assumption that such work was women's work. One of the best-known printed medical works was supposed to have been written by Elizabeth Grey, the Countess of Kent.[70] Another claimed to be the private recreation of none other than Queen Elizabeth.[71]

Katherine Chidley reminds her readers that she is female, despite her fondness for male military metaphors in her battles with Thomas Edwards. It is as if she, Cary, and others constantly play with the instabilities inherent in their transgressions of gender roles, transforming even their supposed lack of power into a kind of power all their own. Chidley notes that 'both I, and my faithful yoakfellow have jointly tasted of the pressures of the Hierarchy above these twenty yeares'.[72] The language of 'yokefellow', drawn from Puritan ideals of marriage, and the word 'jointly' as well as some readers' knowledge of the Chidleys' travails, makes Katherine the equal of her husband. On the next page, she uses her female identity to poke fun at Edwards. Edwards had claimed that his book *Reasons Against the Independent Government of Particular Congregations* was the first published of his books against separation, but not the first or only one he had written. Unfortunately, he used the imagery of conception and birth to describe these writings. Chidley implictly reminds the reader that she, as a woman, knows about matters of reproduction. Edwards claimed that his book was 'the first brought forth, but not the first conceived', to which Chidley replied 'I have waited these three yeares, for the bringing of them [the books already conceived] forth, but now it seemes to

---

[69] Cary, *Word in Season*, 12.

[70] Elizabeth Grey, Countess of Kent, *A Choice Manual of Rare and Select Secrets in Physick and Chyrurgery; collected, and practised by the Right Honorable, the Countesse of Kent, late deceased* (London: printed by G.D. and are to be sold by William Shears, at the Sign of the Bible in St. Pauls Church-yard, 1653), Wing (CD-ROM) K310B. Three different editions were published in this one year. The Countess died in 1651, so the extent of her role in the composition of this text is not known, but it is clear that an aristocratic woman was considered by a publisher to be the right kind of author—and the work went through at least sixteen 17th-c. editions.

[71] *The Queens Closet Opened. Incomparable Secrets in Physick, Chirurgery, Preserving, Candying, and Cookery; as They Were Presented to the Queen by the Most Experienced Persons of Our Times* ([London]: Printed for Nathaniel Brook at the Angel in Cornhill, 1655), Thomason E.1519[1]. This book went through at least thirteen 17th-c. editions.   [72] Chidley, *New-Yeares-Gift*, sig. A2ʳ.

me, It was a false conception.' In addition, if Edwards thought that he had experienced 'painful labouring' in bringing them forth, it 'ariseth out of feare'.[73]

Chidley's arguments also drew strength from her heartfelt descriptions of the depredations of ministers. Her critique of ministerial greed was cast very much in terms of her role as a mother, 'for if a dead child be borne into the world, they will be paid for reading a dirge over it before it shall be laid into the earth'. She continued by scorning the practice of churching new mothers:

> Further, they will yet *have another patrimony for the birth of that childe,* for before the mother dare goe abroad, shee must have their *blessing,* that the *Sun* shall not smite her by *day,* nor the *Moone* by *night,* for which *blessing* of theirs they must have an *offering,* and the like they require for all of the children that be borne into this world, though there live not one of sixe to be men or women.[74]

The language of the sun and the moon was drawn directly from the service of thanksgiving after childbirth in the Book of Common Prayer. Chidley was not unique in her criticisms of it, but the reader's knowledge that she was a woman and had participated in the service herself intensified her critique.

Chidley continues with the theme of ministerial greed in one of the most heart-rending passages in her work, where she describes the costs of burying a child who has died. She says that the poor, suffering great loss already, have to pawn their clothes in order bury a child. She names specific parishes in which the poorest parents will have to pay 7 or 8 shillings for burial, and that in a distant churchyard outside the city.[75] The specificity of her details— which parishes, which churchyards, how much money—suggests that her information was all too painfully acquired. Her children died in frightening succession, and 7 or 8 shillings might be a week's wages for a working man. Here again, Chidley's arguments are made stronger by the reader's knowledge of her sex.

Chidley's main opponent, Thomas Edwards, had no doubt that religious excess, especially by women, would lead to the breakdown of all kinds of social order. In *Gangraena* he tells a cautionary tale. Edwards was at a merchant's house when

> there came in one Mr. Y. who related that in his Family there were but four persons, himself, his wife, a man and a maid-Servant, and saith he, we are of severall Churches and wayes; I am of the Church of *England,* my wife was one of *Mr. Jacies* Church; but she is fallen off from that Church (as many others have) and is now of none, doubting whether there be any Church or no upon the Earth; my Maid-Servant is of *Paul Hobsons,* my man belongs to a company of which there are some twenty or more yong

---

[73] Chidley, *New-Yeares-Gift,* sig. A2ᵛ.   [74] Chidley, *Justification,* 57.   [75] Ibid.

men, who meet together to Exercise, but sing no Psalms, abominate the hearing of our Ministers, keep none of our dayes of Fasting nor Thanksgiving.[76]

This anecdote is cleverly constructed to move the reader from one horror to the next, ever worse. The head of the family's orthodoxy is quickly rendered meaningless by his inability to master his household. His wife does not obey him, but first attended Henry Jessey's congregation, not a parish church (one of Jessey's books is the focus of the next chapter). Worse yet, she now doubts that there are any churches at all. The maid follows her mistress rather than her master in attending an independent congregation although she does not go as far as her mistress in denying the very idea of churches. The manservant is worse—he attends a congregation in which there is not even a ministerial figure of any kind. The young men follow their own guidance and discard all of the apparatus so carefully set up by Edwards and other Presbyterians, such as fast days and their associated sermons.

Elsewhere in his book, Edwards makes his message more abstract, saying 'If a Toleration were granted, they [men] should never have peace in their families more, or ever after have command of wives, children, servants.'[77] Disorder in religion ('toleration') translates immediately into gender disorder in this passage. For Edwards religious difference was truly terrifying. As he notes, 'The armies of heresies, errours among us, are worse than all the Armies of Cavaleers, and Monsters hardlier to be subdued.'[78] Like monsters, religious errors might breed yet more of themselves or devour everything in their path. Edwards's story of the family of four kinds of belief tellingly illustrates his understanding of the way in which proper religion undergirded all other kinds of order, especially the God-given gender hierarchy.

The same patterns structure the evolution of women's political protest. As their critics move from sexual satire to more fundamental critiques of women's ability to act in public, women articulate their understanding of their rights as women in sharper ways. These women remind their auditors and their readers that they are women, even if they are acting in ways not usually sanctioned for women. In 1649, Leveller women presented two petitions to Parliament asking for the freedom of Leveller leaders John Lilburne, William Walwyn, Thomas Prince, and Richard Overton. The Levellers began as radical Independents in London in the mid-1640s. They sought to rework the nature of political rule, arguing for natural law and popular sovereignty. For example, they argued for a written constitution ratified by the signatures of the people of England. An attempted army mutiny by Levellers failed, and the movement's leaders were imprisoned. Lilburne in particular was a dramatic figure; he conducted his own

---

[76] Edwards, *Gangraena*, 89. See also Edwards's recounting of the sexual misdeeds of Independent preachers, for example, pt. 2, p. 9; pt. 3, pp. 185–91.   [77] Ibid. pt. 1, p. 156.   [78] Ibid. 151.

defence in court in 1649 and again in 1653, swaying juries against all odds to free him both times.[79]

In their petitions, Leveller women called attention to their status as women. The first petition asked, with rhetorical modesty, what could be expected of the weaker vessel? A few lines later, however, the women declare 'we have an equal share and interest with men in the Common-wealth'.[80] Just like Katherine Chidley on the title page of her first book, the petition then invokes Jael and Deborah: 'God hath wrought many deliverances for severall nations, from age to age by the weake hand of women: By the counsell and presence of *Deborah*, and the hand of *Jaell, Israell* was delivered from the King of *Canaan, Sisera* and his mighty Host, *Judges* 4.' The petitioners shift from the Bible to the ancient and recent history of the British Isles, describing women who rescued Britain from the tyranny of the Danes, and claiming that the recent war in Scotland was started by women.[81] Women they are, but fearsome women.

The next petition sounded similar themes about women's rights as citizens. The petition is thought to have been written by none other than Katherine Chidley.[82] She asked: 'Have we not an equal interest with the men of this Nation, in those liberties and securities contained in the Petition of Right, and other good Lawes of the Land?'[83] She also threatened that Leveller women would fight to the bitter end:

But if nothing will satisfy but the bloud of those just men, those constant Asserters of the peoples freedoms will satisfy your thirst, drink also, and be glutted with our bloud, and let us all fall together: take the blood of one more, and take all: slay one, slay all.[84]

Here is a gruesome vision of women and men slaughtered for their political ideals. Just after this image, Chidley retreats and reminds the reader yet again that she and her allies are women, chiding Parliament 'not to slight the things therein contained, because they are presented unto you by the weake hand of Weomen, it being an usuall thing with God, by weak meanes to work mighty

---

[79] On the Leveller movement, see H. N. Brailsford, *The Levellers and the English Revolution* (London: Cresset Press, 1961); Richard Gleissner, 'The Levellers and Natural Law: The Putney Debates of 1647', *Journal of British Studies*, 20 (1980), 74–89; Mark Kishlansky, 'What Happened at Ware?', *Historical Journal*, 25 (1982), 827–39. I am much indebted to Hughes, 'Gender and Politics in Leveller Literature', who discusses the complex ways in which Leveller leaders employed gender norms.

[80] *To the Supream authority of this nation* (Imprinted at London, 1649), Thomason E.551[14], 3–4.

[81] Ibid. 4–5. Katherine Chidley may have been the author of this pamphlet or had a hand in its composition; she is considered to be the author of the second 1649 Leveller women's petition. Gentles, 'London Levellers', 292.

[82] On the authorship of this petition, see Higgins, 'Reactions of Women', 218; Gentles, 'London Levellers', 293.

[83] *To the Supream Authority of England The Commons Assembled in Parliament* (London: s.n., 1649), Wing2 T1724A.   [84] Ibid.

effects'.[85] As in many other examples, the rhetoric of female weakness is cross-cut by claims to divine authority.

As women petitioners became ever more articulate about their female identities and what those identities meant politically, responses to them sharpened. No longer were cheap sexual jokes sufficient. Instead, Parliament and others invoked customary gender hierarchies in an attempt to contain the threat of disorder these women represented. After the second Leveller petition was presented to Parliament, the Sergeant at Arms told the waiting women that

> Mr. Speaker (by the direction of the House) hath commanded me to tell you, The matter you petition about, is of a higher concernment then you understand, that the House gave an answer to your husbands; and therefore you are desired to looke after your owne businesse, and meddle with your huswifery.[86]

The House of Commons tried to put women back into their place—the home. Because married women had no legal status separate from their husbands, this statement implies the women's petition, which echoes that of their husbands, is redundant.

Leveller women were very well known in London. Even as newsbook accounts of their petitions and the Commons' response were circulating in London, Leveller women staged a gigantic 1649 funeral procession for Robert Lockyer, executed for his role in an army mutiny over pay. Hundreds or even thousands of women marched, wearing sea-green ribbons denoting Leveller allegiance with black ones for mourning.[87] One of the Leveller women's petitions is supposed to have been signed by 10,000 women and presented to Parliament by 1,000 of them.[88]

Newsbooks revelled in Parliament's reply to these Leveller petitions. Each one chose a slightly different emphasis in their telling of the tale. In each instance, however, the threat to gender hierarchy that these women represent is never far from the surface. One of the first responses was the familiar sexual slander. The newsbook *Mercurius Pragmaticus* makes the petitioners into whores, describing them as 'The Meek-hearted Congregation of *Oyster-wives*, together with the Civill-Sisterhood of *Oranges* and *Lemmons*'. The presentation of the petition was compared to Amazons raping the unmanned 'capons' in the House.[89] Another newsbook, *Mercurius Brittanicus*, reports on the account in *Mercurius Pragmaticus*.

---

[85] *To the Supream Authority of England.*
[86] *Perfect Occurrences of Every Daie Journall in Parliament*, 20 to 27 Apr. 1649, Thomason E.529 [21], 998.   [87] Higgins, 'Reactions of Women', 204.   [88] Brailsford, *Levellers*, 317.
[89] *Mercurius Pragmaticus*, 23 to 30 Apr. 1649, Thomason E.552[12], sig. A1ᵛ–2ʳ. Both oyster-wives and orange-sellers were commonly stereotyped as prostitutes. See Williams, *Dictionary of Sexual Language*.

He tells us of the female Sects, that petitioned the House in behalf of *John Lilburne, Sirrah*, the House returned them a seasonable Answer; which was in effect, that they should go home and look after their own businesses, which was in effect, that they should go home and spin, it being the usuall work of women, either to spin or knit, and not to meddle with State Affaires.[90]

Here unruly women in one context—that of political protest—are elided with unruly women in another, that of religion. The women petitioners are called 'sects'.

Two other newsbooks create a kind of dialogue between the speech of the Sergeant at Arms and the writer of the newsbook. *The Man in the Moone* said:

The Women-Petitioners had their Answer by the Sergeant at *Armes*, it seems the Speaker was afraid, or too good to speak to them; Their *Answer* was this . . . *That the matter of your Petition is of a higher concernment then you understand*, (higher indeed by their own heads, if they had but their deserts) *The House gave an Answer to your husbands* (Uds nails women, what's that to you? Were your Husbands satisfied any more than you? Scratch 'em, I say still) *and therefor you are desired to go home and wash your dishes.*—And bring the dish-water, and scal'd the *Hornetts* out of their Nest for to be sure they will *sting* your friends.[91]

While the Royalist *Man in the Moone* is as critical of the Commons as it is of the women, the parenthetical comments belittle the women's political intervention.

Another newsbook dialogue sounds familiar themes about women's tongues: 'It can never be a good world, when women meddle in States matters. If their tongues must be prattling, they may finde other talke, and their Husbands are to blame, that have no fitter imployment for them.' It concludes by reminding the reader that women petitioners do not belong in public, 'nor civill for Women to prate in Congregations of men, and to aske their Husbands at home; we shall have things brought to a fine passe, if Women come to teach the Parliament to make Lawes'.[92] Although each newsbook took its own characteristic approach to the Houses's replies to the Leveller women, they all suggest that such protest violates fundamental social codes of behaviour. The repetition and retellings of the story from newsbook to newsbook creates a kind of chorus of disapproval, each voice slightly modulated, but in harmony with the rest. Their message is clear: women's place is at home, not in the nascent public sphere created by popular demonstrations and cheap print.

---

[90] *Mercurius Brittanicus*, 1 to 8 May 1649, Thomason E.554[18], 11.

[91] *The Man in the Moon Discovering a World of Knavery under the Sunne*, 23 to 30 Apr., Thomason E.552[8], 22.

[92] *Continued Heads or Perfect Passages in Parliament*, 20 Mar. to 6 Apr. 1649, Thomason E.529[23], 12.

Two interrelated features of the 1640s troubled gender politics. First, as we have seen, women took action in public. Never before had Londoners seen thousands of women marching through the streets to deliver a petition to Parliament. Never before had they seen women confidently asserting their rights to preach in public. These women responded to criticism, not by assuming some kind of gender-neutral identity or claims, but by affirming their female identity, claiming that it did not prevent them from speaking in public. The second feature made those women's words echo throughout the realm: it was the explosion of cheap print that followed the lapse of press censorship in the 1640s. That lapse created something more than just the space for a lot of printed works. The flowering of newsbooks and pamphlets created a kind of public conversation about current events. While newsbooks' stories about women petitioners were not flattering, they did reproduce and disseminate those women's words and deeds. This decade of female activism cast long shadows. Combined with the questioning of all kinds of analogous hierarchies, these women's actions seemed to query many assumptions about the structure of gender relations. In the midst of 'a world turned upside down', some writers turned to the human body itself as a possible producer of stable truths. Before we turn to Nicholas Culpeper and his 1651 attempt to make women's bodies into models of gender relations, we need to look more closely at the difficulties inherent in making bodies produce truths of any kind. The story of Sarah Wight, and Henry Jessey's efforts to tell that story, show us how men continued to struggle to write about women's bodies.

4

Henry Jessey, Sarah Wight, and the Struggle to Make Women's Bodies into Knowledge

Women petitioners and preachers of the 1640s and early 1650s questioned some of the customary limits of female gender roles in early modern England. Noisy and insistent, they proposed new kinds of equality with men. These women emphasized both their spiritual equality with men and their rights to speak out in public. Preaching women, however, were only part of the explosion of religious diversity during the Civil War and Interregnum. Other women burst into prominence as prophets, visionaries, and seekers. Some, such as Anna Trapnel and Elizabeth Poole, took public roles, speaking to members of the government. Many others appeared in public by means of print. These visionaries chose a different means of testing the limits of acceptable female behaviour. Where preachers and petitioners relied on argument, claiming the same kinds of public attention due to men and employing the same rhetorical forms as men, prophesying women took a different approach. They transmuted their inferior gender position into a superior one by a peculiar sort of alchemy. These women made specific claims to weakness, of mind or body or both, and then used that weakness as a kind of guarantor of their spiritual superiority. In this chapter, we will see how one such woman, Sarah Wight, questioned ideas about the female body, and how the minister Henry Jessey struggled to make Wight's body into reliable knowledge in his 1647 text, *The Exceeding Riches of Grace Advanced.*[1]

Sarah Wight was a 15-year-old girl when she was confined to her bed, and so Jessey's book about her is not about motherhood in the same way as many of my sources in earlier chapters. Her story is significant, however, because it shows us how difficult it was to make stable truths from the mutable female

---

[1] Henry Jessey, *The Exceeding Riches of Grace Advanced* (London: Printed by Matthew Simmons for Henry Overton, and Hannah Allen, and are to be sold at their shops in Popes-head Alley, 1647), Wing2 J687. On Wight's story, see Nigel Smith, *Perfection Proclaimed: Language and Literature in English Radical Religion 1640–1660* (Oxford: Oxford University Press, 1989), 45–51; Barbara Ritter Dailey, 'The Visitation of Sarah Wight: Holy Carnival and the Revolution of the Saints in Civil War London', *Church History*, 55 (1986), 438–55; Diane Purkiss, 'Producing the Voice, Consuming the Body: Women Prophets of the 17th c.', in Isobel Grundy and Susan Wiseman (eds.), *Women, Writing, History 1640–1740* (Athens, Ga.: University of Georgia Press, 1992), 139–58, esp. 145–7; on women

body. Much as Edward Jorden struggled to persuade his readers that Mary
Glover was suffering from a natural ailment, so too did Jessey struggle to
persuade his readers that Wight's body was not afflicted in an ordinary way,
because her affliction gave her a powerful connection with the divine. In
both cases, these men struggled with the question of authenticity—were these
girls just faking it? In both cases, these girls' disturbed bodies prompted
questions about what normal female bodies might be. And finally, in both
cases, these girls' weird afflictions served as peculiar commentary on aspects of
motherhood and the maternal body. In the next chapter, we shall see how
Nicholas Culpeper resolved Jorden's and Jessey's struggles to make female
bodies into reliable knowledge by invoking anatomy and, just as important, by
talking about men's bodies. In order to understand the magnitude of his
accomplishment, however, we first need to understand Henry Jessey and Sarah
Wight.

   Wight and the prophesying women of the 1640s and 1650s did not use new
tactics to underwrite the truths they produced. Playing with the tension
between bodily weakness and spiritual strength goes back to the earliest days
of the Christian church. Medieval women who fasted employed a similar
rhetoric of weakness and strength. Two aspects of English life in the 1640s
and 1650s made use of this kind of rhetoric distinctive. As discussed in
the previous chapter, the breakdown in various kinds of authority both
permitted an explosion of religious diversity and created a much more
open print marketplace, so that people all over the country could read
about the many new ways that men and women sought God. These two aspects
were interlinked: printers capitalized on the more sensational aspects of
religious diversity, and thus promoted and encouraged more of the same.
Writers on religious subjects as well as their critics were very sensitive to the
mechanics and structures of the print marketplace, and shaped their writings
accordingly.

   A brief example illustrates how female religious writers claimed that their
weakness as women paradoxically gave them strength as visionaries. Mary Cary
was a religious seer and writer. Her work plays with her identity as a woman,
simultaneously claiming an almost masculine right to speak, but always
coming back to her weaker status as a woman. Cary dedicates her book *The
Little Horns Doom* to three women, noting 'I have therefore chosen (being of

---

prophets in this period more generally see Mack, *Visionary Women*; Hinds, *God's Englishwomen*;
Christina Berg and Phillipa Berry, 'Spiritual Whoredom: An Essay on Female Prophets in the 17th c.',
in Francis Barker et al. (eds.), *1642: Literature and Power in the 17th c.* (Proceedings of the Essex Con-
ference on the Sociology of Literature, Colchester, 1981), 37–54; Elaine Hobby, 'Discourses So
Unsavoury: Women's Published Writings of the 1650s', in Grundy and Wiseman (eds.), *Women,
Writing, History*, 16–32.

your own sex) to dedicate these Treatises to your Ladiships'.[2] In a passage often quoted, Cary emphasizes her female weakness:

for I am a very weake, and unworthy instrument, and have not done this worke by any strength of my owne, but have often been made sensible, that I could doe no more herein, (wherein any light, or truth could appeare) of my selfe, then a pensill, or pen can do, when no hand guides it.[3]

Here she abases herself, claiming merely to be a kind of transcriber or vehicle. However weak she may be, she is nonetheless proclaiming God's word, and as such, her writings are granted immense power. While many critics have emphasized the humility of Cary's comparison of herself to a mere pencil, few have noted that immediately after this figure of speech, she goes on to compare herself with one of Christ's apostles, 'that to use the Apostles expression, and to speak it feelingly, (for I finde it daily true) I must professe, *I am not sufficient to thinke a good thought, but my sufficiency is of God*'.[4] Cary may be like a pencil, but she is also a transmitter of the divine. This tension between female weakness and a godly power that far outstrips any male authority was given intense bodily meaning by women such as Sarah Wight, who fasted for long periods before prophesying. Here the contrast between female weakness and divine power was expressed literally, since these women could not get out of bed but could speak the word of the Lord.[5]

In Cary's text, even her claim to female unworthiness is countered by the addendum by Hugh Peter, an important Puritan preacher who had spent time with independent congregations in New England. Cary cleverly employs one of the most significant tactics in print culture of the period: she invokes authorities, having one such as Hugh Peter write framing documents to endorse the authenticity of her own words. Peter also plays with the rhetoric of weakness and strength by out-doing Cary in assertions of unworthiness. He opens his encomium thus: 'They that have any knowledge of my self, how worthless a worm I am; do also know how unfit I am either to write Books, or to judge of others writing.'[6] He praises Cary, saying that 'she hath taught her sexe that ther are more ways then one to avoid idleness (the devils cushion) on which so many sit and sleep their last. They that will not use the Distaff, may improve a Pen.'[7] Cary is not just a pencil; here she is licensed to abandon traditional female occupations (a distaff, used in spinning, was emblematic of women's work) and

---

[2] Mary Cary, *The Little Horns Doom & Downfall* (London: Printed for the Author, and are to be sold at the sign of the Black-spred Eagle, at the West end of Pauls, 1651), Thomason E.1274[1], sig. A5ʳ.
[3] Ibid. sig. A8ʳ.   [4] Ibid.   [5] See Mack, *Visionary Women*, 115–16.
[6] Cary, *Little Horns Doom*, sig. a1ʳ.
[7] Ibid. sig. a1ᵛ. Peter was not always receptive to women's religious gifts, having denounced Anne Hutchinson in New England.

take up the pen instead. Indeed, according to Peter, Cary's writing is so good that people might think it was really a man's work. Peter draws upon the stereotypical male work of plowing to make this point: 'you might easily think she plow'd with anothers Heifer, were not the contrary well known'.[8] He finally reminds the reader again that Cary is a woman, but does so in the context of abasing himself before her: 'More would I say; but my feeble thoughts or words will adde but little to her labours. Doubtless she had good help from above in her travel for this birth.'[9] It is as if the writing of her books is a process unknown to men, akin to 'travel' or travail, that is, labour and delivery. Peter's encomium thus complicates any easy picture of Cary as a female mystic whose claims of weakness can be read one-dimensionally. Instead, like others, she plays with the associations between her identity as a weak woman and her strength as a religious seeker and visionary, moving the reader back and forth between considerations of her power and her lack of it. And it is Peter who employs the powerful but female metaphor of giving birth to describe Cary's authorship, not Cary herself.

Female visionaries such as Cary and Wight were uncommon but not unknown in English history. In the 1520s Elizabeth Barton prophesied about Henry VIII's chances of having a son and was executed for treason. Such visionary women, however, came into special prominence in the middle of the seventeenth century. Phyllis Mack has documented over 300 of them in the 1640s and 1650s.[10] As with petitioning and preaching women, the boom in cheap print made these women far more visible than were their earlier counterparts. While Elizabeth Barton had had two of her books published, they were suppressed and no copies survive today. By contrast, Henry Jessey's account of Sarah Wight's sufferings and visions went into eight editions by 1700, more than any other book he wrote.[11] Wight stayed in bed, and Londoners came to her for counsel. Jessey's book in effect made Wight's bed her pulpit, creating a different kind of public than those who went to hear women preachers, but a public nonetheless. The breakdown in institutions of state censorship of the press in the 1640s and 1650s meant that many more unorthodox, radical, or critical works by women and men were printed and have survived.

Women who prophesied proposed a very different model of the female body than did those who preached. The men who transcribed, ordered, and published these women's words played upon stereotypes of femininity in the production of their texts and thereby also shaped this model of the female body. The intricate ways in which female prophets and male ministers together pro-

---

[8] Cary, *Little Horns Doom*, sig. a2ʳ.   [9] Ibid. sig. a3ʳ.

[10] Mack, *Visionary Women*, esp. 415–24.

[11] Jessey also published a series of religiously-oriented almanacs for over a decade, which might be considered his other best-seller.

duced this alternative model of a female body are evident in Henry Jessey's account of 15-year-old Sarah Wight and her relationship with God. Jessey, a 46-year-old minister, had been born in Yorkshire and educated at St John's College, Cambridge. He headed an independent congregation in London from 1637 until his death in 1663. Although usually considered a Particular Baptist, Jessey may be better understood as an Independent, since he continued to permit open membership in his church, and remained tolerant of various forms of religious diversity.[12]

Jessey's book is an exploration of the meanings of femaleness, both for Wight and for himself. Sarah Wight's actions and speeches question what it is to be female and to have a female body. She uses and subverts cultural expectations of women as mothers and as daughters as she wrestles with a profound spiritual and emotional crisis. Even through the medium of Jessey's text we can begin to see how Wight employs a rich set of symbols, evidently understood by many of those around her, in her despair and her discovery of salvation. We can only perceive some of these meanings, because Sarah's actions are framed and interpreted through Jessey's text.

In what follows, I begin with Wight's story, mediated by Jessey's text, and then move out to Jessey's actions and writings. However, I do not wish to imply that Wight's is the real or true story and Jessey's just the telling of it. Rather, I see both of them actively involved in producing the book, Wight through her speech and actions, and Jessey through his writing. As we shall see, Jessey's role was complex, and his concerns about Wight's body and its relation to larger cultural practices and assumptions about female bodies produce a tension between Wight's body and his words throughout the book. What results is a book that explores the meaning of femaleness and female bodies as profoundly as any midwifery manual. Jessey, like Thomas Raynalde (author/translator of *The Birth of Mankind*), or Jacob Rueff (author of *The Expert Midwife*), or Edward Jorden (author of a pamphlet about Mary Glover) found it difficult to interpret the female body and difficult to persuade his readers that he spoke authoritatively on a topic that was usually the focus of women's talk rather than men's writing.

In a peculiar way, some of the bodily details that marked Wight's crisis also characterized Mary Glover's possession by demons, discussed in Chapter 2. The two mechanisms—demonic possession, spiritual crisis—were considered very different, but each young woman drew on a kind of repertoire of bodily signs explicable within their culture. Observers struggled to read the signs

---

[12] On Jessey, see Richard L. Greaves and Robert Zaller, *Biographical Dictionary of British Radicals* (Brighton: Harvester Press, 1982–4), ii. 140–1; Bernard Capp, *The Fifth Monarchy Men* (London: Faber and Faber, 1972), *passim*.

correctly and distinguish between possession and despair. Each young woman withdrew from the world by losing her ability to eat and to hear. Wight's loss of vision pointed towards her spiritual seeing just as Glover's fits pointed to her possession. In each case, only the sustained commitment of religious resources enabled these young women to regain physical health.

Sarah was the daughter of Thomas Wight, a member of the gentry who had held a position of responsibility in the Exchequer. He was dead by the time of Jessey's narrative; Sarah is described as living with her widowed mother, Mrs Mary Wight. Mrs Wight had been married previously, and Sarah had a stepbrother Jonathan, who was a fellow of All Souls, Oxford during the period of Jessey's narrative. The Wight family seems to have been comfortably well off, living in Caning or Cannon Street in the London parish of St Lawrence Pountney, in Tower Hill.[13] In 1647 Sarah fasted for seventy-five days, remaining bedridden, deaf, mute, and blind while she was convinced that she was damned. She began to speak about her conversations with God, and women sought her counsel even while she stayed in bed. Finally, she began to eat again and was able to get up and resume a more usual style of life. In the 1650s, devastated by the death of her stepbrother, Wight suffered again but seems to have recovered. In 1656 a lengthy letter of hers about religious matters was published as a book, supposedly without her knowledge or permission.[14]

Jessey's book about Wight is a kind of double production. Both Jessey and Wight draw upon cultural scripts, Wight to structure her actions, and Jessey to make meaning from those actions. As Phyllis Mack has suggested, prophesying women appear to transgress cultural norms about appropriate behaviour for women, but the ways in which they do so profoundly evoke the very norms they seek to disrupt.[15] In the case of Jessey's book, we can see both the highly patterned ways in which Sarah experiences and structures her religious quandary, and Jessey's attempts to make Wight's speech and actions into clear manifestations of the divine by embedding them within culturally specific ideas about the female body.

For example, at one point Sarah hurled her drinking cup against the wall, saying 'As sure as this cup shall breake, there is no other Hell', implying that her torments on earth were Hell itself, and that there might be no afterlife at all. Miraculously, the china cup did not break, although for good measure Sarah threw it at the wall a few more times. Only when a tiny chip broke off from the

---

[13] Jessey, *Riches*, sig. A5ʳ, pp. 5–6.

[14] Sarah Wight, *A Wonderful Pleasant and Profitable Letter Written by Mris Sarah Wight* (London: Printed by James Cottrel, for Ri. Moone, at the seven Stars in Pauls Churchyard, 1656), Thomason E.1681[1].

[15] Mack, *Visionary Women*.

rim did she stop. Wight, however, did not invent this piece of theatre all by herself. As Jessey reminds the reader, Sarah was modelling herself after an Elizabethan woman, Mrs Mary Honeywood, who had thrown a Venetian glass against the wall, saying that she was as sure to be damned as the glass was to break. The glass did not break, proving that God still intervened in the lives of his saints, even in the most tiny detail.[16] A very similar story was told about Mrs Susanna Snow in a 1641 pamphlet. Mrs Snow, who lived in Surrey, was intrigued by rumours about the Family of Love, a group of whom were supposedly meeting near her home. She spent a week with them and returned to her father's home and, in the words of the pamphlet, 'she fell starke mad', convinced she was damned. A minister attempted to reason with her, and she threw a Venetian glass against the floor, saying that it was as impossible for her to be saved as it was for the glass to rebound unhurt.[17] These echoes suggest the ways in which Sarah Wight's actions were both her own and were culturally scripted in ways that made her actions meaningful to her immediate circle of godly family, friends, and ministers.

Jessey made Wight's story his own by adding a homely detail: Sarah continued to drink from her special cup until the family water-bearer broke it by accident.[18] His interpolation functions in a number of ways. First, he gets the chance to present himself as a kind of omniscient narrator, since he mentions the detail about the water-bearer breaking the cup out of the chronological sequence of the narrative he is telling. It is as if he looks the reader in the eye for a moment, and says, 'oh, by the way, the cup did finally break', before returning to the story at hand. Second, by reminding the reader about Mrs Honeywood, Jessey serves as a kind of interpreter of Wight's actions, making a bizarre or peculiar episode into testimony of the divine. For Puritans like Jessey or Wight, no detail seems to have been too trivial to examine for signs of God's purpose.[19] Finally, Jessey's detail about the water-bearer adds a kind of verisimilitude to his narrative; it makes Jessey seem to be an honest and transparent narrator. The china cup was, after all, just an ordinary china cup, broken easily by a careless servant.

[16] Jessey, *Riches*, 11–12. See Patrick Collinson, 'A Mirror of Elizabethan Puritanism: The Life and Letters of "Godly Master Dering" ', in his *Godly People: Essays on English Protestantism and Puritanism* (London: The Hambledon Press, 1983), 289–324 at 318. The printed source Collinson cites is Fuller's *Worthies* (1662), but as we see here, the story obviously circulated in godly circles and in cheap print well before the publication of Fuller's book.
[17] *A Description of the Sect called the Familie of Love* (London: printed 1641), Thomason E.168[2], 5–6, quote on 4. Venetian glass was especially fine and precious.
[18] Jessey, *Riches*, 11–12.
[19] Indeed, Jessey carefully frames the entire incident with reference to Mrs Honeywood. He interrupts his narration of Sarah's cup-throwing almost before it begins with a long parenthetical recital of Mrs Honeywood's case. By the time the reader gets past Mrs Honeywood and back to Sarah Wight, he or she knows just what to expect when Sarah hurls her drinking cup.

Sarah was aged 12 when her troubles began. Like many other children in godly households, her crisis intersected with adolescence, and the struggle to create a self independent of her parents was intimately intertwined with her spiritual despair.[20] Her story is reminiscent of that of Nehemiah Wallington, as analysed by Paul Seaver. Wallington, son of a London wood-turner, underwent his crisis in his late teens, and like Sarah he was convinced that he was damned. Both Wight and Wallington tried to kill themselves, although it seems that Wight did so much more energetically. Both Wight and Wallington had parents who were well aware of their children's travails and who attempted to help them. Sarah's mother, for example, climbed out on the roof of their house to try to prevent Sarah from jumping off. Nehemiah's father set him up in business and got him married off at a young age, evidently trying to create a sense of stability and a loving household for his troubled son.[21]

From Wallington's writings that survive, it seems that he and Wight drew on different cultural scripts regarding the relationship of body and soul. Although Wallington was tempted to kill himself, he seems to have understood his crisis as spiritual rather than physical. For Wight, the spiritual and the physical were utterly intertwined. Her spiritual crisis was manifested in physical symptoms: she could not eat, she was struck blind and deaf, she could not walk. As we shall see, the legitimacy of both Wight's crisis and its resolution was understood by Jessey in profoundly corporeal ways. While we cannot be sure why Wight and Wallington's crises manifested in different ways, these ways were marked by gender role conventions. Women were understood as more fully the prisoners of their bodies, as 'weaker vessels' who were much more easily swayed by emotions that were experienced and understood as bodily functions rather than what we would understand as psychological ones. Perhaps Wight was drawing on a long tradition of fasting girls and women. As Diane Purkiss has suggested, her refusal to eat plays on cultural expectations about women as the providers of food, both literally as nursing mothers, and domestically as the purchasers and preparers of a household's meals.[22]

Wight's spiritual crisis took the form of a struggle over the meanings of her body and of being female. First, her relation to her own body was complex and

---

[20] On adolescence, see Paul Griffiths, *Youth and Authority: Formative Experiences in England 1560–1640* (Oxford: Clarendon Press, 1996); Ilana Ben-Amos, *Adolescence and Youth in Early Modern England* (New Haven: Yale University Press, 1994).

[21] Paul Seaver, *Wallington's World: A Puritan Artisan in 17th-c. London* (Stanford: Stanford University Press, 1985); see esp. ch. 2.

[22] Purkiss, 'Producing the Voice'. On the longer tradition, see Bynum, *Holy Feast and Holy Fast*. Wight is also reminiscent of Hannah Allen, who experienced a spiritual crisis when she was 12 years old in very corporeal terms, including sustained fasting. See Elspeth Graham, 'Authority, Resistance and Loss: Gendered Difference in the Writings of John Bunyan and Hannah Allen', in Anne Laurence, W. R. Owens, and Stuart Sim (eds.), *John Bunyan and His England, 1628–88* (London: Hambledon, 1990), 115–30. Allen's autobiography was published in 1683.

changing, but was structured in part by ideas and practices associated with girls and women. Second, the social patterns within which her crisis was contained and magnified were shaped by gendered norms. Although Wight was visited by men as well as women, her world was largely female. Finally, her crisis was wrapped up with her relationship with her mother. Wight tests the limits of her role as daughter and as a potential mother. However, I do not wish to portray her as the passive prisoner of a set of gender role expectations. Instead, I argue that she questions some of these expectations and reshapes others to her own ends. The book that recounts her experiences thus reinforces some contemporary ideas about what it was to be female, but it questions others. It suggests that, in unusual circumstances, some women could transform their inferior position into a superior one, transmuting one status into another very different one.

Wight's relationship with her own body was troubled. At the very beginning of her travails, her body seemed to betray her when she spoke an untruth. When she was 12, her superior told her to do something that Wight thought was unlawful (Jessey does not specify what this unlawful action was), 'and as she did it, a great Trembling in her hands and body fell upon her'; her conscience spoke through the medium of her body. We do not know to whom Sarah was referring when she mentioned her 'superior', but the context suggests that she was in some kind of informal service in another household, helping out a relative or family friend. A month later she lied to her mother about having lost her hood, telling her that she had left it at her grandmother's house. Perhaps her grandmother was a particularly unfortunate person upon whom to hang such a falsehood, for it was she who had schooled Sarah in Scripture. Sarah's body spoke the truth at once: 'Her heart condemned her instantly, and trembled againe exceedingly.' After these two episodes, Sarah became convinced of her utter sinfulness, and began to try to destroy the body that seemed to defy her words.[23] Over the next two and a half years, she tried to kill herself a number of times, employing a wide range of methods, but in each instance was saved.

In early spring 1647 Sarah's crisis deepened. She took to her bed, unable to eat or drink. Not long afterwards, she was struck blind, deaf, and mute. Understandably, her family was very concerned, calling in a succession of ministers to try to help. Sarah's brother came back from Oxford to see her, and her mother attended to her constantly. When her mother was utterly worn out, she hired a godly maidservant, Hannah Gay, to alternate shifts with her in taking care of her daughter.[24]

[23] Jessey, *Riches*, 7.   [24] Ibid. 7–12, 13.

In some ways, Sarah's refusal or inability to eat can be understood as a denial of her body, a kind of slow means of suicide. Although she was blind, deaf, and mute for long periods of time, her crisis was interspersed with periods when she could talk, during which she tried to interpret her own body to others. She promoted an understanding of her body as a passive receptacle when Jessey asked her about not eating and drinking. Sarah assured him that 'I do not abstaine out of wilfulnesse'; instead, she simply could not eat or drink.[25] She said that she would eat if she could, but the smell of food made her ill.[26] Twice Jessey noted carefully that Wight was persuaded to have a little broth, but that each time she threw up. He added that despite not eating for weeks, 'shee looks better now, then shee did seven or eight weeks agoe'.[27] Although Jessey strove to portray Wight's inability to eat as purely involuntary, there is a hint that she also had some choice about the matter. When she was counselling another troubled young woman, Wight told her that she had not dared to drink anything for a week at a time, '*because I judged, it was a Cup of Devils, and I drank to Devils, if I drank, and if I did eat, I thought I did eat my own damnation*'.[28] It is as though Wight understood her inability to eat as both voluntary and involuntary, depending in part on the person to whom she was speaking. To Jessey, her stepbrother, and other authority figures, she could not eat. However, to another young woman like herself, she admitted that the problem was more complex and had to do with her understanding of herself as damned.

Wight's interpretation of her own body deepened when she construed her inability to eat as a mark of divine favour, for she was fed, not with earthly food, but with heavenly manna. In mid-April, her brother asked her to eat a little and she said no, '*I cannot, I have what I did desire*'.[29] A few days later, when urged to eat, she said:

Doe you think, I doe not eat? How doe you think I live? Being asked, what did shee eat? Shee said, *No eye of man sees it, but the eye of God. None could tast the sweetnesse of the Manna, by looking on it, none but they that eat of it.*[30]

Mrs Palmer, the wife of her minister, asked her 'what promise have you, that any should live without food?', and Wight replied with the scriptural citation 'Man lives not by bread alone' (Matt. 4: 4 and Luke 4: 4). Much the same discussion happened again with Dr Coxe and with Henry Jessey himself.[31] Again, Wight's rejection of earthly food and her claims to be fed with manna echoed her denial of her body and its needs. Instead, she tried to subsist in the realm of the spirit, leaving her body behind as a mere vessel.

---

[25] Jessey, *Riches*, 132.   [26] Ibid. 56, 90–1.   [27] Ibid. 21, 56, quote at 21.
[28] Ibid. 109.   [29] Ibid. 31.   [30] Ibid. 33.   [31] Ibid. 57–8, 117, 132.

On one level, therefore, Wight seemed to be denying her body and its female sex. On a deeper level, she was employing metaphors about the female body even as she denied her own particular body. As Caroline Bynum has shown for the Middle Ages, female saints who fasted were inverting their culture's usual understanding of the links between femaleness and food. Women purchased, prepared, and cooked food and nursed babies; they took in food and trans-formed it into milk. In both the medieval period and in seventeenth-century England women's bodies were understood as the more porous of the two sexes, taking in and giving out, menstruating, lactating, and producing babies.[32] While Wight rejected many of these aspects of her body, on a deeper level she was, like other women, profoundly generative. Her body, by being removed in many ways from the messiness of earthly existence, produced divine revelation. One of Henry Jessey's other books was called *A Storehouse of Provision*, and in some ways Sarah Wight was producing just such spiritual provision.[33]

Sarah's crisis unfolded within a deeply female world, and, as such, high-lighted her own tensions about being female. Although Jessey was careful to list the many godly ministers who came to try to help her, Sarah's daily reality was a world of women. Before the crisis, she lived with her widowed mother and, we presume, a servant or two. When Mrs Wight became exhausted, she hired a female maidservant to watch Sarah. Of the fifty-six people whom Jessey names as Wight's visitors, thirty-five were women. More strikingly, all of the people whom Wight counselled in detail were girls or women. Once she began to recover, she acted as a spiritual guide to others experiencing spiritual suffering. Jessey carefully recorded these conversations in dialogue form in his book. Of the sixteen such 'conferences' he detailed, all were with women. Wight may well have counselled men also, but in Jessey's account, she advised only women. This was not a trivial detail, because in the contests over preaching women, many commentators admitted that there was biblical justification for women to teach other women. It was when women preachers started to preach to men that writers became most upset. Since Wight, and Jessey, took a very different approach to legitimating Sarah's speech as divine than did women preachers, it is not surprising that he depicted her as teaching only other women, remaining within biblical precept.

The effect of this choice (if it was a choice) was to surround Wight with other women. A substantial portion of Jessey's book consists of dialogues between Wight and other women. A pregnant woman, for example, was past

[32] Bynum, *Holy Feast and Holy Fast*; Gail Kern Paster, *The Body Embarassed: Drama and the Disciplines of Shame in Early Modern England* (Ithaca: Cornell University Press, 1993), esp. ch. 1.

[33] Henry Jessey, *A Storehouse of Provision, to Further Resolution in Severall Cases of Conscience* (London: printed by Charles Sumptner for T[homas] Brewster and G[regory] Moule, and are to be sold at the three Bibles in Pauls-Church-yard neere the west-end, 1650), Wing (CD-ROM) J698.

her reckoning (what we would call her due date) and came to Sarah for spiritual guidance because she said that her soul's torment was worse than any labour pains. She almost implied that she could not give birth until her spiritual torment was assuaged.[34] Although Wight transcended some of the norms for a young girl—turning her bed into a virtual pulpit, for example—her conversations often emphasized the customary constraints on women and girls. For example, a young woman with experiences much like Sarah's came to see her, and the two young women engaged in a kind of contest about who was the worst sinner. Each tried to outdo the other in lowness in dialogues such as these:

Maid said: Some kept a fast for me yesterday, and I remaine as I was still, and therefore I am the more terrified, that no prayers shall be heard for me.

Wight responded, as she often did to this young woman, that she had experienced the same, only worse:

Mris Sarah W. So it was with me; I was so terrified when there was no answer of prayers for me, when many dayes were kept for me. But I was rather worse than better; for I knew no prayers should be heard for a damned Creature. I concluded, I was rejected. But the Lords time is the best time to give an answer.[35]

It is as though these two young women were engaging in an adolescent attempt to out-do each other in the depths of their self-loathing. However, perhaps they were also stretching ideas about women's inferiority to the limit, seeking to best each other as damned and worthless.

Another young woman who came to see Wight provided a different opportunity to think about gender role conventions. In this case, Wight employed ideas about women's work that were utterly typical of the period. When the young woman confessed that she had thoughts of sin and misery when she was not working, Wight told her 'Then tis better for you to be imployed in business: For els, the enemy hatth more advantage: And specially because God bids you labour the thing that is good.'[36] 'Business' does not mean commerce in the sense that we use it. Rather, it refers to the business of housewifery; women were frequently advised to make every moment productive, doing needlework when other chores were done. The proverbial expression 'a woman's work is never done' was so well known in England that a ballad used the phrase as its title.[37]

---

[34] Jessey, *Riches*, 99.

[35] Ibid. 44–8, quote at 45. See also a similar kind of abasement in Hannah Allen; Graham, 'Authority, Resistance and Loss', esp. 122–3.

[36] Jessey, *Riches*, 109.

[37] *A VVomans VVork Is Never Done* (London: printed for John Andrews, at the White Lion in Pye-Corner, [1660?]) Wing (CD-ROM) W3326; Tilley, *Dictionary*, W659.

Wight's actions and words can be understood as interrogations of her female role in a third way. In addition to constructing a peculiar relationship with her female body, and exploring the limits of her gender role within a largely female world, her distress centred on her relationship with her mother. In testing her mother's love for her, she seemed to be testing the roles of mother and daughter alike. It is tempting to impose a modern reading about the dynamics of mother/daughter relationships, especially in relation to body issues and food, on this aspect of Sarah's crisis. However, I do not think that we know enough about the ways in which selfhood was imagined and lived in the seventeenth century to justify such an imposition. Instead, I prefer a cautious reading that focuses on Sarah's actions and her mother's responses to them. No historian is truly an innocent reader, and like any other, I bring my own culture's preoccupations to bear on the past. Rather than employ modern psychological theories, however, I wish to try to understand how the participants in Wight's crisis ascribed meanings to her actions and words.

Spiritual crisis was not unknown in Wight's family. Indeed, one might say that Sarah was following in her mother's footsteps. When Sarah was 7, her mother had had some kind of profound spiritual crisis, of such severity that Sarah was sent to live with her grandmother for two years. We can only speculate that this might have been around the time that Sarah's father died. Certainly, during her crisis, Sarah took comfort in understanding God as her Father, and counselled another woman in distress that God was a more perfect father than any earthly man.[38] However, it was her mother who was the pivotal figure for Wight.

Sarah must have tried her mother's patience many times. In Jessey's book, we get glimpses of Wight's sustained efforts to harm herself and her mother's vigilance in trying to stop her. In a kind of bizarre reversal of Paul's epiphany on the road to Damascus, Wight threw herself off a horse on the road to Shrewsbury, and, when she was unharmed, insisted on staying in her cold wet clothes when she got to a nearby inn. While often we still link exposure to coldness and wetness to catching a cold, its meaning was deeper in the seventeenth century. Changing the body's temperature and/or degree of moisture was a significant intervention in the humoral system of medicine which then prevailed. Sarah's actions would have been seen as utter folly by those around her; death might have ensued from such carelessness.[39]

In a detailed recital of some of Sarah's suicidal episodes, we hear how one night she locked her mother out of the buttery, and then crept from it out on the roof tiles, meaning to throw herself off. She heard a voice when she got to the edge telling her she would not fall, so instead she beat her head and hands

---

[38] Jessey, *Riches*, 84.   [39] Ibid. 70.

against the brick chimney. Meanwhile, her mother discovered that she was locked out, got someone to break open the lock, and started to crawl out on the roof to save her daughter. Sarah then rolled off the roof, miraculously avoiding harm as she dropped to the ground. Next, she secretly got a knife, and hid it, in order to kill herself. Sometime in the next few days, she begged her mother to let her stay with a neighbour while Mrs Wight attended a religious lecture. In hopes that Sarah was recovering, Mrs Wight assented. Instead of going to the neighbour's house, Wight took herself to Lambeth Marsh, and considered either throwing herself into the river or knifing herself. While she was crying, two ministers came by and asked her what was the matter. They brought her to where her mother was attending the lecture. Her mother saw her come in. Sarah tried to hide from her mother, because now she planned to go to the dogs' house in Moorfields, 'there to offer her selfe to the Dogs, to eate her up, that her Mother might never heare of her more'. Once again, Sarah's mother intervened: 'But at the Sermon her *Mother* seeking her, espied her: and shee againe hid her self beyond others: but her Mother againe found her, and had her home.'[40]

While she was bedridden, Sarah rejected her mother's attempts to preserve her earthly life once again. In early April, when Sarah was deaf and mute, her mother urged her to take something to eat or drink. Somehow Sarah heard her mother's requests, and 'she spake as one troubled at it and said, "Why do you hinder my communion with God?"'[41] Mrs Wight's role as Sarah's mother prescribed that she nourished her daughter, first with breast milk (either her own or by hiring a wet-nurse) when she was a baby, and then subsequently with food as mistress of the household. Sarah, however, would not let her mother nourish her, instead criticizing her for failing to understand the divine nature of her inability to eat. Perhaps we can also hear a muted rebuke in this exchange— Mrs Wight's spiritual crisis had deprived Sarah of her mother's care for two years, and now Sarah was reversing the situation and not permitting her mother to care for her, making her crisis a mirror image of her mother's own seven years earlier.

After some while in bed, Wight's attitude towards her mother changed utterly. On 15 April, still deaf, and unable to see because her eyelids were in some way gummed shut, Sarah asked, 'Have not I a Mother some where? I pray you pray her to pardon me the murmurings against her.' Sarah requested that her mother be brought to her bedside so that she could tell Sarah that she had forgiven her. Even though she could not see or hear, Sarah said, '*I know a Jacob from an Esau.*' When her mother arrived, Sarah did indeed recognize her, and wept, and asked for water to wash her eyes so that she might see her mother.

---

[40] Jessey, *Riches*, 128–30; see also 24.   [41] Ibid. 19.

Their neighbour Mistress Dupper held her eyelids open for her so she could see her mother, and Sarah's hearing was restored for a brief while so that she was able to hear her mother's voice telling her that she was pardoned.[42] After this episode, Sarah slowly began to understand that she was saved, and commenced her role as religious prophet and counsellor, although she continued to be unable to eat, drink, see, or walk.

By early June, Sarah's physical health had declined so severely that everyone around her feared that she would die. On the night of 10 June, however, Sarah prayed, and was able to consign herself completely to God's will. Then she was finally vouchsafed the knowledge that she was saved, and that, like Paul, she must arise and go to Damascus.[43] While she was filled with joy, she hesitated to wake her mother, who was sleeping with her. Instead, she spent the rest of the night quietly awake, 'enjoying sweet *communion* with God'. Jessey describes how:

And June 11 when her Mother awoke, and was arising, shee spake to her, with teares in her eyes, being grieved that (through that foresaid pensiveness) shee had not spoken a word to her Mother, and thereby might offend her; entreating her pardon; which was sooner granted, then asked.[44]

After the maid read to them from Scripture, Sarah startled everyone by asking for some broiled fish. At this point she had not eaten anything for 76 days. 'Fish was got, and broild, and brought to her: and shee with joy in the Lord, did eat heartily before them.'[45] A few days later, Sarah was able to walk. In early July, Mrs Wight moved her daughter to the country, because so many people had sought her counsel in London that the household was becoming overwhelmed.

This episode, when Sarah finally recovered, is rich with meaning. While she stayed awake in perfect communion with God, she was also in a kind of perfect communion with her mother sleeping next to her. This moment has echoes of a kind of deep bond between a mother and an infant, with the infant barely if at all aware that she is a separate entity from her mother. But Sarah has reversed roles for a moment. Now she is the mother who is quiet so as not to wake a sleeping child. When her mother wakes up, Sarah embraces her role as a daughter in a new way. She not only begs her mother's pardon for a possible offence, but she calls for food, endorsing her mother's role in providing and preparing food. Jessey's passive construction—'fish was got, and broild'—hides the actual domestic work involved. Had Sarah wanted dried fish or bread, or some other less perishable or common foodstuff, her wishes could have been granted

---

[42] Jessey, *Riches*, 23–5. Perhaps Mistress Dupper was related to John Duppa, the well-known Independent who had formed his own congregation in London in the 1630s, a congregation that included Katherine Chidley, discussed in the previous chapter.

[43] Ibid. 133–5.   [44] Ibid. 137.   [45] Ibid. 138.

instantly. Instead, she asks for broiled fish, entailing a trip to a market and the stoking up of a fire.[46] It is almost as if she were a pregnant woman, entitled by bodily cravings to ask for whatever she wished. But it is also one of the last moments when Sarah's peculiar bodily status made her the utter centre of her household. In a few weeks, Mrs Wight tried to restore her daughter to an uneventful life by moving to the country.

The physical nature of Wight's crisis is paradoxical. On one hand, Jessey and others believed the truth of Wight's utterances because of the bodily manifestations of her crisis. On the other, they also believe the truth of Wight's words because they saw her body as utterly lacking in will or any voluntary behaviour. Because Wight's body was completely powerless, her words must be divinely inspired. It is as if her body was just a transmitter for the divine. The title page of Jessey's book describes Wight as an 'Empty Nothing Creature'. If she were truly nothing, there would be no book. Instead, as Jessey said, 'The Lord enabled this weak earthen vessell to utter forth extempore.'[47] Wight's own belief in her utter unworthiness—she said 'What am I? A poor empty, disconsolate, sinfull, vaine, contemptible worme: a poor, wretched, empty, unthankfull, sinfull, vile, contemptible worme'—reinforced Jessey's portrayal of her as the passive instrument of divine will.[48]

While Wight struggled with the relationship between body and soul, and thus with the meanings ascribed to female bodies in her culture, Henry Jessey struggled to reconcile Wight's body and her words. He tried to make her body produce religious truths that would be believed by those who read about them. To put it slightly differently, he tried to show that Wight's words were divinely ordained by closely examining her body and its role in the production of those words. Jessey repeatedly called attention to Wight's body, meticulously cataloguing its disabilities in order to authenticate the divine nature of her speech. In particular, he emphasized Wight's relationship with food, her blindness, and her nearness to death in his discussions of her body. Each of these functions served to assure the reader that Wight was genuine. Jessey's constant insistence on these authenticating details suggest that a great deal was at stake for him and for others in the acceptance or rejection of this 15-year-old girl's experiences. Jessey was wrestling with the same problem, distinguishing genuine corporeal manifestations of the supernatural from fakery, that Edward Jorden struggled with in the Mary Glover case. He was also at odds with Wight about the correct interpretations of her body: was she starving? Or sated with spiritual food? Deaf, or tuned into the divine?

---

[46] Many thanks to Bruce Janacek for pointing out to me that Wight may be echoing two biblical stories: Luke 24: 41–4, when the resurrected Jesus proves to his disciples that he is resurrected in the body by eating broiled fish, and John 21: 9, where he also has a meal of grilled fish with his disciples.
[47] Jessey, *Riches*, sig. A6ʳ.   [48] Ibid. 21.

First, Jessey's book was obsessed with Wight's relationship to food. He returned to the theme again and again and again.[49] As mentioned above, he noted carefully that she had tried to drink some broth twice, but threw up both times. He detailed exactly what she ate when she first recovered—the broiled fish. When people questioned Wight about her inability (or was it refusal?) to eat, Jessey recounted the conversations in detail.

Jessey also emphasized Wight's inability to see. For him, it seems as if her inability to see underwrote the authenticity of her visions and prophecies; she 'saw' the divine because she could not see the earthly. Even after her sight was restored, Jessey noted that her eyes were so weak that she lay in bed with a linen cloth covering them. When Wight was asked about her eyes, which had been covered with a linen cloth for weeks, she said 'Christ hath done a great miracle upon me: he hath made the blind to see.'[50] Even though God had enabled her to see again, it is as if she chose not to exercise this ability, preferring to leave a cloth over her eyes. In a similar fashion, Wight became deaf and mute. Since she could not speak voluntarily, her speech became truly divine in origin; since she could not hear, what she did hear must have been divine.[51]

Third, Jessey used Wight's body to authenticate her speech by pointing out how near to death she was. He prefaces the book by reminding the reader that 'The *Earthly Vessel* of conveyance being most likely to return to earth, within a few daies.'[52] In other words, Wight was just a conduit, a 'conveyance' for the words of God. It was widely believed that those about to die would speak only the truth. For instance, midwives asked unwed mothers to confess the name of the child's father while the mother was at the height of labour pains, because it was thought that the mother would not dare to lie when she was at such great risk of death. Courts accepted this childbed admission, preferring it to other testimony about the likely father, thus reinforcing the belief that a person at risk of death was unlikely to lie.[53]

Jessey thus provided a very close description of certain aspects of Wight's bodily functioning in order to authenticate the divine nature of her suffering and speech. The weakness of her body, demonstrated through her fasting, her loss of speech and hearing, and her nearness to death testified to the paradoxical strength of her spirituality.

Throughout the book, Jessey worried that he would not be believed, and he employed at least three textual devices to assure the reader of his veracity:

---

[49] Jessey, *Riches*, sig. A3ʳ, A8ʳ⁻ᵛ, pp. 15, 19, 21, 32–3, 38, 55–8, 131–2, 138.
[50] Ibid. 88.
[51] Ibid.; turning over in bed: 22; sweetness of speech: 3, 28, 35; blindness and muteness: 3, 15, 23, 25, 28, 55, 59, 136; cloth over the eyes: 35, 39.
[52] Ibid. sig. A8ʳ. See also sig. A3ᵛ.
[53] Ingram, *Church Courts, Sex, and Marriage*, 263.

witnessing, encasement, and an emphasis on the details of textual produc-tion.[54] First, he often referred to himself as a witness and invoked a number of other witnesses who could be believed for a variety of reasons. On the title page and on subsequent pages he assured the reader that he has been 'an eye- and ear-witness' to everything he described. Jessey also listed many other people who witnessed aspects of Wight's story. Some of these people were to be presumed truthful because of their religion. Wight's mother and her maid, for instance, were described as being of 'approved faithfulness' that was 'sufficient' to ensure their veracity. Jessey also evoked social status, describing some of his witnesses as 'persons of note'. He cited many such people by name or title, including two Ladies, numerous ministers, a physician, and a judge's wife.[55] When Jessey said that Wight did not eat anything from 27 March to 21 April, he noted that some people had 'counted it a forgery, or pretence', but that the minsters who were witnesses to it would not have dared to lie.[56] The physician Dr Coxe asked Sarah directly if the divine comfort she received was just a delusion, and even suggested that the people she counselled might have faked their responses to her. He interrogated Sarah, trying to trip her up, but she withstood the test, at least as reported by Jessey.[57]

Second, Jessey used a technique of textual encasement to make his story about Wight's experiences seem truthful. Like many other books of the period, this work has a variety of different textual apparatuses that frame Wight's tale. Before the reader can get to Wight's words, he or she is presented with an epistle to the reader, a dedication to Wight's brother, another epistle (this one to the Christian reader), a postscript to this epistle, a letter from minister John Saltmarsh approving the book, a list of all the biblical citations in the text, and a detailed table of contents. Only then can the reader plunge into the details of Wight's story so tantalizingly mentioned in the prefatory material. It is as if each reader must assent individually to the truthfulness of what follows before he or she can read it.

Finally, Jessey created a text that claimed to be truthful by carefully describ-ing the mode of its production. He said that most of the text came directly from his listening to Wight and writing down what she said: 'Her own very words being here writ down, and kept close unto; the most part of them being first writ whilst shee spake'. Other parts of the text were written down afterwards, 'as they were remembred [*sic*] by the Writer, or by your Mother, or by the Maid'. Sometimes Wight spoke so quietly that no one was absolutely sure of

---

[54] Jessey was far from unique in choosing these devices. See Ann Hughes on Thomas Edwards's *Gangraena* (forthcoming from Oxford), and Steven Shapin and Simon Schaffer on witnessing in a very different context, that of the early Royal Society, *Leviathan and the Air-Pump* (Princeton: Prince-ton University Press, 1985).

[55] Jessey, *Riches*, sig. a1ʳ; pp. 8–10.   [56] Ibid. 55.   [57] Ibid. 114, 119.

what she had said. Jessey told the reader that he has put these few words, or his guess at these words, in a different typeface, so that the reader would be able to gauge the degree of accuracy of any part of the book.[58] In the body of the text, he also calls the reader's attention to the ways in which the written word was produced from its oral enactment. In one case, both he and another listener, Mrs Palmer, took notes while Sarah spoke, and then compared their notes afterwards.[59] Jessey's obsessive attention to the truth-producing details of his narrative point to his anxieties about being believed. However, they also create a kind of tension between his words and Wight's body. For it is Wight's body that produces the ultimate truths in this text. Jessey is the recorder and authenticator of those truths but he does not create them.

Sarah Wight's body, like that of Mary Glover, was troubling to observers on at least two counts. First, as we have seen here, these young women's bodies did amazing things: although they took in no nourishment, they continued to live. They seemed to be in close connection with the supernatural, be that demonic or divine. In the very ways that these young women did not meet the norms of female bodily life, they called attention to those norms. By pushing on the boundaries of appropriate female behaviour, they delineated those boundaries. Second, these were troubling bodies because of the weight of uncertainty attached to them. On the one hand, the truth of these bodies mattered greatly—was Glover possessed? What was the nature of possession? Could it be healed by exorcism? Was Wight, to use our terms, just acting out? Or was she really nourished by the divine? Did God still intervene directly in the lives of his sinners? On the other hand, the truth of these bodily claims was elusive, and the gravity of the men who wrote about them was always on the brink of being disrupted by laughter. Jorden was still smarting from his courtroom failure to persuade a judge that Glover was sick, not possessed, when he wrote his pamphlet. Jessey, a marginal figure in many ways, was skilled in using the medium of print to promote himself, but he risked ridicule if Wight could be shown to be disturbed rather than in touch with the divine. Each of these men was confronted with the messy unknowability of the female body. Leaky, unstable, containing a potentially dangerous uterus that no one could see or touch—female bodies were shaky ground upon which to erect a claim to certain knowledge.

In both cases, Jorden and Jessey had to contend with women's own interpretations of their bodies. Mary Glover, for example, might be understood as rejecting Jorden's medical interpretation of her affliction when she was healed by a group of Puritan exorcists. She claimed her body as a spiritual battleground, rather than a medical problem, when she uttered the same words that

[58] Jessey, *Riches*, sig. A6^r.   [59] Ibid. 58–9.

her ancestor had spoken when burnt at the stake for heresy, and she was healed. At many moments in his book, Jessey tried to square his interpretation of Wight's body with her own. For Jessey, Wight's body was literally starving—but then Wight claimed that no, she was fed with spiritual provision. Neither Jorden nor Jessey could easily rely on the female body as a producer of truths. In the next chapter we shall meet a very different man, who wrote about women's bodies in a new way. Neither embarrassed nor uncertain, Nicholas Culpeper transformed the way men could write about women's bodies and in writing about them, make them the bearers of stable and certain meaning.

5
Culpeper's Radical Book

In 1651 Nicholas Culpeper published a midwifery manual that proposed new ways of thinking about women's reproductive bodies. Many of the ideas in the book were not novel, but the connections he made between women's reproductive bodies and the politics of knowledge were new. Just as Thomas Raynalde's 1545 book was shaped by the turmoil of the Reformation, Culpeper's work was structured by the gender troubles of the 1640s. His book offers readers a model of the relationship between men and women that is grounded in the body itself. In the midst of a world turned upside down by civil war, Culpeper imagined the human body as a source of stability and an image of appropriate relations between men and women. He presented this source of stability in engaging prose that made no apologies for its subject matter. Unlike earlier writers such as Raynalde or Henry Jessey, Culpeper did not worry about male readers or about the improprieties of writing about female bodies. He revelled in them. His book became a model for a new kind of writing about women's bodies that made them representations of larger social relations.

Culpeper's vision of the human body was a part of his larger political vision. Although he is well known as the author of the herbal that bears his name, which has rarely been out of print in the last 350 years, his deeper political commitments have not been fully understood. Before looking at his midwifery book and its radical proposals about the female body and about the social meanings of reproductive bodies, we need to look more closely at Culpeper himself and at his larger goals.

Culpeper's dramatic life shaped his radical politics. He was born in 1616, a month after his father died. He was brought up by his maternal grandfather, a minister in Sussex. While he was at university in Cambridge, he planned to elope with an heiress he knew from home; her name remains unknown to us. While on the way to their rendezvous, she was killed by a bolt of lightning, and Culpeper, broken-hearted, could no longer bring himself to study for the ministry. Instead, he was apprenticed to a London apothecary. Building on a long interest in magic and the stars, he became a kind of unlicensed astrological physician. He married and settled into a productive London practice as an apothecary and healer. Culpeper's treatment of the poor seems to have radicalized him: his writings are full of critiques of wealthy physicians who refused care to the needy. With the advent of war, he joined the Parliamentary army and was seriously wounded in the battle of Newbury in 1643. He returned home to his wife Alice and in 1649 began an immensely productive career in medical and astrological writing. When he died in 1654, he had published eleven books in twenty editions, and is supposed to have left his wife another seventy-nine manuscripts, which she and their one surviving child sold to support themselves. At least another 117 editions of thirty titles, many of them translations, were published up to 1700.[1]

In his own day, Culpeper was well known as an astrologer as well as a healer. During the Civil War, almanacs, like so much else, were polarized into Royalist and Parliamentarian versions, each predicting the future in a kind of wishful politics.[2] From his astrological writings as well as his medical ones, Culpeper emerges as complicated man, whose politics were increasingly shadowed by disappointment and disillusion. Like Katherine Chidley, the petitioner and preacher discussed in Chapter 3, Culpeper was an Independent in religion and had Leveller sympathies. Unlike Chidley, he was not radical when it came to women's roles. As we shall see, he was a radical in politics but a conservative at home, reconstructing hierarchical gender relations even as he criticized hierarchy in other spheres of life.

As Culpeper convalesced from his Civil War wounds and began his writing career in the mid-1640s, Parliament became deeply divided on religious issues. Presbyterians favoured hierarchical church government to ensure uniformity of religious worship and belief, and sought a strict moral reformation underwritten by law. Independents grew out of the experience of separate congregations, such as the clandestine ones attended by Katherine Chidley, or those exiled in the Netherlands or New England. They did not advocate separate churches per se but argued for religious toleration. Independents wanted to

[1] On Culpeper, see F. N. L. Poynter, 'Nicholas Culpeper and his Books', *Journal of the History of Medicine and Allied Sciences*, 17 (1962), 152–67; id., 'Nicholas Culpeper and the Paracelsians', in *Science, Medicine and Society in the Renaissance: Essays to Honor Walter Pagel* (New York: Science History Publications, 1972), 201–20; Charles Webster, *The Great Instauration. Science, Medicine and Reform, 1626–1660* (London: Duckworth, 1975), 268–73. Mary Rhinelander McCarl, 'Publishing the Works of Nicholas Culpeper, Astrological Herbalist and Translator of Latin Medical Works in 17th-c. London', *Canadian Bulletin of the History of Medicine*, 13 (1996), 225–76. Unfortunately, the recent biography by Olav Thulesius cannot be relied upon since it includes fictitious episodes. All scholars of Culpeper draw on a biographical section of a posthumously printed work: *Culpeper's School of Physick* (London: Printed for N. Brook at the Angel in Cornhill, 1659), Thomason E.1739[1]. It has been assumed that the outlines of his life presented here are accurate, since the presumed author was William Ryves, his amanuensis. Recently, McCarl has suggested that the story of Culpeper's failed elopement should be read as a metaphor for his engagement with alchemy. I am sorry that I have been unable to consult Jonathan Sanderson, 'Nicholas Culpeper and the Book Trade: Print and the Promotion of Vernacular Medical Knowledge' (Ph.D. thesis, University of Leeds, 1999). Many thanks to Yvonne Noble for this last reference.
[2] Patrick Curry, *Prophecy and Power* (Oxford: Blackwell, 1989); Bernard Capp, *Astrology and the Popular Press: English Almanacs 1500–1800* (London: Faber, 1979).

ensure that individual churches could worship in their own ways and that each minister was responsible only to his own congregation. Although a Presbyterian form of organization was mandated by Parliament in 1646, it never succeeded in becoming dominant. By 1649 only London, Lancashire, and Essex had the full Presbyterian hierarchy in place. Many of the parishes elsewhere in England were characterized by a kind of residual Anglicanism or were modelled on independent congregations. Much worship took place outside the parish structure, in independent congregations and in the 'free worship' in the New Model Army.

Culpeper was an Independent. He described how, for him, religion came from inside himself rather than from outside church structures:

It is at present my opinion, That true Religion will scarse ever flourish by publick authority, till Jesus Christ be set upon his holy hill of *Zyon* . . . At present, I know not what belongs to that Religion *Presbytery* would establish; all the Religion I know, is *Jesus Christ and him Crucified, and the indwelling of the Spirit of God in me:* this I am sure is real Gospel.[3]

Much more trenchantly, he declared ' 'tis but a scurvy Trade to be a Pyrate, and in truth not much better to be a Presbyterian'.[4] As we shall see, his dislike of the Presbyterian hierarchy was connected to a larger world-view about human nature and governance. His belief that true religious knowledge was a deeply personal gift was shared by many in the 1640s.

Culpeper's ideas also suggest that he was influenced by the Leveller movement. The Levellers were masters of cheap print, their leaders producing hundreds of pamphlets and petitions. Levellers, many of whom worshipped in separated churches, argued for religious toleration and a kind of freedom of conscience. They emphasized reason and natural law as the grounds for human governance rather than the arbitrary powers of oligarchic and monopolistic institutions. For example, Levellers fought for a written constitution, to be signed by every citizen, as the basis for England's government. Ideas such as these have prompted some historians to understand the Levellers as anticipating John Locke's contract model of government, but they are probably better understood in their own context. The Levellers grounded their political beliefs in a powerful set of mythic stories about England's past. Like many others in the 1640s, they insisted that England throw off the 'Norman Yoke'. The yoke referred to the belief that the Norman Conquest in 1066 was the

---

[3] Nicholas Culpeper, *An Ephemeris for the yeer 1651* ([London]: Printed by Peter Cole, and are to be sold at his shop at the sign of the Printing Press in Cornhil, near the Royal Exchange, 1651), Thomason E.1343[1], sig. G3ᵛ. See also his statement on the next page: 'I have as much faith in the Synods *Directory*, as I have in the History of *Bel and the Dragon*, or the fable of *Arion and the Dolphin*.'

[4] Ibid. sig. H4ᵛ.

imposition of French slavery on a free-born Anglo-Saxon people. John Lilburne, the leader of the Leveller movement, was especially intent on law reform. He wanted to put all legal work into English (lawyers used Latin and a kind of creole legal French) and to simplify and codify the law. For Lilburne, as for others, lawyers were but parasites; every free-born Englishman should be able to act as his own lawyer once the law was reformed.

Women, however, were not envisaged as 'free-born' in the same way. Most Leveller writings suggest that Lilburne and others wanted to retain the gender hierarchy intact. As Ann Hughes has elegantly shown, Leveller leaders relied on and manipulated elements of a traditional understanding of gender roles in their depictions of themselves as heads of families.[5] As we have seen in Chapter 3, Leveller women like Katherine Chidley took part in mass demonstrations and wrote petitions. Such women attempted both to transcend the bounds of their gender role and to transform it into a powerful one. However, their actions were portrayed by male Levellers as extensions of their roles as wives.

In 1649 Nicholas Culpeper published an English translation of the College of Physicians' pharmacopoeia, a move parallel to John Lilburne's insistence that all legal matters be discussed in English. This was the book that was supposed to include all the remedies officially sanctioned by the College and was therefore intended for the use of all apothecaries, who made up the medicines prescribed by physicians. The College thought that it should regulate all of medicine, but actual practice was quite different. Apothecaries not only made up medicines, but also acted as general practitioners for a good proportion of the population that could not afford or have access to a learned physician. Nor were the drugs recommended by the College the only remedies patients wanted and apothecaries prepared. Chemical remedies, based on the teachings of the radical sixteenth-century healer Paracelsus, were scorned by the College as unsound innovation. By the 1650s such chemical remedies had attracted a considerable following, and Culpeper saw no reason to exclude them from a healer's stock in trade.[6]

Culpeper was outraged by the College's attempts to dictate which medicines were acceptable and which were not, and he was incensed by its emphasis on expensive imported drugs. He never fully recovered from his war wound, and spent much of his time in bed, dictating translations and original works to an amanuensis. The late 1640s were an ideal moment for his pharmacopoeia, because the College of Physicians was a royally chartered institution, and it

[5] Hughes, 'Gender and Politics in Leveller Literature'.
[6] Allan Debus, *The English Paracelsians* (London: Oldbourne, 1965). On the larger context of the College of Physicians, see Harold J. Cook, *The Decline of the Old Medical Regime in Stuart London* (Ithaca: Cornell University Press, 1986), and Margaret Pelling, *Medical Conflicts in Early Modern London* (Oxford: Clarendon Press, 2003).

spent the war years and the Interregnum very quietly, trying not to call attention to its Royalist heritage and privileges. Members were surely aware that their customary recourse to law would be of little use.

Culpeper saw his pharmacopoeia in a much broader context than just a list of medicines. In the first edition, he used the preface to explain the political import of his work. He said: 'God gave Tyrants in his Wrath, and will take them away in his Displeasure.' King Charles I had just been executed and no one could miss the implications of his remark. He continued by clarifying what the struggle of the war was about: 'The Prize which We now, and They [other European countries] within a few years shall play for, is, THE LIBERTY OF THE SUBJECT.'[7] For Culpeper, this last phrase means something very similar to what Leveller writers referred to as the rights of free-born Englishmen.

Culpeper's bold claims and his engaging writing style brought him to the attention, not just of the College of Physicians, but of the newsbooks that proliferated in London. *Perfect Occurences*, a Parliamentary partisan, trumpeted the publication of the work: 'There come forth an excellent translation of the *London Dispensatory* made by the College of Physitions in *London*, being that Booke by which all Apothecaries in *England*, are strictly commanded to make their Physick.'[8] *Mercurius Pragmaticus*, which baldly proclaimed itself 'For King Charls II', replied in outrage, spending an entire page destroying Culpeper's character and using his words against him. It started by repeating the words of *Perfect Occurences*, but then slid into bad-mouthing Culpeper, saying that he was neither gentleman nor scholar, as he claimed on his title page. He was, the paper pointed out, the son of a Sussex minister—one of the breed who, in Culpeper's words, 'deceives men in matters belonging to their precious Soules'.[9] The newsbook, in other words, accused Culpeper of unfilial or insincere behaviour. A small biography followed that depicted him as running away from his master, marrying a whore, and living by cheating, conjuring, and the practice of astrology.

Worse yet, the paper described his religious affiliations in terms that remind us of those attached to Katherine Chidley by her opponents: Independency, Anabaptism, Seeker, and finally, worst of all, Atheist. The paper described what he looked like, so that readers might avoid him:

he hath got an old black-Cloake lined with Plum, by the meanes of his Stationer [i.e. his publisher], who bought it him in Long-lane, to hide his Knavery, being (till then) a

---

[7] Nicholas Culpeper, *A Physicall Directory or A Translation of the London Dispensatory* (London: Printed for Peter Cole and are to be sold at his Shop at the sign of the Printing-presse near to the Royall Exchange, 1649), Thomason E.576[1], sig. A1ʳ.

[8] *Perfect Occurences*, 21 Aug. to 7 Sept. 1649, Thomason E.532[35].

[9] *Mercurius Pragmaticus*, 4 to 11 Sept. 1649, Thomason E.573[9].

most despicable, ragged-fellow, and yet hee lookes as if hee had been stued [i.e. stewed] in a Tan-pit.[10]

Finally, the paper tried to turn Culpeper's language back on himself, accusing him of monopolizing 'all the Knavery and Cozenage' that an apothecary's shop could muster.[11] The effort that this Royalist newsbook devoted to discrediting Culpeper suggests that his politics were clearly understood in the highly polarized world of London public opinion.

Culpeper fought back in the next edition of his book, noting that some had commented on his criticism of priests. So he made his criticisms more specific and stinging, saying that he honoured moderate divines, 'But if I were to be hanged for my labor I cannot fancy a Priest whose conditions are as like a Weather-cock as a Pome-Water is like an Apple: I pray how dislike to it was our City presbytery a while ago?'[12] He could fill a dozen sheets of paper with 'their Pulpit Lyes and Railings' but focuses on one issue. He opens the epistle to the reader with equally pointed words: 'William the Bastard having conquered this Nation, and brought it *sub jugo*, brought in the Norman Laws written in an unknown tongue, and this laid the foundation to their future, and our present slavery.'[13] He links the Norman Yoke with the fact that scholarship was published in Latin, which was a kind of class barrier, 'unless a man have gotten a very large estate he is not able to bring up his Son to understand Latin'.[14] Like Chidley, Culpeper seems to relish battle with his opponents. His pharmacopoeia was reprinted six times between 1649 and 1654, with new prefaces that fought back at his critics and articulated his political views with wit and directness.

Like the Levellers, Culpeper focused his critique of social power on the three professions: law, medicine, and the clergy. As he put it, 'The Liberty of our *Common-Wealth* (if I may call it so without a Solecisme) is most infringed by three sorts of men, *Priests, Physitians, Lawyers.*' He explains that 'one deceives men in matters belonging to their Souls, the other, in matters belonging to their Bodies, the third in matters belonging to their Estates'.[15] Culpeper echoes Katharine Chidley's complaints about priests who will not bury a child's body when the parents lack the burial fee, no matter how poor they are, but for him the villains are the doctors: 'Send for them to a poor mans house, who is not able to give them their Fee, then they will not come, and the poor Creature for whom Christ died must forfet his life for want of money.'[16] He continued his critiques of doctors and clergymen in the introduction to his *Directory for*

[10] *Mercurius Pragmaticus*, 4 to 11 Sept. 1649, Thomason E.573[9].   [11] Ibid.
[12] Nicholas Culpeper, *A Physical Directory*, 2nd edn. (London: printed by Peter Cole, and are to be sold at his shop at the sign of the Printing-Press in Cornhil, near the Royal Exchange, 1650), Wing (CD-ROM) C7541, sig. B1ᵛ.   [13] Ibid. sig. B1ʳ.   [14] Ibid.
[15] *Physicall Directory* (1649), sig. A1ʳ⁻ᵛ.   [16] Ibid. sig. A1ᵛ.

Midwives: 'For had not the Priests formerly absconded the Mysteries of Truth from us, Sermons would have been so cheap, that they would have been cried about the Streets for three half pence a dozen.'[17] Culpeper was a master of the market for cheap print, and his fertile imagination saw sermons hawked like ballads in the street.

At the centre of Culpeper's dislike of the learned professions was the way in which they kept knowledge to themselves. For him, knowledge was truly power, and he wanted it in the hands of many, not a select few. As he proclaims in his midwifery book,

What an insufferable injury is it, that in a free Commonwealth Men and Women should be trained up in such Ignorance, that when they are sick, and have Herbs in their Garden conducing to their cure, they are so hood-winked that they know not their Vertues.[18]

Culpeper's vision was to have every man or woman able to heal themselves with herbs growing for free at the edges of roads or in common lands—or at least to be able to buy native plants much more cheaply than the expensive imported remedies favoured by elite physicians. He knew that the College of Physicians would argue that popular medical books written in English would lead to a great amount of ignorant practice by untrained people. Culpeper, however, with his years of experience treating London's poor, saw the problem differently: 'All the Nation are already Physitians, If you ayl any thing, every one you meet, whether man or woman will prescribe you a medicine for it.'[19] His goal was to make this multitude of vernacular healers more effective by giving them knowledge written in ways that they could easily use.

Nicholas Culpeper published his own works for only four years, and then he was dead, probably from consumption. His writings are suffused with a kind of sadness and disillusionment characteristic of the late 1640s and early 1650s. He had fought in what is called the first Civil War, from 1642 to 1646, and been wounded. He then saw the seeming triumph of the Presbyterians in Parliament, while he remained an Independent. The King fought and lost a second civil war in 1648, with more suffering and death on both sides. Culpeper did not like those in charge, describing them like those whom 'Widdows and Fatherless Children daily pray against; such as one day shall dearly answer for the Blood that hath been spilt in this Civil War'.[20] Presbyterian ministers who had encouraged men to go to war also came in for criticism: 'forcing men to fight for fear of Hell and Damnation? What was the matter

---

[17] Culpeper, *Directory for Midwives*, sig. A4ʳ [hereafter cited as *Directory*].
[18] Ibid. sig. ¶2ᵛ–3ʳ.   [19] Culpeper, *Physicall Directory* (1649), sig. A2ʳ.
[20] Culpeper, *Ephemeris* (1651), sig. I1ᵛ.

pray? The Bishops must be puld down, and we [i.e. the ministers] up in their places'.[21]

By the end of the decade, Culpeper was profoundly disillusioned about the nation's rulers and their failure to build a godly society: 'Such an Age, that calleth Vertue vice, and Vice Vertue, that calleth Good, Evil, and Evil, Good, that strike at the Devil, and hit Christ in his Saints.'[22] As John Morrill has noted, for those who had thought that they were in the process of building the new Jerusalem in England in the early 1640s, the later years of the decade were full of 'heartbreak and disillusionment'.[23] Such feelings cut across the divide between Presbyterians and Independents. Both shared the Puritan dream of making England a godly nation, but the difficulties inherent in the project were all too apparent by the late 1640s.[24] Like others, Culpeper veered towards millenarian despair, saying 'Certainly the worlds mad, and therefore 'twill not live long.'[25] He dreamed of reforming all of society, but by the late 1640s both hope and time had begun to run out. Perhaps we can understand Culpeper's burst into print as both an attempt to reform a piece of his world and a kind of healing that he could perform despite being an invalid.

In reforming popular medicine, Culpeper was always struggling for a grander reformation. His book about women's bodies is full of political allusion and commentary. He moves directly from a typical critique of priests to a pointed comment about the elite members of the College of Physicians: 'They kill Men for want of Judgment.'[26] He indulged in a long discussion of ants and how they govern themselves, exclaiming 'Ants labor all for the publick good (as you may see if you do but observe them) and mind not private interests. Oh that we could learn to do but so!'[27] He then moved to bees, and again, the bees have a much more admirable commonwealth than does England.[28] Whether writing an almanac, an astrological account of an eclipse's meaning, a popular midwifery book, or his pharmacopoeia, Culpeper developed a consistent vision of the role of popular knowledge and a critique of the abuses of power he saw around him.

[21] Culpeper, *Physical Directory* (1650), sig. B1[v].

[22] Nicholas Culpeper, *Pharmacopoeia Londinensis: or the London Dispensatory* (London: Printed for Peter Cole, at the sign of the Printing-Press in Cornhil neer the Royal Exchange, 1653), Wing (CD-ROM) C7525, sig. B1[v].

[23] John Morrill, 'The Impact of Puritanism', in his *The Impact of the English Civil War* (London: Collins and Brown, 1991), 65. More generally, William Hunt's *The Puritan Moment* (Cambridge, Mass.: Harvard University Press, 1983) remains an absorbing study of the fates of Puritanism in one county.

[24] For example, Culpeper's feelings seem to match those of the Presbyterian Nehemiah Wallington, like Culpeper a London-based artisan much given to reading and writing. See Seaver, *Wallington's World*.

[25] Culpeper, *Ephemeris* (1651), sig. I3[r]. On the larger currency of millenarian ideas, see Capp, *Fifth Monarchy Men*.

[26] Culpeper, *Directory*, sig. A4[v].   [27] Ibid. 42, 42–3.   [28] Ibid. 43.

While Culpeper sought to reform the world around him, and offered trenchant critiques of hierarchical social relations, he was a conservative in gender
relations. As we shall see, his midwifery book emphasized men's superiority to
women and undermined the authority of midwives. His domestic conser-
vatism should not surprise us. Many a political radical has been a conservative
at home. Gerrard Winstanley, for example, was the leader of a radical group
called the Diggers, who called for land to be held in common. Despite his
radical social policies—so radical that the Leveller leaders refused to support
him—he did not question men's authority over women.

Culpeper's midwifery book broke with the past: it describes men's bodies as
well as women's. After the dedication and preface, the first words of the book
are: 'First, for the Genitals of men (for I hope good Women will pardon me for
serving mine own Sex first).'[29] On page 26 Culpeper turns to women: 'Having
served my own Sex, I shall see now if I can please the Women.'[30] Earlier texts,
such as Raynalde's *Birth of Mankind* or Rueff's *Expert Midwife*, did not
describe men's bodies. They saw no need to discuss them in their accounts of
pregnancy and childbirth. Culpeper's stated intentions were the same as those
of earlier works: he wanted to make reproductive processes clear to unlearned
women. But he was the first popular writer to do so by starting with men's
bodies.

By putting his own sex first, Culpeper made women into inferior versions of
men; their bodies were described as variants of male anatomy. For example,
when discussing women's stones (what we would call ovaries) he describes
them only in terms of their differences from men's stones (what we would call
testicles): 'The Stones of Women (for they have such kind of toys aswel as Men)
differ from the Stones of Men.'[31] He lists nine differences, and it is only those
differences that describe this part of women's bodies. A few pages later, he turns
to the 'preparing vessels', again making female bodies just a variant of the male:
'Yet there is some difference between the Preparing Vessels in Men and those in
Women; else I need not have troubled my self about them.'[32] Comments such
as these make women's bodies into second-rate objects, with which a writer
need not trouble except where they differ from the standard, which is male.

Culpeper's is a book about making babies, but it makes male anatomy and
functioning standard, rather than female. This habit, of making male the
standard and female the variant, is a very old tradition that extends up to today.
Medical students are still taught the 'standard' body, which is a 70 kg white
male.[33] Culpeper makes the male body the standard of human perfection in

[29] Culpeper, *Directory*, 3.   [30] Ibid. 26.   [31] Ibid. 35.   [32] Ibid. 37.
[33] Susan Lawrence and Kai Bendixen, 'His and Hers: Male and Female Anatomy in Anatomy Texts
for U.S. Medical Students, 1890–1989', *Social Science and Medicine*, 35 (1992), 925–34.

comments such as this about the structure of the penis: 'you see what a rational piece the Lord made when he made Man'.[34] If he were writing about almost any other body part, it might be possible to construe 'Man' as meaning all humans—but not when he is describing the penis.

The idea that women are but an imperfect version of men dates from classical antiquity. Aristotle, for example, considered men more 'perfect' than women. Perfection, for him, meant not only a kind of flawlessness. It also referred to a teleological understanding of Nature, who always sought to make the ideal version of any organic being. Nature strove to make men, because they were the standard, the ideal, the essential form of human beings. All daughters were the result of a kind of mistake in the womb, an imperfection in formation. They were Nature's second-best. Like other popular medical books, Culpeper drew much from classical learning, mediated by generations of medieval and early modern scholars. However, he chose different aspects of the classical heritage to present to his female readers than had earlier writers.

Like Thomas Raynalde in the 1545 *Birth of Mankind*, Culpeper argued that anatomy was the key to midwifery. However, where Raynalde used anatomy to illustrate the wonders of the female body and to defend a particular understanding of conception in the face of heresies about the Incarnation, Culpeper used anatomy to show the superiority of the male body over the female and to attack the authority of midwives. In each case, the actual anatomy that the authors provided was not especially novel for its time. Each book's novelty lay in the larger claims for which the authors employed anatomy.

Anatomy was the keystone to Culpeper's version of the body. While Henry Jessey emphasized the care with which he listened to and transcribed the words of Sarah Wight, Culpeper privileged vision rather than hearing as the primary means of producing knowledge. He belittled writers who discussed the female body without ever having seen a woman anatomized, saying that they made many errors. As he did so often, Culpeper linked their ignorance to a critique of social power, saying that because these writers 'were famous men' they were treated as 'god-a-mighties' who could not err.[35] Culpeper's readers, on the other hand, were encouraged to be sceptical of all learned authority, even of Culpeper himself. In his introduction to the book, he begs his readers to tell him if they find errors in the work, so that the mistakes 'shall be both acknowledged, and amended', and includes his address: 'Spittle-fields, next Door to the Red Lyon'.[36] Culpeper says that a man who believes a book rather than the evidence of his own eyes is a fool.[37] However, few if any of his male or female readers would have had the opportunity to see an anatomical dissection of a female body, so they had to rely on Culpeper's book rather than their own eyes.

---

[34] Culpeper, *Directory*, 22.   [35] Ibid. 34.   [36] Ibid. sig. ¶8ʳ.   [37] Ibid. 5.

Culpeper does not present anatomy in the usual format by referring to illustrations. Instead, he constantly uses images of vision to persuade the reader that he has seen what he describes. For example, he assures his readers that he has been 'an Eye-witness in all I have written'.[38] He describes looking at the way veins and arteries intermix just before entering the testicles, which 'brings an exceeding deal of delight to the eye, and content to the mind (I could show it [to] any man in the Anatomy of a Dog)'.[39] His comment suggests that dissection, rather than being a messy or difficult process, is a pleasurable one, revealing the beauties of God's handiwork to men. In the midst of a popular midwifery book, Culpeper evokes a homosocial moment, in which men delight in seeing the workings of male bodies. Anatomical dissection was an uncommon practice in early modern England, and as far as we know, neither performed nor usually attended by women, even by midwives. Similarly, Culpeper describes making an anatomical preparation to show that the urethra begins at the neck of the bladder but does not grow from it, 'for if you boyl the bladder, you may see it separate it self from it [i.e. the urethra]'.[40] Seeing is knowing, and the reader is encouraged to believe that he, too, could see what Culpeper saw if he were standing beside him as he dissected. Although Culpeper makes an equation between seeing and knowing, he conceals much of the work involved in connecting the two. Anyone who has dissected a frog in a school biology class or has looked under the bonnet of her car has experienced some of the ways in which seeing is not always knowing.

There is a peculiar tension in the *Directory for Midwives* between its insistence on anatomy and vision and its relative lack of illustrations. Certainly, pictures cost money, and publishers may have been reluctant to foot the bill for a new wood engraving. The most important midwifery text prior to Culpeper's, Thomas Raynalde's *Birth of Mankind*, has a series of illustrations discussed below. Culpeper includes only one illustration in the first edition of his book, a picture taken from Spigelius.[41] It is an image of the position of the baby in the womb (see Fig. 5.1). The baby is curled up, but there is nothing of the mother's body in the image. In the original, the baby is pictured inside the mother's body, with the womb dissected to show the infant's position. In Culpeper's image, this might be a newborn baby, with the umbili-

---

[38] Culpeper, *Directory*. I have added a second 'l' to 'all'; in the original it is spelled 'al'.

[39] Ibid. 10.

[40] Ibid. 23. See also 37–8, where Culpeper describes inflating the spermatic veins with a quill so that 'you may perceive both the right and left sides of the Womb blown up'. The reader, of course, can only 'perceive' this inflation vicariously.

[41] Subsequent editions do include another illustration taken from Spigelius that illustrates female reproductive anatomy, but other midwifery texts provided more. See Adriaan van de Spiegel, *De Formato Foetu Liber Singularis: Aeneis Figuris Exornatus* (Padua: Apud Jo. Bap. de Martinis, & Livium Pasquatum, expensis ejusdem Liberalis Cremae, [1626]).

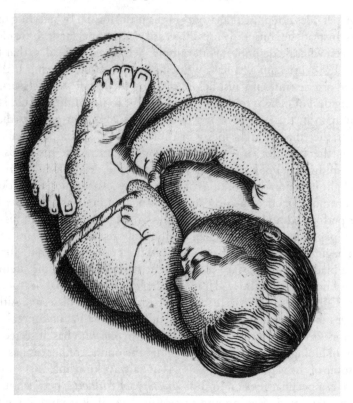

Fig. 5.1. The position of the baby in the womb. Nicholas Culpeper, *A Directory for Midvvives* (1651). Courtesy of the British Library, shelf mark E.1340[1]

cal cord positioned across its body as yet uncut. For all that Culpeper insisted on the primacy of anatomical knowledge, he did not include images to help the reader visualize the structures he discussed. The effect of the lack of illustrations in the book, linked with his insistence on anatomy and vision, is to make Culpeper's knowledge curiously privileged. Although the text is ostensibly for all childbearing women as well as for midwives, Culpeper made himself the only possessor of true knowledge since only he had dissected a pregnant female cadaver.

Again and again, Culpeper insists that 'any that hath seen a Woman Anatomized' would properly understand the structure of the female reproductive body.[42] He laments the difficulty of finding subjects for dissection who would

[42] Culpeper, *Directory*, 34.

illustrate the way the fetus fits into the mother's body, because most women who died while pregnant miscarried before dying.[43] He continues:

My self saw one Woman opened that died in child-bed, not delivered, and that is more by one than most of our Dons [i.e. learned professors] have seen, yet they are as confident as Aesops crow was, that he was an Eagle.[44]

Although Culpeper had dissected only one pregnant woman, that was more than most had.

Culpeper's insistence on anatomical knowledge and its pleasures violated some of the customary norms and practices of childbirth. After getting the baby breathing, the first thing a midwife did was to cut the umbilical cord, or, in their words, the navel-string.[45] Cutting the navel-string correctly was important, because the length of the cord that remained attached to the infant's body affected his or her future sexual performance. Boys' cords were cut long, to ensure a generous-sized penis, while girls' were cut short, to make their vaginas tight-fitting. Raynalde euphemistically says: 'some say that of what length the reste of the navel is lefte / of the same length shal the childs tonge be, if it be a man childe'.[46] In 1612 Jacques Guillemeau distanced himself from these beliefs by prefacing his discussion with 'some do observe', and put words in the mouths of the gossips:

Some do observe, the Navell must be tied longer, or shorter, according to the difference of the sexe, allowing more measure to the males: because this length do make their tongue, and privie membres [*sic*] the longer: whereby they may both speake the plainer, and be more serviceable to Ladies . . . the Gossips commonly say merrily to the Midwife; if it be a boy, 'Make him goode measure'; but if it be a wench, 'Tie it short'.[47]

Even the piece of the string that was cut had magical properties, being still linked sympathetically to the baby's body from which it came. If it touched the floor, for example, the baby would grow up to be incontinent, never able to control urination.

Culpeper describes the anatomical structure of the navel-string, and then instructs his readers: 'Women may, if they please, when they have cut it off, take

---

[43] Culpeper, *Directory*, 55. Characteristically, Culpeper goes on to attack learned authorities, in this case Galen and Vesalius, for never having dissected a pregnant woman.

[44] Ibid. 55–6.

[45] Jacques Guillemeau uses the cutting of the navel-string to claim that surgery was the oldest profession: 'For the Antiquitie: without doubt the first work in Chirurgery, that ever was in the worlde, was the cutting of the Navell which (as saide before) Adam practised uppon his first borne.' Guillemeau, *Child-birth*, sig. ¶3ᵛ. Part of Guillemeau's purpose in his text is to encourage women to call in male surgeons when labour goes awry. Despite his portrayal of a male surgeon cutting the navel-string, it is clear that this procedure was very rarely done by anyone other than the midwife; in the body of his text, Guillemeau gives very careful instructions to the midwife on just how to cut the string (pp. 98–9).

[46] Raynalde, *Byrth of Mankind* (1545), fo. 109ᵛ.   [47] Guillemeau, *Child-birth*, 99.

the pains to open it, and see for their own content, and those about them, that what I have written here is the truth.'[48] For him, this body part had no magical meanings; it could be cut open and examined for women's 'content'. Rather than ensuring the baby's successful adult control of urination and sexual function, it was to be used to demonstrate the truth of his words.

While the *Directory* makes women's bodies into passive objects of consumption by male readers, its most fundamental critique of contemporary practices lies in its attitudes to midwives, and, by implication, to all women. The book appears to be pro-midwife, since it is dedicated to the midwives of England. Culpeper proclaims that if midwives follow his rules, they need never call in a man-midwife, 'which is a disparagement, not only to yourselves, but also to your Profession'.[49] At this time, men only intervened in childbirth in dire circumstances. Calling in a male surgeon meant that the midwife and the women with her had decided that the baby's life was lost already or that it would have to be sacrificed in order to save the mother. The surgeon's job was to extract the baby, usually in parts. Not surprisingly, this gruesome exercise often resulted in the death of the mother as well.[50]

While Culpeper praises the midwives of England and assures them that he considers their work a profession, that is, a calling, he quickly reminds them of the religious implications of their profession. God committed the life of an infant to a midwife, 'even at the very first Minute that he allots it to draw its breath; and at your hands He will have an Accompt of it another day'.[51] Humility was to be the keystone of a midwife's knowledge: 'All the Perfections that can be in a Woman, ought to be in a *Midwife*; the first step to which is, To know your ignorance in that part of Physick which is the Basis of your Art.'[52] Here Culpeper cleverly makes midwifery a branch of physic and thus subject to male

---

[48] Culpeper, *Directory*, 50.

[49] Ibid. sig ¶4ᵛ. Culpeper's use of the word 'man-midwife' is quite early, especially for a popular medical book. Adrian Wilson has argued that the term is related to the Chamberlen family's use of three secret obstetrical tools: the forceps, the vectis, and the fillet. Each enabled a practitioner to deliver an obstructed birth. Unlike all other male surgeons called into an emergency birth, the Chamberlens were able to deliver a living child rather than extract a dead one—in other words, they acted as midwives rather than surgeons. Adrian Wilson, *The Making of Man-Midwifery: Childbirth in England, 1660–1770* (Cambridge, Mass.: Harvard University Press, 1995), see esp. 47–67. It is possible that Culpeper knew Dr Peter Chamberlen, since both practised in London and had not incompatible politico-religious allegiances, or knew of his ability to deliver a living child with secret tools. According to the *OED*, however, the earliest 17th-c. uses of 'man-midwife' were on the London stage, where the term was used metaphorically by Ben Jonson and others.

[50] On these points, see Adrian Wilson, 'Childbirth in Seventeenth- and Early Eighteenth-Century England' (D.Phil. thesis, University of Sussex, 1982). Wilson's book *Making of Man-Midwifery* deals primarily with the post-1660 period.

[51] Culpeper, *Directory*, sig. ¶5ʳ.   [52] Ibid. sig. ¶5ᵛ.

authority.[53] While obstetrics is a part of medicine today, such was not wholly the case in the mid-seventeenth century. The only form of licensing to which midwives were subject was episcopal. When a midwife applied for a bishop's licence, she called worthy matrons to testify to her skills rather than physicians and surgeons.[54] Culpeper moves from admonition to threat in his discussion of the religious imperatives of midwifery. He tells the midwives: 'Many of you are Ancient, but if you be too old to learn, you are as much too proud.'[55] Midwives who did not heed Culpeper's words were guilty of the sin of pride, and God would call them to account for it.

More specifically, Culpeper's book attacks the basis on which midwives and all women know things about female bodies. He sets up a new epistemology of female bodies, one in which women can learn only from men, not from each other. Culpeper starts the main part of his text by arguing that midwives and all women 'should be well skil'd in the exact knowledge of the Anatomy of these Parts'.[56] He does not think that midwives have much if any anatomical knowledge. For example, he claims that most midwives have been poisoned by the idea that the womb has seven cells, so that a woman might give birth to up to seven children at once, but no more. As Culpeper says in his vivid and vernacular way, 'and this is just as true as the Moon is made of a Green Cheese'.[57]

To claim that seeing was knowing was an implicit critique of customary midwifery practices, and thus of the female culture of the birthing room, with its ritual practices and invocations of supernatural aid. Midwives' knowledge was grounded in touching, not seeing. Indeed, 'to touch' was synonymous with 'to examine'. Books written before Culpeper all stress the manual aspects of midwifery practice. To be anachronistic for a moment, a midwife's hands were her diagnostic tools and medical instruments. For example, the midwife used her hands to know if a woman's pains were true or false labour. As one book explains, 'But for more certainty, the Midwife may put up her hand, being anointed with fresh butter, & if she perceive the inner neck of the womb to dilate it self, 'tis a certain sign.'[58] Rueff's *Expert Midwife* describes the midwife's task during labour:

Let the Midwife instruct and encourage the party to her labor, to abide her paines with patience, and then gently apply her hands to the worke as she ought, by feeling and

---

[53] In his warning to midwives about their religious duty, and in his claim that midwifery is a branch of medicine, Culpeper echoes the German editions of *The Birth of Mankind*; see discussion in Ch. 1.

[54] Evenden, *The Midwives of 17th-c. London*; Hilary Marland (ed.), *The Art of Midwifery: Early Modern Midwives in Europe* (London: Routledge, 1993).

[55] Culpeper, *Directory*, sig. ¶6ʳ.   [56] Ibid. 1.   [57] Ibid. 34.

[58] *Compleat Midwifes Practice* (1656), 80. Although the first edition of this work was published in 1656, it is almost all a compilation of older works, including those by Jacob Rueff and Louise Bourgeois. See the next chapter for further discussion of this text.

searching with her fingers how the child lieth, and by relaxing and opening the way and passage conveniently for him, while the mother is in paine.[59]

It is the midwife's fingers that 'see', figuring out how the baby will present. This 'seeing' tells her how to proceed. If the baby is not presenting correctly, it is the midwife's hands that must remedy the situation, turning the baby to the best position possible for delivery. As Raynalde said, 'But when the birth commeth not naturally, then must the midwife do all her diligence and pain, if it may be possible, to turn the birth tenderlye with her anointed hands, so that it maye be reduced againe to a naturall birth.'[60] A so-called 'natural' birth, in which the infant presented head-first, was always desirable.

Images such as those in Fig. 5.2 illustrated for a midwife the very many dangerous positions in which an infant might present. For twentieth-century historians, such images are often irreverently known as 'babies in bottles'.[61] These pictures, which have their origins in medieval manuscripts, seem peculiar to us because they abstract the womb from the body of the labouring woman. However, the images of babies-in-bottles need to be understood within their own context—namely, a book on midwifery that emphasizes the multiple dangers to which a labouring woman is exposed. While these images seem odd to us because they specifically ignore the body of that woman, within texts such as Raynalde's they serve as a kind of mnemonic, a brief visual summation of elaborate directions to the midwife and labouring woman. For example, Fig. 5.3 depicts a baby who presents with one foot forward. The text emphasizes the body of the labouring woman:

And in this case it behoveth the laboringe woman to lay her upright uppon her backe, holding up her thighes and belly, so that her head be the lower part of her body: then let the midwife with her hand returne in againe the fote [foot] that commeth out first, in as tender maner as may be, and warne the woman that laboureth to stere [stir] and move her selfe, so that by movinge and steringe, the birth may be turned the head dounward, and so make a naturall birth of it.[62]

Thus, while the picture seems to remove the labouring woman from the birth process, the text does quite the reverse. These images in Raynalde's text remind us that an emphasis on anatomy did not necessarily imply a negative view of the skills of midwives. Raynalde sings the praises of anatomical knowledge just as does Culpeper. However, he leaves the anatomy of labour and delivery in the realm of touching—the midwife's way of knowing—endorsing the knowledge and skills of midwifery.

---

[59] Rueff, *Expert Midwife*, 81.   [60] Raynalde, *Byrth* (1545), fo. 62[r].

[61] See Karen Newman, *Fetal Positions: Individualism, Science, Visuality* (Stanford: Stanford University Press, 1996).

[62] Raynalde, *Byrth* (1545), fo. 63[r–v].

Fig. 5.2. Raynalde's image of a
natural birth (lower right).
Thomas Raynalde, *The Birth of
Man-kinde* (1626). Courtesy of
the Folger Shakespeare Library

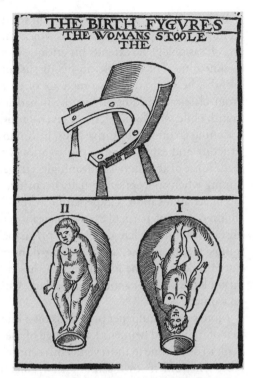

Fig. 5.3. An unnatural birth.
Thomas Raynalde, *The Birth of
Man-kinde* (1626). Courtesy of
the Folger Shakespeare Library

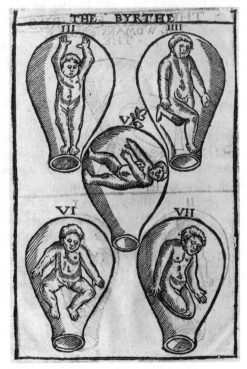

By contrast, Culpeper's emphasis on seeing as the correct way to know was an implicit critique of the ways in which midwives learnt and practised their art. Occasionally, he extends his critique to all women, faulting their capacity for knowing. For example, in his discussion of children born early at eight months, he suggests that women are often ignorant about their own bodies. From classical antiquity onwards, it had long been believed that an eight-month child was doomed, but a seven-month child might survive. While this reasoning is counter-intuitive to us, historians have suggested that it gave some structure and explanation to the vagaries of the survival of newborn babies: it made sense of an otherwise meaningless tragedy. Given the difficulties in determining when conception actually occurred, such a belief could be quite flexible in its application. Culpeper, however, did not believe that eight-month children were at particular risk. Instead, he argued that mothers were often mistaken about the lengths of their pregnancies. A woman might 'be a Month mistaken of their time, that is as easily done, and as often by some, as a Woman can mistake one Shoe for another in the dark'.[63] While presumably men also mistook one shoe for another in the dark, Culpeper's homely metaphor focuses on women.

More subtly, Culpeper placed his own knowledge of the female body above that of individual women's knowledge of their own bodies. Pregnancy was difficult to determine in the seventeenth century, and many of the early indicators relied on women's own sensations. Guillemeau's 1612 book warns that surgeons have to be very careful in determining pregnancy:

For there is nothing more ridiculous, then to assure a woman that shee is with childe; and afterward, that her natural sicknesse [e.g. the menses], or store of water should come from her: and in stead of a childe, some windie matter should breake from her, and so her belly fall, and grow flat againe.[64]

The sex act itself might provide clues to conception. If a woman experienced 'extraordinary delight', if no fluid issued forth from her privy parts, if she felt a kind of yawning and stretching all over her body, and a kind of shaking or quivering, and a chill between the shoulders—all of this just after sex—she might have become pregnant.[65] Guillemeau provides many other symptoms and signs of pregnancy, but the cardinal one is the moment of quickening—when a woman feels the baby move within her for the first time. Guillemeau describes it as 'not unlike the stirring of a flie when he flieth'.[66] For Guillemeau, as for most other writers, the best determination of pregnancy was that which

---

[63] Culpeper, *Directory*, 67–8.   [64] Guillemeau, *Child-birth*, 2.
[65] Ibid. 4. Guillemeau also thought that the man's experience of sex might provide clues about conception.
[66] Ibid. 6.

came from the woman herself. Determining pregnancy was very much a female act, and in denigrating women's abilities to do so accurately, Culpeper was attacking female bodily knowledge more generally.

The *Directory for Midwives* is a curious book. Although it is addressed to women, and dedicated to midwives, it attacks ways of knowing the body most often associated with women. It presents a model of the female reproductive body that, as we have seen, makes it inferior to the male body. By anatomizing the female body, Culpeper's book implicitly denies that a female body might be the producer of knowledge itself. Only an anatomically trained person (which in mid-seventeenth-century England almost always meant a man) could make truths about the female body, truths that were hidden from view and inaccessible to the body that contained them. Only another person could see into the secrets of the female body, and if the seeing were that of an anatomical dissection, the female body was dead, completely without agency.

Finally, Culpeper writes in a style that both undermines female authority and creates a new kind of vernacular voice. His lively and witty style contributed to the huge popularity of his books. It also broke with traditions of writing about women's bodies and made those bodies into a topic through which gender relations could be articulated. First, he wrote in a demotic style, full of humble proverbs and turns of phrase that linked the written word with the spoken word. Second, he wrote about women's bodies in an almost playful way, asserting his right to speak about them unashamedly, unlike prior writers. The structure of his text sexualizes the reading process, implicitly making women's bodies into objects to be consumed by men. Finally, Culpeper appropriated the metaphor of motherhood for his own production of his book.

The *Directory* is full of colourful expressions and homely metaphors. As cited above, Culpeper compared the idea that the womb had seven cells to the idea that the moon was made of green cheese. Most doctors, he said, were afflicted with covetousness that outweighed their wit as a millstone outweighed a feather.[67] Another opinion was 'as probable as that a Millstone can swim'.[68] On occasion, Culpeper addressed the reader directly, as if speaking to him or her. When he notes that many good midwives were ignorant, he rhetorically asks, 'What then? The more is the pity, say I.'[69] When he discusses the testes he writes: 'The Stones are called in Latin, Testes, that is, Witnesses, because they witnes one to be a Man: Ask the Pope else, he will tel you I say true.'[70] That gleeful reference to the Pope, the very last authority a radical Protestant such as Culpeper would be likely to invoke, and the direct address to the reader, are characteristic of his playful and engaging style. One final example will have to serve to illustrate this demotic style. In one of his frequent attacks on reliance

[67] Culpeper, *Directory*, sig. A¶3ʳ.   [68] Ibid. 79.   [69] Ibid. 1.   [70] Ibid. 11.

on tradition, Culpeper says: 'for I assure you, he that builds his faith upon Tradition all day, may sit down in the Chimny-corner at night and scratch his Head with a pair of Fools Nails'.[71] No other writer of popular medical books tickled readers with images such as these.

Earlier writers of midwifery manuals fretted about male readers. Raynalde, as discussed in earlier chapters, spent half his preface warning men not to read the book in the wrong way, and worrying that the wrong sort of male reader would be prompted to make jokes about the female body. In the *Directory*, it is Culpeper who does the joking, inviting male readers to jest with him. After the remark about the Pope cited above he continues by discussing the anatomical situation of the testicles, saying 'I need not tell you where they are placed, for every Boy that knows but his right hand from his left, knows that'.[72] Again, he addresses the reader directly, with a kind of nudge and wink. Culpeper was not being frivolous. His writing was part of his larger critique of entrenched privilege and useless learning. The effect of his desire to make knowledge available to all, however, was to make women's reproductive bodies a fit topic for male discussion.

Culpeper's way of describing male and female reproductive bodies creates an unusual effect by sexualizing the reading process. His discussion of male anatomy, echoed by many subsequent writers, starts with the vessels that bring the blood to the stones in order to make seed. The reader follows the path of the formation and use of the seed. We start with the blood vessels, tracing seed's distillation from blood, moving through seed-vessels, stones, and prostate, continuing to the penis and ejaculation. Women's bodies do not follow a similar sequence. Instead, it is as if the reader is still following the male seed. First, women's exterior genitals are described, then we move inside to the neck of the womb by way of discussions of the hymen, then to the womb itself. Finally, there is mention of women's stones.[73]

This pattern of descriptive penetration is underscored by the ways in which images of seeing and sensation are used. Culpeper describes the female genitals in a way that imaginatively creates a (male?) viewer of female anatomy: 'The lips, which are visible to the eye at first sight.'[74] Other texts of the 1650s echo Culpeper's pattern of moving from the inside of the male body to the outside, but going in the reverse order for the female body. For example, a 1656 text says: 'This is also further to be noted in the neck of the womb, that as soon as

---

[71] Culpeper, *Directory*, 59. See also 'A man had as good put his Wits Apprentise to a man in Bedlam, as make them slaves to TRADITION', 69, for the same kind of colourful writing that sounds like speech.   [72] Ibid. 11–12.

[73] Culpeper, *Directory*, see discussion of female genitals that starts on p. 26; for comparison, see *Compleat Midwifes Practice* (1656); discussion of female genitals starts on p. 25.

[74] Culpeper, *Directory*, 27.

ever your sight is entered within the female fissure, there do appear to the view, two certain little holes, or pits.'[75] Culpeper may not have been conscious of the effect he was creating, where reading becomes analogous to the sexual penetration of a woman's body. However, the text hints at its own sexual allusions. For instance, the phrase 'Having served my own Sex, I shall see now if I can please the Women', plays upon sexual connotations of 'serve' and 'please' in Culpeper's characteristically light-hearted tone.[76]

On the one hand, Culpeper's text suggests a male reader, one who would look over his shoulder at a dissection, or snicker at his comments about the location of the testicles, 'ask the Pope else'. On the other, he plays with gender roles, describing his own work as like a mother's production of a baby. At the very end of the book, he includes a list of errors, a glossary, and a table of contents (in the seventeenth century it was not unusual to place the contents at the end of the book, rather than the beginning, as it simplified the work of the printers). Playful as ever, he wrote a parody of the usual errata list before including the serious version. The parody is an attack on potential critics, including 'For Neglect of my Rules, read Death of Infants' and 'Raging against me, read Covetousness'.[77] At the beginning of the real errata list he writes: 'Although it seem very improbable to Nature, that a Generation should be gotten by absence; yet hath my absence from the press beget a generation of errors, thus to be corrected.'[78] It was customary for authors to read the proof copies of their books in the printer's shop, as the sheets came off the press. Culpeper, by now largely bedridden, played with his absence from the print shop, making the book his 'generation' or his progeny. In this image, he might be the father or the mother of his book. Earlier in the text, he slides from mother to father, saying 'If it [the book] be childish, tis like its Mother: before you dispraise my work, put forth your own like a Man.'[79] Culpeper adopts a female persona when he writes 'I conceived a few thoughts, and I hope to bring them to perfect birth.'[80] He compares his writing to milk for babies, as if he were a mother providing for her offspring.[81] Culpeper was not the first author to compare writing to conception and birth. However, in the context of a book on midwifery, these comparisons suggest that the processes of generation are not mysterious and are not just women's business.

The *Directory for Midwives* was very successful. Historians of medicine have tended to focus on William Harvey's 1651 Latin text on generation, but for any bookseller in that decade, the 1651 item to copy was Culpeper's text. And copy it they did. The book went into four more editions by 1660. More important, its success, and the new model it propounded for writing about women's

[75] *Compleat Midwifes Practice* (1656), 30.   [76] Culpeper, *Directory*, 26.
[77] Ibid. [218].   [78] Ibid. [219].   [79] Ibid. sig. A5ᵛ.   [80] Ibid. sig. ¶3ᵛ.
[81] Ibid. sig. A5ʳ.

bodies, prompted many others to try their hands at a midwifery book. At least eight other texts were produced in the 1650s alone (compared to three in the previous century).

Two strands of Culpeper's work were widely imitated. First, he made women's bodies into microcosms of gender relations. He made male reproductive anatomy superior to female anatomy, and by implication underscored men's superior relation to women. Second, he made women's bodies something men could talk about unashamedly—indeed, something that men were uniquely qualified to discuss. No longer was the knowledge of women's bodies the stuff of midwives' talk. It was the subject of men's printed books.[82] Two final quotes from his book sum up the larger implications of his epistemological project. In his jokey errata list, Culpeper says: 'For *Discovering Womens Matters* read *Encrease of Knowledge*.'[83] This phrase encapsulates the transformation he wrought: women's bodies were not the stuff of women's gossip, or of men's jokes, but could be made a part of a larger project to increase the sum of knowledge. For Culpeper, that project was always part of his religious and reforming agenda. It is too easy to paint him as a simple kind of anti-feminist, wresting knowledge from midwives and giving it to men. He was more complex than that. He thought that increasing human knowledge, even of women's reproductive bodies, was a godly project.[84]

But Culpeper was also responding, whether consciously or not, to the changed gender dynamics of the 1640s and proposing a model of the body that would not allow women such latitude in making political and spiritual statements. Indeed, he specifically criticized prophesying women: 'God speaks not now by voice to Men and Women as formerly he did; but he speaks in, and by Men, and tis no part of wisdom for Men and Women to stop their ears against it.'[85] Here he directly attacks visionary women such as Sarah Wight, claiming that God no longer spoke to women or men in this way. Instead, God spoke through men—but not through women. In the context of the 1640s and 1650s, his words were loaded. All around him, women were claiming to be God's instruments. For Culpeper, however, these women were wrong; God no longer worked that way. In his explication of the anatomy of the female reproductive body, he made men the authoritative makers of knowledge of all kinds.

---

[82] On this larger point, see Crawford, 'Sexual Knowledge in England'.
[83] Culpeper, *Directory*, [218].
[84] On the larger Puritan project, see Webster, *The Great Instauration*, esp. 246–323.
[85] Culpeper, *Directory*, sig. ¶6ʳ.

6

Reforming the Family and Refiguring the Body in the English Revolution

Early in 1652 George Horton published a pamphlet called *The Ranters Monster*. It told the story of Mary Adams, of Tillingham in Essex, who blasphemously declared that she was the Virgin Mary, pregnant with the Saviour. The father of the child, she added, was the Holy Spirit itself. Mr Hadley, the local minister, had her arrested and thrown into prison. Local women aided the midwife when Adams went into labour. She 'lay in exceeding great misery and torment' for eight days, and gave birth to a hideous monster on the ninth day. The monster was born dead but terrified the women nonetheless, who buried it with great haste. As the pamphlet explains, the women's hearts trembled when they saw it, because 'every part was odious to behold'. Mary Adams came to an equally hideous end. Suffering from 'botches, blains, boils & stinking scabs', she told the women that she had no ability to repent of her sins, and having borrowed a knife, ostensibly to pare her nails, she stabbed herself to death.[1]

Mary Adams's story thus far could have been told at any point in the previous century. The elements of blasphemy met by divine punishment and monster births as signs of God's displeasure were commonplaces in English culture, as discussed in Chapter 2. However, when the pamphlet tells how Mary Adams came to her dreadful fate, the story becomes one specific to the upheavals of the 1640s and 1650s. In this telling, her life became a slippery slope of religious and sexual deviance. Although born of good parents and living an exemplary life for a number of years, Adams lost her way when she became a Baptist, and 'desired to participate with them in their watry Element'. The hint of sexual feeling implied in the word 'desire' developed further in this story as Adams joined the Family of Love, a heretical sect associated in cheap print with sexual excess from its origins in the sixteenth century. Next she became a Ranter, characterized in this text by beliefs that there was no God nor any heaven or hell, and by the idea that 'it was no sin to lie with any man,

---

[1] *The Ranters Monster: Being a True Relation of One Mary Adams, living at Tillingham in Essex* (London: printed for George Horton, 1652), Thomason E.658[6], 3–4.

whether Batchelor, Widdower, or married; but a thing lawful, and adjured thereunto by Nature'.[2] In the 1640s and 1650s, old and new radical religious groups such as the Baptists and the Ranters flourished. Church courts were closed, and such groups were rarely prosecuted by the government. Cheap print pamphlets and newsbooks publicized the doings of genuine sects, such as the Baptists, and wholly imaginary ones, such as the Adamites. At the close of Horton's pamphlet, the writer adds 'one thing I had almost omitted', namely, that Mary Adams was very set against the Independents in religion, and she said that rather than give birth to a child who would be a Roundhead (a supporter of the Parliamentary side in the Civil War) or Independent, she would prefer the child have no head at all.[3]

As we shall see, this detail links Mary Adams's story to a number of other pamphlets about headless or beheaded babies. In miniature, her story, and those to which it refers, point to some of the ways in which the customary regulation of family and gender relations was challenged and reworked during the 1640s and 1650s. Her story makes a terrifying connection between those reworkings and the actual mechanics of reproduction. The politics of the family and the mechanics of reproduction were connected in a variety of ways in the 1650s; monstrosity was only the most extreme way in which gender relations and the body itself were reimagined.[4]

The detail about Mary Adams's curse on her unborn baby refers to a number of other cheap sensational pamphlets that connected political and religious upheaval to headless babies. In the first, published in 1642, the central issue was the tension between Anglican and Puritan views of baptismal services. Mary Wilmore, of Mears Ashby in Northamptonshire, was eight months pregnant when she conferred with her minister about the ceremony of baptism, and, in particular, the use of the sign of the cross. Her minister, named John

[2] *Ranters Monster*, both quotes on p. 5.
[3] Ibid. 8. 'Independent' refers both to conflicts about religion and to two different groups in Parliament who disagreed about the conduct of the war and other issues. In both cases, 'Independents' were opposed to 'Presbyterians'. See pp. 136–7 above.
[4] The literature on monstrosity is now substantial. I have found the following to be the most helpful: Park and Daston, 'Unnatural Conceptions'; Huet, *Monstrous Imagination*; Dennis Todd, *Imagining Monsters: Miscreations of the Self in 18th-c. England* (Chicago: University of Chicago Press, 1995). On monstrosity in the mid-17th c. in particular, see David Cressy, *Travesties and Transgressions in Tudor and Stuart England* (Oxford: Oxford University Press, 2000), 29–50; Jerome Friedman, *The Battle of the Frogs and Fairford's Flies* (New York: St. Martin's Press, 1993), esp. 48–54; William E. Burns, 'The King's Two Monstrous Bodies: John Bulwer and the English Revolution', in Peter G. Platt (ed.), *Wonders, Marvels, and Monsters in Early Modern Culture* (Newark, Del.: University of Delaware Press, 1999), 187–202. For the decline of such beliefs, see Todd, and Lisa Cody, ' "The Doctor's In Labour; or a New Whim Wham from Guilford" ', *Gender and History*, 4 (1992), 175–96. The case of Anne Hutchinson in New England has also been the subject of historical attention: Anne Jacobson Schutte, ' "Such Monstrous Births": A Neglected Aspect of the Antinomian Controversy', *Renaissance Quarterly*, 38 (1985), 85–106.

Locke, sent her husband to the next parish to confer with the minister there, who told him that the sign of the cross was an 'ancient, laudable, and decent ceremony' although it was not necessary for salvation.[5] Mrs Wilmore, whom Locke accused of consorting with sectarians, was still not satisfied. Like others, she saw the sign of the cross as a remnant of Catholicism, and she declared that she would rather have a baby with no head than one whose head would be signed with the sign of the cross. Subsequently, she gave birth to just such a headless babe, which Locke saw as a dreadful warning to all who might deviate from the Anglican church or who might challenge God.[6]

Three years later, the pamphlet narration of the production of another headless baby was used to demarcate the boundary between Catholic and Protestant rather than that between Anglican and Puritan. The devoutly Catholic Haughten family lived in Kirkham, Lancashire, a county that the pamphlet reminds the reader was a hotbed of both witchcraft and papistry. Mrs Haughten, a gentlewoman, uttered another variation of the curse while she was pregnant, saying that she would rather give birth to a baby with no head than a Roundhead. She too gave birth to a headless infant. The pamphlet that recounts the story uses the woodblock illustration later adopted by the publisher of the Mary Adams pamphlet (see Fig. 6.1).[7]

The story of Mary Adams also refers to another sensational pamphlet that combines concerns about baptismal practices with headless babies. In this story, published in 1647, the conflict is not between families, as it was in Kirkham, but within the family, between husband and wife. Mary Champion disagreed with her husband John about baptizing their infant. In the title page woodcut she is identified as an Anabaptist and he as a Presbyterian (see Fig. 6.2). In the text, however, no such labels are used, and the husband is portrayed as a moderate who merely wants to follow 'the ancient Custome of the Kingdome' in having his child baptized. While her husband was away, Mary Champion cut off the head of her infant, and when her husband returned, she

---

[5] John Locke, *A Strange and Lamentable Accident That Happened Lately at Mears Ashby* (printed in London for Rich: Harper and Thomas Wine, and are to be sold at the Bible and Harpe in Smithfield, 1642), Thomason E.113[15]; quote at sig. A3^r. On the larger issues about the sign of the cross in baptism, see Cressy, *Birth, Marriage and Death*, esp. 173–5.

[6] Locke, *Strange and Lamentable Accident*, sig. A3^v.

[7] *A Declaration of a Strange and Wonderful Monster* (London: printed by Jane Coe, 1646), Thomason E.325[20]. Like other characters in such pamphlets, this family seems almost to look for trouble. Mrs Haughten's mother, Mrs Browne, cut off the ears of the family cat and renamed him Prynne, after the Puritan William Prynne who was punished with similar mutilation in February 1640 for publishing anti-Arminian tracts. Prynne, along with his fellow sufferers John Bastwick and Henry Burton, had been Puritan heroes since 1637, when they were prosecuted in the Court of Star Chamber for seditious libel. When they were freed by Parliament in late 1640, and returned to London, they were met by thousands of supporters. Mrs Browne's act must have seemed like a deliberate provocation to many readers of this pamphlet.

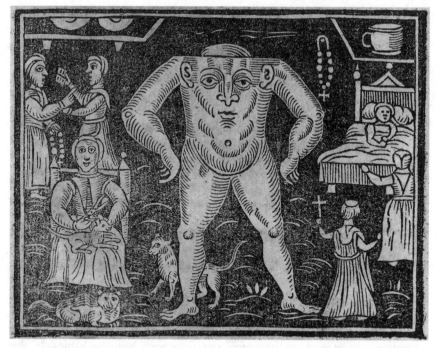

Fig. 6.1. A headless baby. *A Declaration of a Strange and Wonderful Monster* (1646). Courtesy of
the Folger Shakespeare Library

said to him: 'behold husband, thy sweet babe without a head, now go and
baptize it; if you will'. As is often the case in pamphlets about murder, Mary
Champion repented and was much troubled by visions of her headless baby.[8]

   The basic plot of these stories about headless babies is not new: irreligion is
punished in swift and bodily ways. However, the details of the stories—how
the protagonists erred, for example—are very specific commentaries on contemporary affairs. The density of inter-reference, from the use of the same
woodblocks to the ways in which the women in these stories seem to echo each

---

   [8] *Bloody Newes from Dover* ([London]: Printed in the Year of Discovery, 13 Feb. 1647), Thomason
E.375[20]; quotes at [3]. On the genre of murder pamphlets and their meanings, see Lake, *Antichrist's
Lewd Hat*, which includes two of his previous articles, 'Deeds against Nature: Cheap Print, Protes-
tantism, and Murder in Early Modern England', in Peter Lake and Kevin Sharpe (eds.), *Culture and
Politics in Early Modern England* (Stanford: Stanford University Press, 1994), 257–83; Peter Lake,
'Popular Form, Puritan Content? Two Puritan Appropriations of the Murder Pamphlet from Mid-
17th-c. London', in Anthony Fletcher and Peter Roberts (eds.), *Religion, Culture and Society in Early
Modern Britain: Essays in Honour of Patrick Collinson* (Cambridge: Cambridge University Press,
1994), 313–34, and the literature cited in Ch. 2.

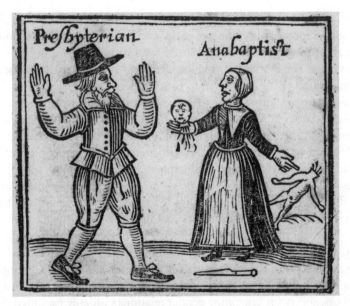

Fig. 6.2. Infanticide makes a headless baby. *Bloody Newes from Dover* (1647). Courtesy of the British Library, shelf mark E.375[20]

others' curses, is also characteristic of the 1640s and 1650s. It was only in these decades that sufficient numbers of sensational pamphlets were produced to permit the kind of theme-and-variations analysed above.

So too, these stories remind us that cheap print was a kind of imaginative space, a place in which a wide range of fantasies could be rehearsed and revised. Like the female body itself, cheap print was a capacious medium for the making of meaning. In what follows, I employ many such pamphlets that claim to be true—the headless baby ones often include lists of witnesses—yet I would not venture to hazard any opinion about their veracity. Historians have tended to employ some of these pamphlets as if they were truthful witnesses to real events, and to dismiss others as fiction.[9] Instead of emphasizing these texts' production in relation to some real events, I understand them as stories whose value to the historian lies in their popularity. People wanted to read these pamphlets, and the producers of them seem to have been responsive to the market.

---

[9] See e.g. the debate about the existence of the Ranter movement. Hill, *The World Turned Upside Down*; A. L. Morton, *The World of the Ranters: Religious Radicalism in the English Revolution* (London: Lawrence and Wishart, 1970); J. C. Davis, *Fear, Myth and History: The Ranters and the Historians* (Cambridge: Cambridge University Press, 1986). The Ranters in pamphlet literature seem to have little connection with the men arrested as Ranters.

Sexual excess and monstrous births, combined in the story of Mary Adams, had long been powerful symbols of social and theological disorder. Both were complex figures that could be mobilized for a wide array of purposes. When these two themes were used during the Civil War and Interregnum, they functioned in a number of ways. First, of course, these images connoting disorder were quickly pressed into service to depict and explore the world turned upside down—the chaos of civil war and breakdown of social controls. Second, these two themes became especially significant because of women's activities during the 1640s and 1650s. As discussed in Chapters 3 and 4, women claimed new kinds of authority in a nascent public sphere. They petitioned, preached, and prophesied, and their words and deeds circulated in cheap print as never before. Thus the older set of meanings that linked sexual excess and monster births with social disorder were given new impetus at a time when women were challenging the limits of their roles, moving beyond those of wife and mother.

There is a third layer of significance to these themes in the 1640s and 1650s. During these decades, a range of discussions erupted about the meanings of the family and the gendered relations at the heart of the family. It is as though the range of possibility for imagining gender relations suddenly exploded. English men and women who could read were afforded a plethora of cheap pamphlets and newsbooks offering everything from discussions of divorce and fantasies about complete sexual freedom to new laws that made adultery punishable by death and marriage a civil ceremony. Cheap print capitalized on two different challenges to norms of family life. First, when Parliament enacted a variety of legislation concerning family life, cheap print both described these laws and revelled in satirical accounts of their potential effects. Second, as in the case of Mary Adams's monster, cheap print provided sensational accounts of sexual licence supposedly associated with the boom in diverse religious groups.

Central to the boom in cheap print in the 1640s and 1650s was the development of sexual satire.[10] Dreadful jokes, puns, and sexual slanders became a language used over and over again to describe events in Parliament, radical religious groups, and just about every other current event. As described in Chapter 3, early women preachers and petitioners were quickly slandered as whores. By the 1650s, such sexual satire was commonplace. As we shall see, one of the effects of such writing was to put gender relations at the heart of all kinds of political and religious debate. Even events that seemed to have little to do with relations between men and women came to acquire a kind of gendered edge when they were repeatedly described in the language of sexual satire.

[10] See Achinstein, 'Women on Top'; Underdown, *A Freeborn People*, ch. 5, '*The Man in the Moon*: Loyalty and Libel in Popular Politics, 1640–1650', 90–111; Potter, 'The *Mistress Parliament* Dialogues'; Williams, ' "Magnetic Figures" '; Wiseman, ' "Adam, the Father of All Flesh" '.

Having accomplished a political revolution, the parliamentarians attempted a cultural revolution as well. They sought to make England a godly nation. They wanted to rid their country of superstitions, rituals, idle recreations, and moral failings. Perhaps their project was doomed from the start; perhaps legislation can rarely accomplish the magnitude of attitudinal change sought by the Puritans in power in the late 1640s and 1650s. However, their efforts to remake their nation's culture were prodigious, and the aftershocks of their attempts were felt long after the Restoration. The best-known aspects of the Puritan cultural revolution were the attacks on popular recreations and rituals: no more may-poles; no more Christmas.[11] Less well understood were the Puritans' attempts to remake family and gender relations. While historians have discussed many of the individual aspects of this attempt, such as the Adultery Act of 1650 or the transformation of marriage from a church to a civil ceremony, we have yet to understand the ways in which these different pieces fitted together in a concerted attack on the customary regulation of marriage and family relationships. As the usual mechanisms through which family relations were reproduced and represented were dismantled, people tried out a wide range of other ways to think about those relations, including sexual satires, moral panics, and reworkings of the body. Perhaps only a small proportion of the population was directly and individually affected by new laws about marriage, adultery, and the like, but shifting representations of the family were the subject of a vast cheap literature, suggesting that these issues were of concern to a great many people whether or not they experienced the effects of specific changes personally.[12]

Cheap print subverted the construction of godliness in a second way. From 1641 pamphlets described all kinds of behaviours directly antithetical to the tenets of reformed religion. The rash of pamphlets about Ranters in the early 1650s played on the customary association between religious deviance and sexual licence, creating a moral panic centred on gender relations. The figure of the Ranter was a sort of anti-Puritan, the inverse of the kind of person parliamentary legislation was designed to create. While the writings of individual Ranters contributed to their reputation as sexually transgressive, the cheap

[11] Underdown, *Revel, Riot and Rebellion*; David Cressy, *Bonfires and Bells: National Memory and the Protestant Calendar in Elizabethan and Stuart England* (London: Weidenfeld and Nicolson, 1989); see esp. ch. 3; Hutton, *The Rise and Fall of Merry England*, chs. 5 and 6.

[12] See e.g. Keith Thomas, 'The Puritans and the Adultery Act of 1650 Reconsidered', in Donald Penington and Keith Thomas (eds.), *Puritans and Revolutionaries: Essays in 17th-c. History Presented to Christopher Hill* (Oxford: Clarendon Press, 1978), 257–82. Here I take issue with Christopher Durston, *The Family in the English Revolution* (Oxford: Basil Blackwell, 1989), who argues that the overall impact of the Puritan attempts to restructure the family were not substantial, despite providing the most detailed account of these attempts. Durston makes this claim because he argues that the actual number of people directly affected was small (pp. 164–5).

sensationalist pamphlets about Ranters seem to have far outweighed any actual Ranter writings in the creation of the panic. While ostensibly condemning Ranter excesses, these pamphlets also subversively enticed readers into imagining communities in which gender relations were barely regulated at all.

Both legislative acts of Parliament and the proliferation of satires and stories of sexual transgression in cheap print thus challenged customary ideas and practices through which the English understood and represented the family to themselves. A third kind of challenge to family life happened in January 1649. Eyewitnesses to the execution of Charles I claimed that after the King's head was cut off, the watching crowd uttered a long and deep communal groan.[13] In that wordless moment, we can begin to imagine the cultural consequences of regicide. Almost every writer on marriage and family for the previous century had drawn the usual equation between a father's rule of his family and the king's rule of his subjects.[14] Each mirrored the other, and each functioned to underwrite the authority of the other. For us, metaphor is just a comparison, but in the early modern period, similarities still spoke of some common or shared identity. To say that the family was like the State and vice versa implied a kind of connectedness between the two that we can no longer fully imagine. Executing the king implied a challenge to the domestic rule of fathers throughout the land.

Perhaps it stretches interpretation too far, but the obsession with headless babies in the 1640s and 1650s seems to echo these grander narratives of State and monarchy.[15] These women repeatedly refuse to be ruled, to accept the head of their household as their ruler. Instead, they provide examples of the anarchy that results from the absence of patriarchal order. That absence takes bodily form in the bodies of their babies born without heads, without rulers. Details of Mary Adams's story suggest how deeply the body figured as the State/household and vice versa. In her story, she rules herself, choosing to participate in a succession of deviant religious sects despite having spent her early years as a model of godliness. However, she is female, and her tongue betrays her. She utters her curse, and doom follows. Her suicide is described in especially gruesome terms: she repeatedly stabs herself in the abdomen. Her baby's headless state speaks to her own inability to be ruled, and she kills herself by attacking the part of her body that produced that witness. In a well-ordered family, the

[13] Philip Henry, *The Diaries and Letters of Philip Henry, MA, of Broad Oak, Flintshire, 1631–1696,* ed. Matthew Henry Lee (London: Kegan Paul, Trench & Co., 1882), 12.
[14] Susan Amussen, *An Ordered Society: Gender and Class in Early Modern England* (Oxford: Oxford University Press, 1988); Margaret Ezell, *The Patriarch's Wife: Literary Evidence and the History of the Family* (Chapel Hill, NC: University of North Carolina Press, 1987).
[15] On other metaphors of headlessness at this moment, see Burns, 'King's Two Monstrous Bodies', esp. 190–1.

husband functioned as the head and the wife as the womb, the source of the generation of the family.

Cheap print created another model of gender relations in its exploration of the body itself. The 1650s boom in books about pregnancy and childbirth afforded readers a range of ways of thinking about relationships between men and women. As we have seen, Nicholas Culpeper's 1651 text proposed that women were inherently inferior to men, implying that sexual subjugation was grounded in natural fact. Other books that followed, however, proposed other ways to imagine gender relations. Some texts, such as *The Childbearer's Cabinet* (1652), adopted the format of women's manuscript remedy books, which minimized men's roles in reproduction. Others, such as *The Compleat Midwifes Practice* (1656), restructured discussions of pregnancy and birth to assign new and important roles to fathers and fetuses, roles that by their very prominence diminished the prior centrality of women to reproductive processes.

The parliamentary challenge to customary structures of family life was twofold. First, Parliament reshaped the regulation of sexuality. In 1641 the system of ecclesiastical justice was abandoned. No longer would sexual sinners risk prosecution in church courts. Nine years later, Parliament tried to regulate sexual behaviour by passing the Adultery Act, which made adultery punishable by death. Second, Parliament sought to replace or reinvent the church's celebration of life-cycle events. As various radical sects challenged the meanings of ceremonies like baptism and marriage, the state tried to make itself rather than the church the source of authority in such moments. At every turn, Parliament's efforts to remake the institutions of family life were challenged both by radical religion, which sought greater changes, and by the subversive weapon of satire. In the longer term, Parliament's project to remake family life foundered upon people's attachment to the older ways of celebrating and marking crucial moments in a family's history. The effect of the parliamentary challenge to the structures of family life, however, was acute in the 1640s and early 1650s. Legislative efforts and their inverted representation in satire provoked a wealth of questions and challenges to family life and the gender roles at the heart of the family.

In May 1641 Parliament moved towards disbanding two much-hated courts: the Court of Star Chamber and the Court of High Commission. In July a bill abolishing both was sent to Charles I. Star Chamber was a much-feared royal prerogative court, where a wide range of offences against the state were tried. High Commission was the capstone of the national system of church courts. These ecclesiastical courts heard cases involving a range of moral offences, from fornication to Sabbath-breaking. As historians Martin Ingram and Laura Gowing have shown, these courts were places where fairly ordinary people could pursue what they believed to be justice and local communities could seek to regulate irregular sexual behaviour.[16] Gowing and Ingram both argue that these courts were not obscure features of an arcane ecclesiastical structure but rather were widely understood and utilized by a broad range of the population. These arguments are given added support by the responses to the abolition of church courts. Pamphlets that attacked the functions of these courts or mocked the results of their closures assumed that many readers were familiar with the personnel and function of the courts.

In May 1641, for example, the pamphlet *The Proctor and the Parator their Mourning* made fun of two church court officials. The proctor was an ecclesiastical lawyer who acted for individual clients while the apparitor (parator) was a travelling court official who served papers and delivered orders.[17] In the pamphlet, the two mourn the loss of their lucrative and corrupt employments. Hunter, the apparitor, recalls the days when he just had to look at chandlers, ale-houses, taverns, tobacco shops, butchers, comfit-makers, gunsmiths, bakers, brewers, cooks, and weavers to be offered bribes not to report them for Sabbath-breaking.[18] Such corruption seems to have been well known. In another satirical pamphlet published in the same month, Nick Froth the tapster and Rulerost the cook bemoan the Puritan crackdown on Sabbath-breaking but find minor comfort in the fact that they no longer have to bribe the apparitors.[19] Hunter the apparitor continues by describing other targets of ecclesiastical justice, such as 'Brownists, Anabaptists, and Familists, who love a Barne better then a Church', and Sponge the proctor tries to outdo him by recalling the country wenches who would sell their petticoats in order to pay fines rather than face public penance.[20] The woodcut on the title page shows a woman evidently brought into court by the apparitor (Fig. 6.3). As Sponge notes, 'wee feared no vacation as long as women could talke', meaning that lawyers benefited when women sued and were sued for defamation. Women's inability to control their speech quickly slid into another lack of control: 'wee got great imployment by womens tongues, too much talking and lying (I meane) on their backes.'[21]

The following month another satirical pamphlet on the demise of the church courts was published, this one entitled *The Spirituall Courts Epito-*

---

[16] Ingram, *Church Courts*; Gowing, *Domestic Dangers*. These courts have often been understood as a kind of expression of Protestant efforts to accomplish a reformation of manners. However, see also Marjorie Keniston Mcintosh, *Controlling Misbehavior in England, 1370–1600* (Cambridge: Cambridge University Press, 1998).

[17] On the function of church courts, see Ingram, *Church Courts*, esp. ch. 1.

[18] *The Proctor and Parator their Mourning: Or, the lamentation of the Doctors Commons for their downfall* ([London]: Printed in the year 1641), Thomason E.156[13], sig. A2ᵛ.

[19] *The Lamentable Complaints of Nick Froth the Tapster and Rulerost the Cooke* ([London]: Printed in the year 1641), Thomason E.156[4], 7.

[20] *Proctor and Parator*, sigs. A3ʳ, A3ᵛ.   [21] Ibid. sig. B1ʳ.

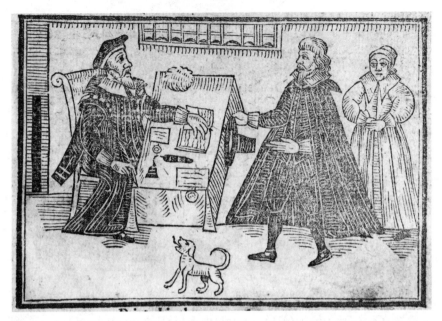

Fig. 6.3. Church courts as prosecutors of women. The man in black on the right is the apparitor, the court official who issued the summons to the woman behind him. *The Proctor and
Parator their Mourning* (1641). Courtesy of the Folger Shakespeare Library

mized. Two proctors, named Busie Body and Scrape-all, similarly lament the
end of a good income. As one says, 'I got very well by a wench that has been
undone in a darke entry. Sir John would commit her penance into ten pounds,
towards the repaire of Pauls [i.e. St Paul's Cathedral], and then we would share
it.'[22] The woman was happy to pay a large sum of money, ostensibly for a good
cause, in order to avoid the humiliation of doing public penance. Like the
earlier pamphlet, the woodcut on this title page shows a woman brought into
court (see Fig. 6.4). In this case, she is presumably accused of fornication or
some other sexual sin since she is depicted holding a baby.

A few months later, yet another pamphlet emphasized the corruption of the
courts. Two whores bemoan their loss of income now that ecclesiastical lawyers
are out of work. Like the tapster and the cook, however, the whores cheer up for
a moment when they recall how those lawyers used the mechanisms of ecclesiastical justice to mulct them. As Mrs Bloomsbury explains,

[22] *The Spirituall Courts Epitomized, in a dialogue beetwixt two Proctors* ([London]: Printed 1641),
Thomason E.157[15], 3.

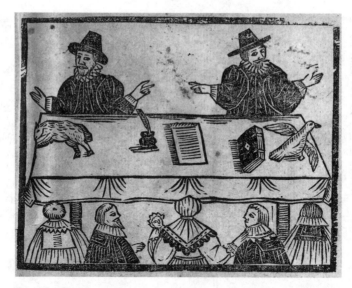

Fig. 6.4. Church courts regulating female sexuality. The woman with the
baby is presumed to be an unwed mother or an adulteress. *The Spiritual
Courts Epitomized* (1641). Courtesy of the Folger Shakespeare Library

The very next day they would send an Apparator, who would warne both me and my
whole harmlesse houshold to appeare in Pauls the next Court day, to answere for
keeping a common bawdy-house, ready furnished with mercenary whores, who daily
commit the carnall act of incontinency, and for many other misdemeanors.[23]

After paying the apparitor's fees and bribes, the madam is faced with larger
bribes to the proctors to avoid having to close her house. The way Mrs Bloomsbury ironically reuses legal phrases, such as 'the carnall act of incontinency',
makes the dialogue funny and also underlines the message of the pamphlet,
which is that the lawyers are the biggest sexual offenders.

   These pamphlets, full of greedy apparitors, irreverent whores, corrupt proctors, and lamenting tapsters, make it clear that ordinary readers found much to
laugh at in the process of ecclesiastical justice. Their laughter, or the pamphlets
designed to invoke it, suggests that Parliament's attempts change the mechanisms through which behaviour was policed were widely known. Indeed,
Hunter the apparitor claimed that apprentices everywhere were laughing at

---

[23] *The Sisters of the Scabards Holiday: or, A dialogue between two reverent and very vertuous Matrons*
([London]: Printed, 1641), Thomason E.168[8], 3. This is the pamphlet whose woodcut is reused to
illustrate the first pamphlet about women preachers, linking religious and sexual transgression yet
again.

'those ragges and reliques of Romes superstition' such as the courts. Hunter concluded by considering working for the hangman instead: 'better live by a Rope then by the Pope', he said cheerfully.[24]

These pamphlets all take the same approximate position regarding the courts. Each makes fun of the courts' corrupt officials and arcane procedures. In this sense, they might be considered almost as propaganda, advocates for the Parliament's decision to disband the spiritual courts. However, they are better understood in relation to the London mobs who forcefully demonstrated their dislike of many of the church's ecclesiastical functions. The attack on ecclesiastical courts was a part of the much larger agitation against bishops embodied in the Root and Branch petitions of 1640 and 1641 submitted not just by Londoners but by half the counties in England.[25] In October 1640 a mob attacked the Court of High Commission, which was meeting at St Pauls. The judges fled, some of them through windows, and the crowd ripped up papers and books, broke open desks, tore down benches, and proclaimed an end to bishops and ecclesiastical courts.[26] The title-page woodcut to *The Spirituall Courts Epitomized* (above, Fig. 6.4) reminds its readers of these events. On the courtroom table are a duck and a lamb, who are advised 'Runne Lambe' and 'Fly Duck'. Dr Arthur Ducke, the Bishop's Chancellor, was one of the officials who had fled the courtroom via the window. He had already been humiliated the month before when he was run out of two London parishes during visitations and had to be rescued by sheriffs from the mob. 'Lambe' was an even more threatening reference. Dr John Lambe, magician in the employ of the Duke of Buckingham (despised as the king's favourite), had been killed by a mob in 1628. In May 1640 a seditious rhyme circulated that threatened to kill William Laud, Archbishop of Canterbury, just as Lambe had been killed.[27] Rioters stormed Lambeth Palace on 11 May, although Laud had been forewarned and escaped via the river. Thus, although these satires on church courts make their cases with humour, the violence of London mobs to which the woodcut refers rendered ecclesiastical justice more than a laughing matter. Satire proved to be a powerful agent in cheap print, destabilizing the efforts of Parliamentarians and Royalists alike throughout the 1640s and 1650s.

Parliament disbanded the church courts, and sought to make the regulation of morals the business of the State rather than the church. Perhaps the

---

[24] *Proctor and Parator*, sigs. B3[r]; B4[v].

[25] As mentioned in Ch. 3, these petitions sought to abolish church hierarchies 'root and branch', doing away with bishops and other church officials. For the context of Root and Branch, see Fletcher, *The Outbreak of the English Civil War*, 91–124; Lindley, *Popular Politics*, 4–91.

[26] See Lindley, *Popular Politics*, 11, 37.

[27] Keith Lindley, 'Riot Prevention and Control in Early Stuart London', *Transactions of the Royal Historical Society*, 5th ser., 33 (1983), 109–26, esp. 114–15. It has been suggested to me that 'lambe' may also refer to Lambeth Palace, the home of the Archbishop of Canterbury.

best-known example of these attempts is the passage of the Adultery Act in 1650. Adultery, like other sexual transgressions, had formerly been the purview of church courts. Now adultery, fornication, incest, brothel-keeping, and other such sins became crimes. Adultery and incest became capital crimes, carrying death sentences. Although very few individuals were executed, the severity of the punishment reveals the intensity with which the Puritans sought to police gender relations and family life.[28] Just as in the case of the abolition of church courts, however, the draconian new law was not the only voice to be heard. Satirical accounts of the Act accompanied its passage, undercutting the gravity of punishment and drawing on a rich reservoir of sexual jokes.

By 1650, satire came in twice-weekly instalments in newsbooks. While some reported the news soberly, other Royalist ones invented an entire satirical language to lampoon the doings of Parliament.[29] An Act became a 'Knack' or a 'Crack'; Oliver Cromwell became 'His Noseship', 'the Nose', 'Nose-almighty', or 'Copper-Nose' (a reference not only to Cromwell's outstanding facial feature but also to his supposed family trade of brewing); the Mayor of London and Common Council became 'Mayor and Common Cuckolds', and so on.[30] The Adultery Act became just another point of reference, another focus for never-ending sexual jokes.

Historians have tended to focus on the adultery part of the Adultery Act, but the text of the act is more complex. It opens with a long section on incest, specifying that marriage or carnal knowledge between a person and his/her grandparents, parents, siblings, children, aunts, uncles, parents-in-law, sib-lings-in-law, or children-in-law is deemed incest. It is a felony punishable by death without benefit of clergy.[31] Only after detailing incest does the act describe adultery, also punishable by death.

Incest was already the subject of prohibition in England. Ever since 1563, each parish church was supposed to display a table of kindred and affinity, that is, a list of the degrees of relatedness within which it was forbidden to marry. When bishops conducted visitations, detailed interrogations of the function-ing of individual parishes, they often enquired about marriages performed within the prohibited degree. As historian David Cressy has remarked,

---

[28] My discussion builds on Keith Thomas's germinal article on this subject, 'The Puritans and the Adultery Act'.

[29] On these newsbooks and their use of inversion, see Underdown, *Freeborn People*, 90–111.

[30] On the range of images of Cromwell, see Laura Lungers Knoppers, *Constructing Cromwell: Ceremony, Portrait, and Print, 1645–1661* (Cambridge: Cambridge University Press, 2000).

[31] For the text of the Act, see *Acts and Ordinances of the Interregnum*, ed. C. H. Firth and R. S. Rait (London: H.M. Stationers Office, 1911), ii. 387–9. On some of the contemporary meanings of incest, see Susan Wiseman, ' 'Tis a Pity She's a Whore: Representing the Incestuous Body', in Lucy Gent and Nigel Llewellyn (eds.), *Renaissance Bodies: The Human Figure in English Culture, c.1540–1660* (London: Reaktion Books, 1990), 180–97.

'Reading the records of episcopal administration one might think that the table of degrees of kindred and affinity was almost as important to some bishops as the table of the ten commandments.'[32] While this attention to the potential sin of incest might seem excessive to us, we might think about the complex families of our own time, created by divorce, remarriage, adoption, surrogacy etc., and recall that many marriages in early modern England were remarriages consequent upon the early death of a partner. There were thus many complicated families in seventeenth-century England, made up of stepchildren, remarrying parents, and the like. Perhaps a clear table of the prohibited degrees was not superfluous. When the Parliament took upon itself the task of defining and punishing incest, it was making a bid to take this aspect of the church's jurisdiction for itself. Since the table of degrees was supposed to be posted in every parish church, Parliament's decision to take on the responsibility of defining incest was not an obscure measure.[33]

As Keith Thomas has discussed, the Adultery Act had a long prehistory in Puritan attempts to create legislation that would promote the reformation of manners and make England a godly nation. Indeed, as recently as 1626 and 1628 Parliament had considered acts against adultery and other sexual failings, and the Long Parliament began discussing an act against whoredom in 1641.[34] Thomas highlights the curious gender inequality of the Act. Adultery is defined as sexual intercourse between a married woman and a man not her husband. While both parties are subject to the death penalty, nowhere does the Act consider that a married man might be guilty of adultery if he had sex with a woman not his wife. Instead, men are used as the defining example of fornication. If any man shall 'have the carnal knowledge of any Virgin, unmarried Woman or Widow', he and the woman could be tried for fornication.[35] The punishment for fornication was three months in jail, and the offenders had to post a bond for their good behaviour for a year thereafter.

On first glance, the severity of the penalty for adultery overshadows the entire Act. However, the Act is not solely about Puritan imposition of stricter controls on expressions of sexuality. Rather, it is part of a larger project to remove authority over family life from the church and grant it to the State. The Act states that the death penalty 'shall not extend to any woman whose

[32] Cressy, *Birth, Marriage and Death*, 313.
[33] Indeed, so well known were the prohibited degrees that the Westminster Assembly's revision of the Book of Common Prayer did not even list them; it merely alluded to 'the degrees of Consanguinity or Affinity prohibited by the Word of God', implying that these were sufficiently well known as not to require specification. *A Directory for the Publique Worship of God, Throughout the Three Kingdoms of England, Scotland, and Ireland* (London: Printed for Evan Tyler, Alexander Fifield, Ralph Smith, and John Field; and are to be sold at the Signe of the Bible in Cornhill, neer the Royal-Exchange, 1644), Thomason E.273[17], 58.
[34] Thomas, 'The Puritans and the Adultery Act', 273–6.   [35] *Acts and Ordinances*, 388.

Husband shall be continually remaining beyond the Seas by the space of three years, or shall by common fame be reputed to be dead'.[36] Men who did not know that a sexual partner was married were also not guilty of adultery. The satirical Royalist newsbook *Mercurius Pragmaticus* immediately interpreted these features for its readers:

three yeers absence of a husband from his wife beyond Seas or elsewhere, she not knowing him to be living (at less if she know it she may say no) may marrie, and sure after she is married, he may take the same libertie; a fine cleanly way of Divorce of such who love not their wives, or such wives who will blaze abroad their Husbands deaths, because they love them not.[37]

All a woman has to do is plead ignorance—and she can be free of an absent husband. Although the Act said nothing about marriage in this case, merely about sexual relations, the writers of newsbooks connected the agitation of the 1640s about divorce to this clause of the Act. In the larger sense, this satire is correct. Both the discussion of divorce and the provisions of the Adultery Act reflect Puritans' attempts to remake marriage into a concern of the State rather than the church. As we shall see, Parliament redefined marriage twice, once in 1646, next in 1653.

The same newsbook points to the central weakness of the Act. Proof of adultery was very hard to obtain, and no one was specifically empowered to initiate prosecution. As the newsbook had it, 'But for their Knack against Incest, Adultrie; &c. No doubt it will make it selfe void, for Ile warrant there will bee but few prosecutors unlesse some reward were set down for the discoverers thereof, and then there would be knaves enow . . .'[38] The Act protected the rights of the accused: they could call witnesses to defend themselves, spouses could not testify against each other, and even one participant in adultery could not provide evidence against the other participant. The only ways in which adultery could be proven was through an individual's own confession or by eyewitnesses. As a critic of the Act pointed out, people were very unlikely to confess, 'to the taking away of their own Lives'.[39]

---

[36] *Acts and Ordinances*, 388. Previously, church courts could decide after seven years of absence that a women's husband was dead and grant her the right to remarry, another instance of the ways in which the Adultery Act sought to make functions that had belonged to the church part of the State.

[37] *Mercurius Pragmaticus*, 14 to 21 May 1650, Thomason E.601[10], sig. Hhh3ʳ.

[38] Ibid. sig. Hhh3ʳ. Most newsbooks quickly incorporated the Act into their ongoing characterizations of some members of Parliament as libertines. See e.g. *Mercurius Pragmaticus*, 30 Apr. to 7 May 1650, Thomason E.600[6], sig. Fffʳ⁻ᵛ; *Mercurius Elencticus*, 6 to 13 May 1650, Thomason E.600[12]; *The Man in the Moon*, 29 May to 5 June 1650, Thomason E.602[24], 427. The density of these references, and the ease with which they were incorporated into the newsbooks' long-standing themes, suggest that the Act was well known to many.

[39] D. T., *Certain Queries, or Considerations Presented to the View of All That Desire Reformation of Grievances* (London: printed for Giles Calvert, and are to be sold at the Sign of the Black spread-eagle

The necessity of an eyewitness provided more grist for the mill of satire. Less than two months after the Act was passed, a pamphlet dialogue between two whores and their usher bemoaned its effect on their trade. The Act specified that anyone keeping a bawdy house or being a common bawd would be whipped, set in the pillory, and branded with the letter B. The Act implied, albeit somewhat vaguely, that second offenders could be punished by death. The whores quickly contrast these punishments with those of the church courts, or penances. One asks the usher 'what pennance is allotted us in the late Act'? The usher Pimpinello sarcastically replies 'Pennance, say you, a small slight punishment, I wot, hanging, burning, carting, whipping, or so, matters of small moment, triviall things these.'[40] But the quick-thinking bawd Mistris Macquerella saves the day. She notes that the Act requires eyewitnesses and concludes that the whores can double their doors so that no one can be a witness, and triple their prices. The usher is so taken with her scheme that he says 'O rare Projectresse, let me kisse the sole of thy shooe'.[41]

Thus the Adultery Act, while appearing to uphold family life by punishing extra-marital sex, is better understood as redefining the source of authority over family life. While its draconian imposition of the death penalty and its highly gendered definition of adultery were particularly harsh for women, it also opened a curious window for women whose husbands had abandoned them, permitting them to remarry after three years. Its rigorous legal standards in the requirement for eyewitnesses or self-indictment also mitigated the Act's severity. Scholars have shown that very few people seem to have been prosecuted under the Act. Like the church courts it sought to replace, however, the Act's significance lay not in the few offenders it punished. Rather, it must be understood as a kind of public proclamation of the State's authority over marriage and family. While the church courts provided a kind of theatre of penance, demonstrating to all the boundaries of appropriate behaviour, the Adultery Act reduced the sacramental qualities of marriage by permitting remarriage under ambiguous circumstances that had the potential to function as a form of divorce. Similarly, the Act enabled the State to assume a particular authority over family life—that of defining incest and the boundaries of acceptable family formation.

The Adultery Act is just one example of the ways in which the structures and institutions of family life were questioned and restructured in the 1640s and 1650s. Parliament engineered the rewriting of the Book of Common Prayer,

at the West end of Pauls, 1651), Thomason E.647[10], 10. The author of this text is not known, but Calvert issued works by almost every seeker, Leveller, Ranter, and other kind of free-thinker.

[40] *A Dialogue between Mistris Maquerella, a Suburban Bawd, Ms Scolopendra, a noted Curtezan, and mr Pimpinello and Usher &c.* (London: Printed for Edward Couch, 1650), Thomason E.607[13], 3.
    [41] Ibid. 5–6.

including ceremonies of family life such as baptism and marriage, by setting up the Westminster Assembly, whose new prayer book, the *Directory of Publique Worship*, was first published in 1644.[42] The *Directory* was not a great success. Many parishes continued to use their copies of the older prayer book while individuals evaded its grasp by choosing their minister carefully or getting married or baptized in private.[43] Nonetheless, the *Directory* represents an important attempt by the State to reorganize crucial ceremonial moments in individual families' lives.

Some of the ways in which the *Directory* sought to reformulate family life were anticipated in radical religious circles and in the satires about them. One of the first wave of pamphlets in 1641 about the seeming explosion in religious diversity focused on the rituals of family formation. It alleges that a group of Brownists, Separatists, and Non-Conformists in the Welsh county of Monmouthshire instituted very different rituals for christenings, marriages, and burials. Baptism was performed by cutting the baby in the ear until it bled and declaring the child's name. As the pamphlet emphasizes, 'they use neither the sprinkling of water, signe of the crosse, Godfathers nor Godmothers, nor any of the prayers in the Common prayer booke appointed to be used for that purpose'.[44] Whether or not there really were Brownists in Monmouthshire, this was an account designed to shock the reader. The account of baptism carefully lists the most important features of orthodoxy in baptism that this group denied: the water, the sign of the cross (so contested in the headless baby pamphlets that were to follow), the provision of godparents, and the use of prayers.

Four years later, Parliament's prayer book did away with the sign of the cross and with godparents. So too, the doom-laden questions formerly addressed to the godparents were gone. No longer did they have to assent to a list of the central tenets of the faith, including that God would come again at the end of the world to judge the living and the dead. Instead, the *Directory* emphasized that the ceremony of baptism was but a representation of true baptism. The minister was to ask God to join the outward baptism with water to an inner baptism of the spirit.[45] Indeed, 'the inward Grace and virtue of Baptisme is not tyed to that very moment of time wherein it is administred'.[46] Some of the

---

[42] On conflicts in London over the use of the Book of Common Prayer, and its replacement by the *Directory of Publique Worship*, see Lindley, *Popular Politics*, 260–5.

[43] See discussions in Durston, *Family in the English Revolution*, 71–5, 119–20; Cressy, *Birth, Marriage and Death*, 175–80.

[44] Edward Harris, *A True Relation of Brownists, Separatists, and Non-Conformists in Monmouthshire in Wales* ([London]: Printed in the yeare 1641), Thomason E.172[31], sig. A2ᵛ. 'Brownist' refers to followers of the 16th-c. minister Robert Brown, some of whom emigrated to the Netherlands to avoid religious persecution. By the 1640s, the term is often synonymous with 'separatist'.

[45] *Directory of Publique Worship*, 44.

[46] Ibid. 42. On the larger context of baptism, see Cressy, *Birth, Marriage and Death*, chs. 5–8.

magical and sacramental elements were purged from this ceremony, such as the sign of the cross and the sense in which the ritual accomplishes its purpose. After all, in the Presbyterian world-view, baptism was not sufficient; only the elect would be saved, and so baptisma had somewhat more limited role to play in an individual's salvation.

The *Directory of Publique Worship* was only one challenge to the ritual of baptism. Far more consequential was the evolution of the sects known as Baptists. They originated in the separatist congregations that fled to the Netherlands to avoid persecution from the 1580s onwards. Between 1640 and 1642 both Particular and General Baptists adopted the dramatic ritual of adult baptism by total immersion. Although very different theological impulses underlay these two sects' adoption of the new ceremony, its dramatic potential quickly attracted the makers of cheap print, and both kinds of Baptists became known as 'Dippers'.[47] The London bookseller George Thomason collected at least 125 works about baptism in the period 1641–60, evidence of the intensity of debate. Like other radical religious groups, Baptists were often characterized as sexual rebels. For Mary Adams, whose story opens this chapter, joining the Baptists was the beginning of the long slide into heresy. After participating in Baptist groups, she was led to the Family of Love and then to the Ranters, becoming more radical in doctrine and in sexual licence with every move.

Like baptism, the ceremony of marriage was profoundly questioned during the 1640s and 1650s. The practices of various radical religious groups, legislative actions of the State, and cheap-print satirical accounts all destabilized the meanings of matrimony. The first accounts that challenge marriage are satirical accounts of new religious groups published in 1641. For example, in the pamphlet about the supposed Brownists in Monthmouthshire, the reader was presented with their new service of matrimony. According to the pamphlet, the person who served as minister asked the groom if he would have the bride to be his wedded wife, and usually asked the equivalent question of her. Then the minister would usually say 'goe forth and multiply' and the wedding was over, without 'the plighting of the troth, ring, praiers, or ceremonies whatsoever'.[48]

---

[47] J. F. McGregor, 'The Baptists: Fount of All Heresy', in J. F. McGregor and Barry Reay (eds.), *Radical Religion in the English Revolution* (Oxford: Oxford University Press, 1984), 23–63. General Baptists denied the Calvinist doctrine of election, stressing that anyone could attain salvation. Their adoption of adult baptism stemmed from a rejection of the ceremonies of the Church of England. Particular Baptists retained Calvinist election, and chose adult baptism because, like many other independent churches, church membership was restricted to those who made testimony to their conversion experience. Membership could not, therefore, be granted to an infant via godparents. Despite the profundity of doctrinal difference, the two groups were lumped together in sensationalizing cheap print.

[48] *True Relation*, sig. A2ᵛ.

Here the importance of aspects of the Anglican ceremony, such as the giving and receiving of the ring and the plighting of troths, were underlined by their absence.[49] Instead, the minister blasphemously referred to the sexual aspects of marriage ('go forth and multiply') and the ceremony was over.

In cheap print, there was a plethora of such challenges to marriage, particularly in sensational accounts of religious difference. Baptists might be characterized as disapproving of marriage altogether. In the *Anabaptists Catechisme*, the Baptist says that he can marry a fellow-believer 'without the abominable ceremony of Marriage', but later in the text, the Baptist ceremony is described. Unlike in Anglican weddings, the bride is not given away, rings are not exchanged, and a minister does not officiate. Instead, both parties join hands in front of the congregation, promise to live and die together, and kiss each other—and they are wed.[50]

In 1644 the *Directory of Publique Worship* also did away with rings, giving the bride away, and other features of the usual Anglican ceremony. The *Directory* was uncompromising about the status of the marriage service, noting that 'Marriage be no sacrament' but rather 'of Publique interest in every Commonwealth'. Because people getting married needed 'Instruction, Direction, and Exhortation', the *Directory* judged it 'expedient' for marriages to be performed by a minister.[51] Nine years later, the State no longer found it 'expedient'. In 1653 Parliament passed an act making marriage a civil ceremony, removing it from the context of religious worship entirely. Localities elected 'registers', individuals whose job it was to publicize upcoming marriages and to record them. The actual marriage ceremony was overseen by a Justice of the Peace, but couples in effect married each other by exchanging vows themselves.[52] Newsbooks printed the new form of the marriage service, which was not unlike that in the satirical account of the Anabaptists, as well as the text of the Act.[53]

The satirical newsbooks revelled in the consequences of Parliament's attempt to remake marriage. The Act was passed on 24 August, but did not take effect until 29 September, permitting a month-long window of opportunity for those who wished to be married in church. *Mercurius Democritus*

[49] Cressy, *Birth, Marriage and Death*, chs. 10–12.

[50] *The Anabaptists Catechisme* ([London]: Printed for R.A., 1645), Thomason E.1185[8], 2, 12. See also *The Cony-catching Bride* (Printed at London by T. F., 1643), not in Thomason, in which a bride outwits her father by fleeing after one of these newfangled marriage ceremonies (which lacked the legal formulae that would have made the ceremony binding) and marries her true love.

[51] *Directory of Publique Worship*, 58.

[52] On the background and functioning of the Act, see Durston, *Family in the English Revolution*, 69–84. Durston makes it clear that Parliament was wrestling with problems about marriage repeatedly from 1641 all the way until the Restoration.

[53] For the complete text of the Act, see *Several Proceedings of Parliament*, 23 to 30 Aug. 1653, Thomason E.711[18]; for just the text of the service, see *The Moderare* [sic] *Intelligencer*, 22 to 9 Aug. 1653, Thomason E.711[17], 180–1.

claimed that 500 young women, seamstresses, knitters, lacemakers, cookmaids and the like advertised for speedy husbands, 'because their tender Consciences will not permit them to be married after the New way'.[54] While this particular story sounds improbable, historical demographers have noted that the number of marriages performed in September 1653 is the highest monthly total in all of the 1650s, and that many fewer weddings were performed in October of that year than would be expected.[55] While newsbook accounts owe much to sensational fiction, the demographics suggest that many people in England were well aware of the provisions of the Act, and some hastened their own weddings in order to avoid complying with it. Those not immediately affected by the Act encountered its provisions in the pages of newsbooks or in their own parishes when they were asked to elect an official to register marriages.

Like baptisms and the public penances inflicted on sexual sinners by church courts, weddings were public demonstrations of the forms of family life. Weddings were supposed to be public events, in part in order to assure that the couple were actually eligible to be wed. The *Directory of Publique Worship* maintained the Anglican tradition of asking about 'just impediments' to the marriage, although the minister asked only the couple, not the assembled witnesses. When Parliament instituted the civil ceremony of marriage, it further removed weddings from the supervision of local communities. Instead of a wedding in church, with opportunity for community members to dispute the legitimacy of the proceedings, the civil ceremony merely empowered the Justice of the Peace to call witnesses if he had doubts about the match. No longer was marriage, like baptism, a public ceremony marking its participants' transition from one status to another. Parliament's reworking of marriage and baptism, and its abolition of the church courts, challenged these public representations of the boundaries and forms of family life. As the many satirical comments on these changes suggest, Parliament's efforts to remake the family were not welcomed by all.

The outpouring of satirical responses to Parliament's changes created a broad spectrum of ideas about the family in cheap print. While parliamentary Puritans struggled to remake the family to their own design, the free-wheeling popular press provided readers with a wealth of other ideas. Satirical responses to Parliament's acts were one way in which cheap print broadened any discussion of the meanings of the family. Another, as suggested already, was the

---

[54] *Mercurius Democritus*, 14 to 21 Sept. 1653, Thomason E.713[10], 578. See also *Mercurius Democritus*, 24 to 31 Aug. 1653, Thomason E.711[20], 559, where prostitutes lament the Act.

[55] E. A. Wrigley and Roger Schofield, *Population History of England and Wales 1541–1871: A Reconstruction* (Cambridge: Cambridge University Press, 1981), 521. See Durston's discussion of this point, Durston, *Family in the English Revolution*, 80–1. Durston puts more weight on newsbook accounts than I do.

profusion of pamphlets about radical religious groups. These sets of pamphlets echo each other, with the Adamites and the Family of Love and the Baptists all pronouncing similarly unorthodox ideas about the relationships between sex and marriage. In the early 1650s, pamphlets about these groups were super-seded by those about the Ranters, who were accused of much the same scandalous behaviours as the Adamites and other earlier groups. In all cases, these groups were represented as providing a radically different version of family life from that known by most English men and women and underwritten by the church.

In 1641 pamphlets about the Family of Love and about the Adamites chal-lenged customary sexual norms.[56] As Patricia Crawford has noted, the associa-tion between religious diversity and sexual licence was already a commonplace when it was invoked in pamphlets of the 1640s.[57] In September 1641 a pam-phlet claimed to describe a sect called the Adamites, who attended services naked, like Adam before the Fall. The title-page woodcut depicts the group's meeting, as does another pamphlet published the following month.[58] The Adamites are given a lengthy pedigree in the pamphlet, with citations from various learned works on heresies, but the keynotes are always their nakedness and their sexual freedom. Both pamphlets portray the world of the Adamites as a kind of inversion of sexual norms of mid-seventeenth-century England. The Adamites despised marriage and men were allowed to couple with any women they fancied. In one example, a leader of the sect performs a kind of blasphe-mous parody of the marriage ceremony,

as first he [the group's leader, Mr Pickard] allowed promiscuous copulation any man with any woman, whom he best liked, yet it must be done by his assent; if any had any motions to lust, hee might take any woman, by the hand and come to Mr Pickard and say, I desire this woman then Pickards word was, goe, increase, and multiply . . .[59]

Both pamphlets focus on male desire, describing how men in the sect could have intercourse with any women they chose, but totally ignoring female

[56] For the Family of Love, see *A Description of the Sect called Family of Love With their common place of residence* (London: printed 1641), Thomason E.168[2]. Historical scholarship on the Family of Love has focused on the 16th-c. appearance of the sect in England. Alasdair Hamilton, *The Family of Love* (Cambridge: J. Clarke, 1981), but see the later chapters of Christopher W. Marsh, *The Family of Love in English Society, 1550–1630* (Cambridge: Cambridge University Press, 1994), for a fascinating discussion of early 17th-c. stereotypes about the Family of Love.

[57] Crawford, *Women and Religion*, 120–4; 129–30.

[58] *A Nest of Serpents Discovered. Or, a knot of old Heretiques revived, called the Adamites* ([London]: Printed in the yeare 1641), Thomason E.168[12]; Samoth Yarb [Thomas Bray], *A new Sect of Religion Descryed, called Adamites* ([London]: Printed anno. 1641), not in Thomason. See also Obadiah Couchman, *The Adamites Sermon: Containing Their Manner of Preaching, Expounding, and Prophesy-ing* ([London]: Printed for Francis Coules, in the Yeare, 1641), not in Thomason. See also Cressy, *Travesties and Transgressions*, ch. 15.

[59] *Nest of Serpents*, 4.

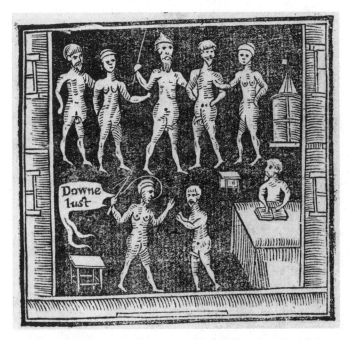

Fig. 6.5. Adamites imagined as sexual hypocrites. *A Nest of Serpents Discovered* (1641). Courtesy of the British Library, shelf mark E.168[12]

desire. Although the 1641 pamphlet did not mention the detail in its text, its woodcut and that of the second pamphlet refer to a prurient detail that again emphasizes male desire (see Fig. 6.5). If a man's penis became erect during one of the sect's services, the clerk was to subdue him or it with a long staff. The illustrations portray this moment in part because it highlights the group's hypocrisy. On the one hand, men were supposed to ignore the sexually stimulating sight of naked women during the services, but they were also free to have sex with any woman they desired. This peculiar dichotomy echoes the many satirical representations of Puritans who proclaim their high-mindedness but are guilty of sins of the flesh.[60] These pamphlets thus provide a sensational account of a supposed new sect, but their presentation relies on a combination of inversion (nakedness; sexual licence) and familiar tropes (religious diversity equals sexual deviance; proclamations of purity often imply their opposite).

---

[60] See Patrick Collinson, 'The Theatre Constructs Puritanism', in David L. Smith, Richard Strier, and David Bevington (eds.), *The Theatrical City: Culture, Theatre and Politics in London, 1576–1649* (Cambridge: Cambridge University Press, 1995), 157–69. Many thanks to Lori Anne Ferrell for this reference.

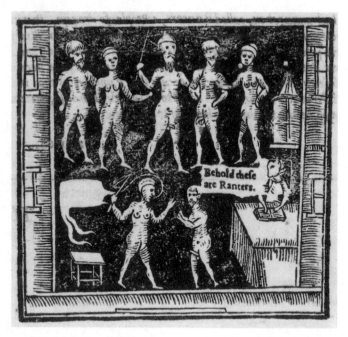

Fig. 6.6. An image of the Ranters that reveals their ancestry in fantasies about Adamites. *The Ranters Religion* (1650). Courtesy of the British Library, shelf mark E.619[8]

Many of the themes of the stories about the Adamites reappear in pamphlets about the Ranters that erupted in late 1650 and early 1651. Parliament had taken action against specific men identified as Ranters and the texts written by them months before the appearance of these pamphlets. Jacob Bauthumley, Abiezer Coppe, and Laurence Clarkson were investigated and punished for blasphemy and heresy in the spring and summer of 1650, but the sensationalist accounts of a supposed Ranter movement begin with the publication of *The Ranters Religion* in October of that same year.[61] At least six more pamphlets followed before Christmas, offering readers a heady mix of sexual licence and religious antinomianism.

The title-page woodcut of *The Ranters Religion* suggests the ways in which the Ranters were like Adamites, only more so (see Fig. 6.6).[62] It is a slightly altered version of the same woodcut used nine years earlier to illustrate *A Nest*

---

[61] *The Ranters Religion. Or, A Faithfull and Infallible Narrative of Their Damnable and Diabolical Opinions* (London: printed for R.H., 1650), Thomason E.619[8].

[62] See also Cressy, *Travesties and Transgressions*, ch. 10.

of Serpents . . . Called the Adamites (see Fig. 6.5). *The Ranters Religion* echoes earlier pamphlets by emphasizing that the Ranters think that all women should be held in common, and describing feasts at which men coupled with any woman they chose, first uttering the blasphemous phrase 'increase and multiply'. At times, the Ranter pamphlet is more explicit about its own inversion of norms than was earlier cheap print. For instance, God supposedly holds the key to liberty, 'whereby he Authorizes us to fulfill our owne Lusts, and sensuall appetites, opening the doores of liberty and licentiousnesse, which were fast locked to the men of former ages . . .'[63] The whole pamphlet is a catalogue of inversions and transgressions. Ranters swore and blasphemed; they 'canonized' the woman among them who had sex with the most men; they debated whether the Virgin Mary was free of original sin or was of illegitimate birth; they conducted parodies of the Eucharist with pieces of boiled beef, and so on.[64]

Subsequent Ranter pamphlets add further details to the same kinds of stories. Ranters danced naked at their services, a feature often included in the woodcut title pages (Fig. 6.7). In this illustration, the Ranters added insult to injury by celebrating Christmas, like other holidays abolished by Parliament since 1644.[65] Ranters were alleged to worship the former Archbishop of Canterbury, the despised William Laud.[66] Many of these Ranter pamphlets include texts as evidence of their truthfulness. Several include blasphemous songs, while another claims to reproduce the text of a verse found in the pocket of an imprisoned Ranter, and another a letter dropped by a Ranter hurrying to escape the constable.[67] It is almost as if the extravagance of the inversions and transgressions attributed to the Ranters needed to be balanced by some form of seemingly truthful witness provided by texts.

Stories about Adamites, Ranters, Familists, and others played on long-familiar links between religious and sexual deviance. What was new in the 1640s and 1650s was the density and intensity of reference—the flood of cheap print providing sensationalizing accounts of these groups in cheap eight-page formats illustrated with scandalous woodcuts. The proliferation of these texts, combined with the profusion of satirical accounts of Parliament's attempts to reformulate family life, created a kind of theatre of opposites. For every moralizing tract, every Parliamentary act against blasphemy or adultery, there was a colourful account of an imagined world in which these kinds of godly rules

---

[63] *Ranters Religion*, 5–6.   [64] Ibid. 6, 8.

[65] *The Routing of the Ranters* (n.p., n.d.), Thomason E.616[9], 2. This is the second Ranter pamphlet, dated 19 Nov. by Thomason.

[66] *The Ranters Declaration* (Imprinted at London, by J.C. MDCL), Thomason E.620[2], 4. This is the sixth Ranter pamphlet, dated by Thomason as 17 Dec.

[67] Texts of songs are included in *The Ranters Ranting* (London: Printed by B. Alsop, 1650), Thomason E.618[8], the third Ranter pamphlet, dated by Thomason as 2 Dec.; *Ranters Declaration*; the verses are in *Ranters Religion*; the letter is in *Routing of the Ranters*.

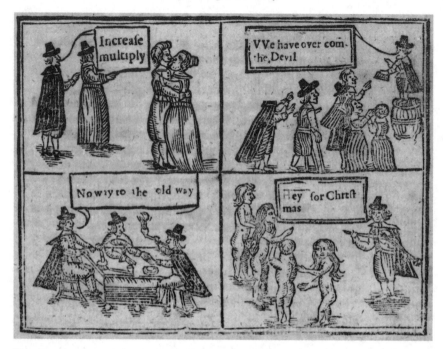

Fig. 6.7. Ranters misbehaving, including celebrating Christmas, a forbidden holiday. *The Ranters Declaration* (1650). Courtesy of the British Library, shelf mark E.620[2]

were turned upside down. Royalist newsbooks suggested that even members of Parliament, who had taken upon themselves the task of reforming the nation's morals, were rakes and libertines. Stories of Adamites and Ranters offered readers a world in which sexual licence was the rule and the family almost non-existent.

It is as if the spectrum of possibilities for imagining family relationships was suddenly expanded way beyond anything that had come before. At the same moment, the instantiation of satire as a routine way of interpreting current events meant that even familiar parts of the spectrum were now haunted by their opposites—for every Puritan, there was a Baptist or a Ranter or a libertine MP. For every reworking of a godly marriage ceremony, there was the spectre of an Adamite preacher leering 'increase and multiply'. For the Adultery Act, there were imaginary whores celebrating its unintended beneficial effect on their trade.

As the customary ways in which ordinary people celebrated and enacted representations of family life were attacked both by Parliament and by the spectacles afforded by radical religion, writers of popular medical books began to offer another way to imagine family relationships. Rather than ground the institution of the family in social structures, these books reinterpreted the female body in ways that made family life seem to arise naturally from the body itself. In the very act of making new members of a family—in pregnancy itself—lay the blueprint for the institution of the family. Pregnancy was reimagined in ways that brought the fetus and the father to new prominence. However, as with everything else in these troubled decades, naturalizing the family was contested. Some small books continued to offer their readers a different vision of pregnancy that emphasized the mother's body and ignored the father and the fetus.

In 1656 a group of London doctors published a book called *The Compleat Midwifes Practice*. The four authors, who are identified only by their initials, describe themselves as 'practitioners' on the title page and claim that they were motivated to write because the books on pregnancy and delivery available in English were 'strangely defficient, so crowded with unnecessary notions, and dangerous mistakes'.[68] All the available popular books devoted to midwifery come in for criticism. Thomas Raynalde's *The Birth of Mankind*, the first such work in English, is described as 'the most antient, but much unfurnished', as is Jacques Guillemeau's *Child-birth* and Jacob Rueff's *The Expert Midwife*. The authors are especially scornful of the main competitor for their book, Nicholas Culpeper's *Directory for Midwives*. It is 'the most desperately defficient of them all, except writ it for necessity he could certainly have never been so sinfull to have exposed it to the light'.[69] The authors actually rely on one of the books they criticize: substantial portions of their book come from Rueff's *Expert Midwife*. Other portions of the book are translations of works by the French midwife Louise Bourgeois; her portrait serves as the frontispiece to this and almost every subsequent edition of the *Compleat Midwifes Practice* (Fig. 6.8).

Like Culpeper's text, the *Midwifes Practice* emphasizes the anatomy of reproduction. The book opens with a discussion of male anatomy and then moves to the female. Like Culpeper, the book suggests that female midwives may be deficient because they do not understand anatomy: 'And it may be lawfully feared

[68] [T.C., I.D., M.S., T.B.], *Compleat Midwifes Practice* (1656), sig. A2ʳ. I have not been able to identify these practitioners, although T.C. is often considered to be Thomas Chamberlayne. The book claims to be 'published with the approbation and good liking of sundry of the most knowing Professors of Midwifery now living in the City of London, and other places'. Evenden claims that the authors were midwives; see *Midwives of 17th-c. London*, 8–9.
[69] *Compleat Midwifes Practice* (1656), sig. A2ᵛ. The authors see Culpeper as otherwise worthy of respect; it is only his midwifery volume that comes in for scorn. Culpeper's midwifery volume had already gone into three editions since its first appearance five years earlier and a fourth was published in 1656. Nathaniel Brooke was well known to Culpeper; when his grandfather left him a paltry 30s. in his will, the will directed Culpeper to collect his inheritance at Brooke's shop. Brooke published many of Culpeper's purely astrological works, such as his ephemerides.

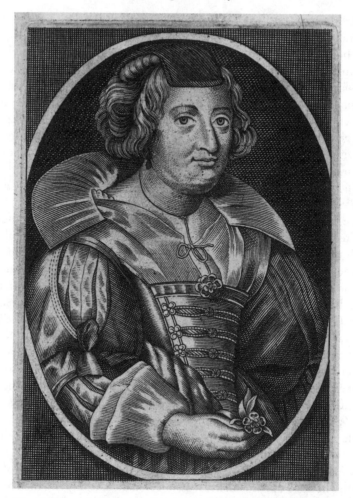

Fig. 6.8. Louise Bourgeois, the French midwife. Frontispiece to *The Compleat Midwife's Practice* (1680). Courtesy of the Folger Shakespeare Library

that many women do miss their design because they know nothing but the outside of things; so that in matters of extremity, because they are ignorant of the structure of the parts, they cannot tell how to go about their work.'[70] While it may be true that midwives were not educated anatomically, it is difficult to see how 'matters of extremity' in childbirth could be remedied by a detailed knowledge of *male* anatomy, a discussion of which follows this passage.

[70] *Compleat Midwifes Practice* (1656), 1.

Although this emphasis on anatomy makes the *Midwifes Practice* appear to be similar to Culpeper's *Directory for Midwives*, the works differ substantially in their account of reproduction and in the social meanings attributed to bodily facts. The *Midwifes Practice* emphasizes the roles of sexual desire in reproduction and foregrounds the roles of fathers and of fetuses in pregnancy. In so doing, the authors of this work make the female body a microcosm of social relations, a kind of fleshly theatre of appropriate gender roles and relations.

As the book explicates anatomy, it constantly refers to the sexual act itself. This emphasis is easy to understand in terms of male anatomy—when else would male anatomy figure in the story of pregnancy? However, women's bodies are remade too, so that the sexual act, rather than fetal development or childbirth, becomes the central drama of reproduction. The structure of male bodies is constantly explained with reference to sex. The ways in which the male determines the sex of the baby are related to sexual pleasure: the left emulgent vein from which 'female' seed is drawn is also the source of a humour that might 'stir up venery by its salt and acrimonious substance', and therefore men whose left testicles are larger than their right ones are 'most prone to venery'. The stones, or testicles as we would call them, are outside the male body in order to keep men chaste, as those creatures 'which carry their stones within their bodies are more salacious'.[71]

Again and again, male anatomy is described in sexual terms that make social precept into biological fact. For example, the substance of the human penis is not like that of the dog or wolf, always hard or erect, since that would 'hinder men from all businesse but the act of venerie'.[72] The structure of the 'yard', or penis, is discussed at great length, and always in terms of the sexual act. Thus the yard has no fat in it lest the fat melt during the heat of sex; the muscles of the yard are designed to erect it and bend the forepart of it for insertion into the womb; the nerves of the yard are the source of 'pleasure and delight' that causes erection; the situation of the yard in between the thighs is to strengthen it for copulation, and so on. The correct size of the yard is discussed in two different sections, the answer being 'the bredth of nine thumbs'.[73] In this text, the yard is such a complex and intricate structure that it takes nine whole pages to describe it while the womb, usually the focus of midwifery books, is disposed of in six pages. The emphasis on male sexual anatomy and on the wonders of the production of male seed serve to valorize men's roles in reproduction.

Women's bodies are also described in terms of sexual pleasure, but that pleasure is as much male as female. In particular, the neck of the womb is reconfigured as a 'sheath' that embraces the yard during sex. The Latin word 'vagina', which means 'sheath', was not yet in vernacular use at this time. Instead, the

---

[71] *Compleat Midwifes Practice* (1656), 4–5.   [72] Ibid. 16.
[73] Ibid. 17, 19–20, 20, 21, 22.

part of the female body that we designate as the vagina was called the neck of the womb—in other words, it was understood in relation to reproduction as much as to sex. The *Midwifes Practice* remakes this body part, emphasizing its role in male pleasure. The structure and size of the neck of the womb are due to the fact that it must be

> fil'd with an abundance of spirits, & to be extended and dilated for the better taking hold of the yard; there is required a great heat for these kind of motions, which growing more intense by the act of frication, doth consume a great quantitie of moisture, so that great vessels are requisite . . .'[74]

Again and again, this text emphasizes sexual pleasure in ways that reconstruct the female body as a site of male pleasure that is only secondarily related to reproduction.

Similarly, the structure of the neck of the womb is explicated in sexual terms. First, 'all this passage is erected and made streight, for the better conveyance of the yard to the womb'. It is then filled with spirits and blood 'whereby it becomes narrower for the more streight embracing of the yard'.[75] The text continues by explaining why the neck of the womb becomes erect in this way: it is so that the yard may have a 'convenient passage' to the womb; to better promote 'affrication', without which seed would not be emitted, and to protect the woman against 'any hurt or damage which might be done by the violent force of the yard'.[76] Women's bodies, in other words, are made for men; their design is built around accommodating a penis. Making babies is treated almost like an afterthought in this part of the text.[77]

This emphasis on male sexual pleasure is all the more startling in comparison with other midwifery texts. The most significant book before Culpeper was Raynalde's *Birth of Mankind*, which did not discuss male anatomy. Indeed for Raynalde, the only mention of men was as problematic readers of his text. As discussed in earlier chapters, he worried that light-headed men would read his book for all the wrong reasons and lose respect for the wonders of conception. While Culpeper describes male reproductive anatomy, he does so in order to render female anatomy second-rate. Nowhere does he consider sexual pleasure as a primary function of these organs, or discuss the ways in which the female body is made for male pleasure.

---

[74] *Compleat Midwifes Practice* (1656), 29. On this issue, see also Laqueur, *Making Sex*, 159–60.
[75] *Compleat Midwifes Practice* (1656), 38, 39, 39.   [76] Ibid. 39.
[77] See e.g. the paragraph on p. 40, in which the function of the vessels of the neck of the womb is explicated in terms of the sexual act. At the very end of the paragraph, mention is swiftly made of the reproductive, rather than sexual, function: 'Another cause of the plenty of these veins, is nourishment of the birth, and the exclusion of the flowers [e.g. the menses].'

The *Midwifes Practice* emphasizes the importance of men in reproduction in a second way. In addition to the focus on male sexual pleasure, the text also considers the complexities of the formation of seed. Culpeper chose not to tackle this subject, saying that too many authors had spilled too much ink on such 'trifles' as whether or not women made seed, how the seed was formed, how the seed formed the infant, and other such questions.[78] This omission makes sense in the light of Culpeper's emphasis on the anatomical inferiority of women compared with men. When the *Midwifes Practice* describes seed-making, its account of male and female seed makes women only slightly inferior to men. Although the text wavers occasionally about the sources of female seed—is it menstrual blood or actual seed?—the pairing of male and female seed emphasizes male and female equivalence, albeit an equivalence always shaded by hierarchy. Thus male seed is 'the effective original of the creature' and therefore hotter than female seed—and hence, again, the text explains that is why the testicles hang outside the male body.[79] The wonders of the male body are further elaborated in the discussion of the seminary bladders, 'the stores and magazines' of seed, which are constructed so that men may have sex repeatedly yet have a ready supply of seed.[80]

Female seed is like male seed only not quite as good. The text poses the age-old question: 'whether the seed of woman be the efficient; or the material cause of generation?' This question, framed in Aristotelian terms, refers to the two conflicting theories of generation that the early modern period inherited from classical antiquity. One model posited that men provided the form, that is, the blueprint or plan of the new being, while women only provided the raw material—the bricks and mortar, as it were—of their offspring. The other model suggested that both men and women provided seed with some kind of plan or form to it, which combined with each other to make a new being.[81] In popular texts such as the *Midwifes Practice* evidence was sometimes offered for both cases, without apparent contradiction. This particular text finesses the answer to its question: 'to which it is answered, that though it have a power of acting, yet that it receives the perfection of that power from the seed of man'.[82] Thus

---

[78] Culpeper, *Directory*, 72.   [79] *Compleat Midwifes Practice* (1656), 10.
[80] Ibid. 13.
[81] Joan Cadden, *The Meanings of Sex Difference in the Middle Ages: Medicine, Science, and Culture* (Cambridge: Cambridge University Press, 1993).
[82] *Compleat Midwifes Practice* (1656), 35–6. See also p. 43, where the stones of women are softer than those of men, 'because they should not perfect so substantial a seed'. The two-seed model in vernacular medical books seems to be derived from Helkiah Crooke, *Mikrokosmographia: A Description of the Body of Man* ([London]: Printed by William Iaggard dwelling in Barbican, and are there to be sold, 1615), STC2 6062, a thousand-page anatomy text. See Crawford, 'Sexual Knowledge in England, 1500–1750', esp. 86–7.

female seed, like male seed, is active, but it is secondary to male seed, evidently deriving some of its powers from male seed.

The book emphasizes the importance of the seed in relation to the female body. While earlier texts highlighted the importance of the womb in making the messy goo of sex into a new, perfectly formed human being, this text lists the functions of the womb, but then summarizes its list: 'The chiefest action of the womb and most proper to it, is the retention of the seed, without which, nothing of other action could be performed for the generation of man.'[83] Here the womb does not have that miraculous forming faculty granted to it in earlier texts. Its most important act is the fairly simple one of retaining seed.

Thus this 1656 text rewrites contemporary accounts of reproduction by emphasizing and valorizing the role of the male. It situates the crucial moment of pregnancy right at the beginning—at the sexual act—and focuses on sexual desire as the underlying cause of anatomical structures. In the remainder of the text, another person assumes new importance: the fetus.

Birth is reimagined with the role of the fetus given a new centrality. Babies are born because of their own needs, not because of the mother. Three things cause birth: first, 'the want of respiration and air, for the infant'; second, 'the want of nourishment, of which when the infant finds a defect in his mothers womb, he is forced to seek it in another place'; and third, 'the narrowness of the place where the infant lies, so that he is forced to seek room other-where'. The birth process is started by the infant, who breaks the membranes that constrain him. Once the waters that surround the infant are loosed, they provoke the mother into labour.[84] In no other account of birth do we see the baby as the chief actor. Earlier texts portrayed the mother labouring to give birth, rather than as merely the container from which the child must escape. Indeed birth is described here as a 'combat' between mother and baby when the mother is 'delicate and timourous' or lacking in patience or because she lives a bad life and eats bad food.[85]

This image, of the baby fighting its way to freedom, is a startling one. No longer is the mother the central actor in birth. Instead, it is the baby. Just as the beginning of pregnancy in this text is dominated by an account of the father, so too the end of pregnancy and the beginning of labour is dominated by an account of the baby, here gendered male. This combination, of father and son, which frames the pregnant female body, creates a new vision of the family, one grounded in bodily fact. It is as if the family is constructed by means of the female body, through its very anatomy, designed for male pleasure, and designed (imperfectly) to house the fetus. Earlier accounts understood the

---

[83] *Compleat Midwifes Practice* (1656), 41.
[84] Ibid. 73. The mother is described as doing her duty for the baby's release.   [85] Ibid.

female reproductive body as complete in and of itself, with no mention of male pleasure or of fetal agency. Rather than seeing it as a temporary residence for the fetus, earlier texts understood the womb as central to the creation of the fetus. This new account, in which the social structure of the family seems to arise from the bodies of women, was especially attractive in the troubled years of the Interregnum. As this chapter has shown, the social institutions that guaranteed and reproduced the institution of the family were under almost constant challenge. This midwifery book suggests that the family might be imagined as corporeal fact rather than social institution, a very powerful and appealing model in times of social upheaval.

Of course, in such troubled times, this was only one account. Other books gave readers a very different model of the female body, contained in a very different format. Culpeper's *Directory for Midwives* or the *Compleat Midwifes Practice* represent only one way to convey information about women's bodies. Equally popular were books that list recipes without much of the didactic exposition originated by Raynalde and favoured by Culpeper and others. In 1652 Leonard Sowerby published his *Ladies Dispensatory*, which includes remedies for all kinds of ailments, ordered from head to foot. A few months later, Gartrude Dawson printed a book called *A Rich Closet of Physical Secrets*, which includes a section called *The Childbearers Cabinet*.[86] Books such as these were often oriented towards women, who were the primary providers of domestic medicine.[87] The *Rich Closet* claims to include recipes presented to Queen Elizabeth, while a subsequent work, the *Queens Closet Opened*, suggests that its remedies were those made by Queen Henrietta Maria in her spare time.[88] In both cases, the figure of the 'closet' or the 'cabinet' might suggest a physical space within which a good housewife kept her collection of preserves, distilled waters, medicines, and the like.[89] The format of such texts is often similar to those of seventeenth-century women's manuscript remedy books, household books in which women recorded recipes over time, often noting

[86] [Leonard Sowerby], *The Ladies Dispensatory* (London: Printed for R. Ibbitson, to be sold by George Calvert at the Halfe-Moon in Watling street, 1652), Thomason E.1258[1]; *A Rich Closet of Physical Secrets* (London: printed by Gartrude Dawson and are to be sold by William Nealand, at the Crown in Duck-Lane, 1652), Thomason E.670[1].

[87] Linda Pollock, *With Faith and Physic: The Life of a Tudor Gentlewoman, Lady Grace Mildmay, 1552–1620* (London: Collins & Brown, 1993); Lucinda McCray Beier, *Sufferers and Healers: The Experience of Illness in 17th-c. England* (London: Routledge & Kegan Paul, 1987).

[88] W. M., *The Queens Closet Opened. Incomparable Secrets in Physick* (London: Printed for Nathaniel Brook at the Angel in Cornhill, 1655), Thomason E.1519[1]. The long title claims that these recipes were honoured by the Queen's 'own practice, when she pleased to descend to these more private recreations'.

[89] This figure of speech goes back to at least 1641: *A Closet for Ladies and Gentlewomen Or, the Art of Preserving, Conserving, and Candying. . . . Also Divers Soveraigne Medicines and Salves for Sundry Diseases* (London: printed by Richard Hodgkinson, 1641). Not in Thomason.

from whom the recipe derived and sometimes noting if it worked.[90] Such books were popular, with the *Rich Closet* going into at least three editions in the 1650s alone and the *Queens Closet* into at least five.[91]

These small books of remedies present a different picture of the relationship between mother and fetus than does the *Compleat Midwifes Practice*. The *Rich Closet* derives much of its advice from earlier books on midwifery, including Jacques Guillemeau's *Child-birth*. In this account, the mother 'shall easily know' when she is pregnant, and the older view of labour and delivery—that the mother labours to give birth—is promulgated.[92] In another section of the work, a possible abortifacient is recommended. The remedy is titled 'To cause a woman to have her Flowers', that is, to make her menstruate. Since pregnancy was definitively established only at quickening, there was much potential for ambiguity between early pregnancy and delayed menses. This recipe acknowledges such ambiguity, stating 'But you must have a special care that no woman being with child have this Medicine administred to her'.[93] The actual remedy would have been fairly simple to make: it consists of iris roots boiled in vinegar or wine.

The *Ladies Dispensatory* provides many remedies for sexual and reproductive ills, including recipes 'to cause standing of the yard' and 'to hinder standing of the yard', those for genital inflammations and warts, as well as a range of ailments of the womb. It offers 133 different recipes to provoke the menses, most of which consist of one or two ingredients only. Some would have been very easy to use, such as putting cinnamon in a drink, or employing unwashed wool as a pessary, or using goose-grease liniment, or eating radishes or leeks, or applying wild or garden rue to the genitals.[94] Many of the same remedies reappear in the section baldly titled 'To cause abortion'. These forty-five recipes include some that we understand today to have the potential to cause miscarriages, such as the herb pennyroyal.[95]

---

[90] For published examples of this kind of manuscript notebook, see Patricia Crawford and Laura Gowing (eds.), *Women's Worlds in 17th-c. England* (London: Routledge, 2000), 25, 26, 27, 29, 30–1. This format is also similar to that of books of secrets, on which see Eamon, *Science and the Secrets of Nature*.

[91] *The Queens Closet* became a bestseller, going into at least seventeen editions in the 17th c.

[92] *Rich Closet*, 1, 9–10. Indeed, this text advocates prayer in difficult labour, constituting Christ as 'Assistant to the wretched party in travail', 10. Both the *Rich Closet* and the *Compleat Midwifes Practice* draw upon Guillemeau's text, but it is striking to see which parts each adopts. The *Practice* takes the part of Guillemeau that emphasizes a mother's responsibility to her unborn baby in terms of diet and lifestyle, that is, emphasizing the well-being of the unborn child as the duty of the mother. The *Rich Closet* ignores this part of Guillemeau's advice, emphasizing instead the part of his text that focuses on the mother's role in labour.

[93] *Rich Closet*, 135.   [94] *Ladies Dispensatory*, 146–53.

[95] Ibid. 158–61. The following section, 'To hinder Conception', includes a number of herbal remedies, both applied internally and ingested. On the larger topic of herbal and other contraceptives

These small books of remedies thus provide a different account of the relationship between a mother and her fetus than that suggested by the *Compleat Midwifes Practice*. Where the latter reimagines family relationships within the female body itself, describing pregnancy as a relationship among three people, a mother, father, and unborn child, remedy books emphasize the primacy of the mother. The recipes for abortifacients, many of which could have been used without anyone else's knowledge, construct pregnancy as the mother's concern. In these remedy books, women might bring on delayed menses or even procure an abortion within the framework of so-called 'kitchen-physick' or domestic medicine.[96] These women's bodies are not imagined as families in miniature or as under the control of men. While infanticide had become a crime punishable by death in 1624, abortion per se was not illegal.[97] More important, the substantial ambiguity about early pregnancy and its relation to delayed menses meant that many women could have used such remedies without ever fully deciding whether they were pregnant or not.

Popular medical books thus provided a range of ways to imagine the relationships among mothers, fathers, and their unborn children. While the *Compleat Midwifes Practice* imagines the pregnant woman's body as a kind of blueprint for the family, books like the *Ladies Dispensatory* draw on an older model that centres on the pregnant woman, largely ignoring the roles of fathers and fetuses. Although reprinted often, none of the popular midwifery books discussed here created a female body that became culturally dominant in the 1650s. Throughout the 1650s, the pregnant female body remained a powerful metaphorical resource for all kinds of issues.

One of the reasons that the female body remained such a site of imaginative contest was the development of sexual satire as a routine means of commenting on current affairs. Throughout this chapter, we have seen how Parliament's actions were immediately parodied in cheap print, often in sexual terms. Leading MPs were satirized as libertines and the Adultery Act was reimagined as a boon to prostitutes. The entire parliamentary process was transformed into sexual comedy by Royalist writers. A series of pamphlets about the so-called Parliament of Ladies satirized both the activities of petitioning women and male MPs. In this imagined Parliament women discuss a law that would give

in this period, see Riddle, *Contraception and Abortion*; ead., *Eve's Herbs: A History of Contraception and Abortion in the West* (Cambridge, Mass.: Harvard University Press, 1997).

[96] Jennifer K. Stine, 'Opening Closets: The Discovery of Household Medicine in Early Modern England' (Ph.D. diss., Stanford University, 1996).

[97] Hoffer and Hull, *Murdering Mothers*; Mark Jackson (ed.), *Infanticide: Historical Perspectives on Child Murder and Concealment, 1550–2000* (Burlington, Vt.: Ashgate, 2002). On abortion, see McLaren, *Reproductive Rituals*, 89–112; Riddle, *Eve's Herbs*, 94–100, 128–31.

every woman two husbands.[98] This image combines an older trope about the lustiness of the female sex with two topical references: the political activities of petitioning women, and Parliament's attempts to reconstruct the framework of family life. While Parliament did not pass laws giving women two husbands, subsequently the Adultery Act did enable a woman to remarry merely on the presumption that her husband was dead.

The Parliament of Ladies pamphlets inspired another round of satire, grounded even more deeply in the female body. In 1648 a series of pamphlets that made Parliament itself into a pregnant woman's body were published under the Royalist pseudonym Mercurius Melancholicus. Mistress Parliament struggles to deliver a baby, lies in, and entertains her gossips to a feast.[99] Mistress Parliament, a whore, is struggling in labour but cannot deliver her baby. In despair, she makes a virtual deathbed confession, and then

the room was strangely overspread with darkness, the candles went out of themselves, and there was smelt noysome smells, and heard terrible thunderings, intermix'd with wawling of catts, howling of Doggs, and barking of Wolves against the Windows flew ill-boading screech Owles, Ravens, and other ominous Birds of night . . .

Finally the whore gives birth to a horrible headless monster.[100] As Lois Potter has shown, every detail of the whore's delivery is a reference to Parliament's struggle to create a uniform national church.[101]

This particular childbed scene was clearly meant to be read metaphorically. The whore's gossips include Mrs Schisme, Mrs Universall Toleration, and Mrs Leveller, references so basic that no reader could miss the point. However, in the context of all the other pamphlets about monstrous births and headless

---

[98] *A Parliament of Ladies* ([London]: Printed in the yeer 1647), Thomason E.388[4], see esp. sig. A3ᵛ. See also *The Ladies, A Second Time Assembled in Parliament* ([London]: Printed in the Yeare 1647), Thomason E.406[23]; *(Het Hoe, for a Husband,) or, The Parliament of Maides* ([London]: Printed in the Yeare 1647), Thomason E.408[19]. These were answered by yet another satirical pamphlet that touched on the fact that John Lilburne mobilized many female supporters: *Match me these Two: or the Convicton* [sic] *and Arraignment of Britannicus and Lilburne. With An answer to a Pamphlet, entitled, The Parliament of Ladies* ([London]: Printed in the Yeere 1647), Thomason E.400[9]. The Parliament of Ladies pamphlets are supposed to have been written by Henry Neville.
[99] *Mistris Parliament Brought to Bed of a Monstrous Childe of Reformation* ([London]: Printed in the yeer of the Saints fear, 1648), Thomason E.437[24]; *Mistris Parliament Presented in Her Bed* ([London]: Printed in the yeer of the saints fear, 1648), Thomason E.441[21]; *Mistris Parliament her Gossipping* ([London]: printed in the yeer of the downfall of the sectaries, 1648), Thomason E.443[28]; *Mrs. Parliament, her invitation of mrs. London, to a Thanksgiving dinner* ([London]: Printed in the year. 1648), Thomason E.446[7]. All historians of the period are indebted to Lois Potter's fine-grained analysis and editions of these four pamphlets: Potter, 'The *Mistress Parliament* Dialogues'. The childbirth theme wanes over the course of the dialogues; the third pamphlet's title implies that it will depict a gossip's feast, but it does not do so, and the fourth one employs the Mistress Parliament name but does not use the childbirth theme.
[100] *Mistris Parliament Brought to Bed*, 8.
[101] Potter, 'The *Mistress Parliament* Dialogues', 111–15.

babies that proliferated in the 1640s and 1650s, satire and 'reality' begin to blur. Whether fiction, satire, or supposed truth, women's fecund bodies produced disorder and monstrosity. Of course, women's reproductive bodies and the monsters they produced had long been used in cheap print to signify disorder.[102] Three aspects of the 1640s and 1650s made the rhetoric of female bodies especially powerful. First, as discussed in Chapters 3 and 4, women took new roles in a public sphere newly created in cheap print. Preaching, prophesying, or petitioning, these women disrupted traditional gender norms and their doings circulated widely in the explosion of cheap print from 1641 onwards. Second, the theme of monstrosity so clearly resonated with the often repeated idea that all customary usages were called into question. Finally, as this chapter has shown, gender relations at the heart of the family were under attack in the 1640s and 1650s.

An early satire on news pamphlets called *Pigges Corantoe, or Nevves from the North* ('coranto' was a contemporary name for a news-sheet) conveyed the confusion people felt about the sources of disorder:

That a great inquiry is made what should be the cause of this distemper, the userer layes the fault on the prodigall, the prodigall on the Scrivener, the Scribe on the broker, the broker on the Gallant, the gallant on the Citizen, the citizen on the courtier, the courtier on the projector, the projector on the common wealth, the common wealth on the ambitious, he upon the drunkard, the drunkard upon the whoremonger . . .[103]

The same kind of rhythm of uncertainty pervades the Pigge's description of his world. In the old times, the pamphlet explains, the cycle ran from peace to plenty to spiritual pride to temporal war back to peace again. But now, the pamphlet continues, 'the world is turned upside downe', and young boys command old soldiers, wise men appeal to fools, married women rule their husbands, and masters obey their servants.[104] This theme of inversion is utterly commonplace in the 1640s, although I would call attention to the fact that these sources date from 1641 and 1642. Before most of the upheavals that we emphasize in the 1640s—war, regicide and the like—cheap print already imagined and circulated an image of utter confusion and inversion.

---

[102] On the earlier use of monstrous births in England, see Katherine M. Brammall, 'Monstrous Metamorphosis: Nature, Morality, and the Rhetoric of Monstrosity in Tudor England', *16th-c. Journal*, 27 (1996), 3–21 as well as references in n. 4.

[103] *Pigges Corantoe, or Nevves from the North* (London: Printed for L.C. and M.W., 1642), Thomason E.153[7], 6. For other examples of this kind of language, see *The Dolefull Lamentation of Cheap-side Crosse* (London, printed for F.C. and T.B. 1641), Thomason E.134[9], 1; Ryhen Pameach [Henry Peacham], *A Dialogue between the Crosse in Cheap, and Charing Crosse* ([London]: printed Anno 1641), Thomason E.238[9]. Both refer to the assaults on Cheapside Cross, which culminated in its destruction in 1643. See Cressy, *Travesties and Transgressions*, ch. 14.

[104] *Pigges Corantoe*, 7.

The *Pigges Corantoe* is an obscure source, but full of absolutely typical images and language. Its very typicality points us towards an understanding of another way in which women's bodies came to represent so much in the 1640s and 1650s. If the world had already been turned upside down by 1642, it should not surprise us that old and powerful images of female bodies and sexuality were pressed into service to explain and describe the wrenching experiences of civil war and the Interregnum. Gender order was one of the most fundamental ways in which early modern English men and women organized their world, and it provided a wealth of metaphors for disarray and disorder. However, I do not mean to imply that understandings of male and female and the relations between them were straightforward or unproblematic. Whether we look at insults hurled on London streets, or the oft-repeated injunctions of ministers about wives' submission to their husbands, or gruesome murder pamphlets about wives who killed their husbands, we see a gender order that was fragile, always in need of being re-enacted and reinforced. This very fragility made gender order such a powerful way of emblematizing disorder. It was as if gender relations were compounded in part of gunpowder, liable to explode if handled the wrong way.

This chapter has argued that there was a third way in which women's reproductive bodies became especially powerful symbols of disorder. Women's new political actions and the symbolic relationship of inversion to gender order were strong enough incentives to exploit the metaphorical potential of female sexuality and reproduction. But then Parliament undertook to change key components of gender relations in family life: the creation of families in marriage; the sanctification of childbirth in churching; the incorporation of babies into church and culture in the ceremony of baptism; and the regulation of extra-marital sexuality. No wonder that gender relations were the stuff of endless political satire, and women's reproductive bodies, the very centre of family life, were used symbolically by hack writers of every political shade.

In this moment, when any piece of news was transformed into sexual satire and hawked in the streets for tuppence or less, popular medical books can be seen as only a small part of the cacophony about women's bodies. The 1650s saw the publication of more popular medical books about women's bodies than any other decade from the advent of print in England up to the 1720s, suggesting that vernacular medical writing was fully a part of the larger cultural obsession about female reproductive bodies.[105] But some of these texts run against the tide in their attempts to circumscribe the meanings of female

---

[105] This figure comes from my ongoing study of popular medical books. In the 1720s, a series of publishers begin to produce multiple editions of the runaway bestseller *Aristotle's Masterpiece*, itself compiled from texts originally published in the 16th c.

bodies. In a world in which Parliament itself was imagined as a pregnant whore, and the births of headless babies signified every kind of religious and sexual deviance, medical books were relatively tame. Most such books from the 1650s eschew discussions of monstrosity per se. Instead, in their various ways, they attempt to counter disorder. As discussed in Chapter 5, Nicholas Culpeper makes female bodies subservient to male ones, and denies that female bodies can produce meaning unmediated by men. *The Compleat Midwifes Practice* adopts a different strategy to contain disorder: it makes women's bodies into microcosms of appropriate familial relations instead of producers of monstrosity and inversion.

Eventually the experiment failed, and England became a monarchy again. Baptisms, marriages, and churchings were celebrated according to the rites of the Anglican church, and adulterers no longer risked execution. However, as we shall see in the next chapter, the events of the 1640s and 1650s cast long shadows. Women's bodies were freighted with a variety of meanings but problematic reproduction continued to be associated with political trouble long after 1660.

7

The Restoration Crisis in Paternity

The process of making babies continued to be a site for arguments about gender relations and political disorder in the 1660s and 1670s. Although Charles II was restored to the throne in 1660, political stability did not follow. His marriage to Catherine of Braganza proved childless, and concerns about who would succeed Charles were coloured by the all too fresh memories of the traumas of the two previous decades. Again and again, people feared the return of the upheavals of 1641. Their fears were amplified by a series of crises, plots, and scandals whose narratives were told and retold in various forms of political propaganda. From the Exclusion Crisis, a parliamentary attempt to change succession by law, to the Popish Plot, a convoluted narrative about a Catholic treason, to Monmouth's Rebellion, in which Charles's illegitimate son attempted to take the throne, English men and women saw the transfer of power from one monarch to the next as a fragile and potentially dangerous process. Some historians now speak of the 'Restoration Crisis' to describe the troubled politics of the period.[1] We can no longer unpack fully the layers of truth, propaganda, and falsehood in these plots and conspiracies, but we can appreciate how fragile political stability seemed in the 1670s and 1680s.

Discussions of reproduction came to focus on the transfer of characteristics from one generation to the next—the problem of succession writ small. Where popular texts of the 1650s used anatomical differences and similarities between men and women as a way of talking about gender relations, those of the 1660s and 1670s emphasized the processes of making seed and mixing seeds at conception. Medical books asked how a baby came to resemble his or her parents.

---

[1] The phrase is Jonathan Scott's. Jonathan Scott, *Algernon Sidney and the Restoration Crisis, 1677–1683* (Cambridge: Cambridge University Press, 1991); id., 'Restoration Process, Or, If this Isn't a Party, We're Not Having a Good Time', *Albion*, 25 (1993), 619–63, and the various commentaries on it. See also Alan Houston and Steve Pincus (eds.), *A Nation Transformed: England after the Restoration* (Cambridge: Cambridge University Press, 2001); Tim Harris, Paul Seaward, and Mark Goldie (eds.), *The Politics of Religion in Restoration England* (Oxford: Basil Blackwell, 1990); Tim Harris, *Politics under the Later Stuarts: Party Conflict in a Divided Society, 1660–1715* (London: Longman, 1993); and the review article by Tim Harris, 'What's New about the Restoration?', *Albion*, 29 (1997), 187–222. In general, historians' debates centre on the timing, location, and forms of the emergence of political parties and the extent to which the period 1660–1715 was punctuated by crises.

In so doing, they cast doubt on women's marital fidelity by making paternity a contested issue. Concerns about political stability and the transfer of power from one monarch to the next were articulated in discussions about the transfer of characteristics from fathers to children.

In other kinds of cheap print, such as broadside ballads, the same questions were framed in discussions of cuckolds and of unwitting men who raised children who were not biologically theirs. In the 1660s and 1670s, ballads reworked older notions of masculinity, redefining the nature of men's relationships with women and with children. No longer was a wife's sexual infidelity assigned to her husband's incompetence. Instead, ballads made every woman a sexual suspect, and advised men to, as we would say, get over it.

In popular medical books, in ballads, and in political propaganda, paternity was in crisis. Medical books problematized any easy assignment of paternity, showing how easily disrupted paternal inheritance could be. In ballads, men were repeatedly deceived by women, cuckolded constantly and never sure about which children were truly theirs. On the national level, questions about monarchical succession quickly turned into scandalous rumours about the king's mistresses and the paternity of his acknowledged illegitimate sons. This crisis in paternity resounded or echoed in these different arenas, thereby becoming louder and more significant than if it had been confined to one site alone. In this chapter, I stay within the bounds of cheap print, because I think that the most significant representations of the body were those that circulated most widely in English culture. However, any reader of this chapter familiar with the histories of high politics and political philosophy will find much that sounds familiar. The later seventeenth century saw a crisis in patriarchal theory, a crisis that echoed in ideas about kingship and in practices of inheritance. The crisis of patriarchy was enacted in cheap print through a very corporeal set of issues about contested paternity, but it obviously took other forms in other discourses.[2]

Popular medical books of the Restoration emphasize the complexities of seed formation and of the relative weight of male and female contributions to the formation of the fetus. I focus on three texts: the 1663 expanded version of *The Compleat Midwifes Practice*; Peter Chamberlen's version of that text, called

---

[2] Carole Pateman, *The Sexual Contract* (Stanford: Stanford University Press, 1988). On a wide range of issues about the relations between language of the family and high politics, see Rachel Weil, *Political Passions: Gender, the Family, and Political Argument in England 1680–1714* (Manchester: Manchester University Press, 1999). On patriarchal thinking, see Steven Zwicker, *Lines of Authority: Politics and English Literary Culture* (Ithaca: Cornell University Press, 1993); Gordon J. Schochet, *Patriarchalism in Political Thought: The Authoritarian Family and Political Speculation and Attitudes Especially in Seventeenth-Century England* (New York: Basic Books, 1975). On some of the ways in which patriarchy erased maternity, see Susan C. Greenfield, 'Aborting the "Mother Plot": Politics and Generation in *Absolom and Achitophel*', *ELH*, 62 (1995), 267–93.

Dr. Chamberlain's Midwifes Practice, and a small book called *A Discourse on Generation.*[3] Each had a complex history, being made of earlier texts. In 1659 the second edition of *Compleat Midwifes Practice* included a new section on the secrets of reproduction, supposedly those which Nicholas Culpeper considered so important that he never published them. This was a clever marketing ploy— Culpeper had died in 1654, and his widow had been publishing a succession of his works ever since. What could be better than Culpeper's best secrets? In actual fact, the secrets were derived from Jacob Rueff's *De Conceptu et Generatione Hominis*, published in Latin and German in 1554 and once in English in 1637 (see Ch. 2 above). Peter Chamberlen's 1665 book billed itself as a critique of Culpeper's *Directory for Midwives*, but it was also an attack on *The Compleat Midwife's Practice Enlarged*, providing a great deal more information about female anatomy and removing metaphors of sexual penetration. *A Discourse Touching Generation* was a selection of chapters on sexual matters from a much larger work, Levinus Lemnius's *The Secret Miracles of Nature.*[4] This hefty folio volume was a 1668 translation of a Latin work written a century earlier by a Flemish physician. It examins a range of natural philosophical issues, including questions about human reproduction.

Neither Chamberlen's critique of the *Compleat Midwife's Practice Enlarged* nor the publisher John Streater's redaction of Lemnius's text became best-sellers in their own right. However, both texts are particularly significant

---

[3]   *The Compleat Midvvife's Practice Enlarged . . . With a Full Supply of Those Rare Secrets Which Mr. Culpeper in His Brief Treatise of Midwifry, and Other English Writers, Have Kept Close to Themselves, Concealed, or Wholly Omitted* ([London]: Printed for Nath. Brooke at the Angel in Cornhill, 1659), Wing2 C1817D, Thomason E.1723[1]. *The Compleat Midvvife's Practice Enlarged . . . the Third Edition Enlarged, with the Addition of Sir Theodore Mayern's Rare Secrets in Midwifry* (London: Printed for Nath. Brooke at the Angel in Corn-hill, 1663), Wing2 C1817E. All subsequent references to this text are to the 1663 edition unless otherwise noted. Peter Chamberlen, *Dr. Chamberlain's Midwifes Practice: Or, a Guide for Women in That High Concern of Conception, Breeding, and Nursing Children* (London: printed for Thomas Rooks at the Lamb and Ink-Bottle, at the East-end of S. Pauls; who makes and sells the best ink for records 1665), Wing (CD-ROM) C1817H. Both are based on Jacob Rueff's *De Conceptu et Generatione Hominis*. Levinus Lemnius, *A Discourse Touching Generation. Collected out of Lævinus Lemnius, a Most Learned Physitian. Fit for the Use of Physitians, Midwifes, and All Young Married People* (London: printed by John Streater, 1664), Wing (CD-ROM) L1043A; see also the 1667 edition held at the National Library of Medicine: *A Discoruse* [sic] *Touching Generation* (London: By John Streater, 1667), Wing (CD-ROM) L1043B.

[4]   Levinus Lemnius, *The Secret Miracles of Nature* (London: printed by Jo. Streater, and are to be sold by Humphrey Moseley at the Prince's Arms in S. Paul's Church-Yard, John Sweeting at the Angel in Popes-Head-Alley, John Clark at Mercers-Chappel, and George Sawbridge at the Bible on Ludgate-Hill, 1658), Wing L1044. This large book full of scholarly references might not seem destined to find a wide audience. However, Sarah Jinner, the first female almanac-writer in English, recommended it to her reading public in 1659, saying that 'The reason why I recommend this piece, is, that our Sex may be furnished with knowledge: if they knew better, they would do better.' Sarah Jinner, *An Almanack and Prognostication for the Year of Our Lord 1659. Being the third after bissextile or leap year . . . By Sarah Jinner student in astrology* (London: printed by J.S. for the Company of Stationers, [1659]), Wing2 A1845, sig. B1ᵛ.

because they lingered on in curious fashion, buried in other texts. Chamberlen's work was one of the most important components of the first English manual on midwifery written by a woman, Jane Sharp's 1671 *The Midwives Book*.[5] Lemnius's work was extensively borrowed in the anonymous best-seller *Aristotle's Masterpiece*, first published in 1684.[6] By peculiar coincidence, then, some of the most significant books about reproduction in late seventeenth-century England were actually composed of selections from the works of two physicians, one Dutch (Lemnius) and one German (Rueff) first published in Latin a century earlier.

As discussed in the previous chapter, the 1656 *Compleat Midwifes Practice* inaugurated discussion of what we might call the physiology of conception in popular texts, examining how men and women make seed and how male and female seed combine to make a new person. Like much else in popular medical books, the core of these discussions of seed dates back to classical antiquity. Medieval and early modern readers were offered two basic models for conception. Either men and women each produced seed which united to form a fetus (the so-called 'two-seed' model) or women provided the matter and men provided the seed that contained within it the plan of the fetus (the Aristotelian or one-seed model).[7] In popular books of the 1660s, however, the debate is not between a one-seed vs. a two-seed model. Instead, this age-old tension about the relative contributions of mothers and fathers to their children becomes an issue about the nature of women's seed.

The *Compleat Midwife's Practice Enlarged* (hereafter referred to as the *Compleat Midwife*) envisages the womb mixing the female seed into the male seed, 'so that there is now but one mixture made of the Seed of both Sexes'.[8] This section of the book moves back and forth between different ideas about the significance and virtue of female seed. Yes, the text admits, there is female seed. But having granted that point, the book then seeks to diminish the importance of female seed by showing how much better male seed is than

[5] Jane Sharp, *The Midwives Book. Or the Whole Art of Midwifry Discovered. Directing Childbearing Women How to Behave Themselves in Their Conception, Breeding, Bearing, and Nursing of Children* (London: printed for Simon Miller, at the Star at the west end of St. Pauls, 1671), Wing2 S2969B. In Elaine Hobby's excellent modern edition of Sharp's work (Oxford: Oxford University Press, 1999), other less significant sources are noted, such as Culpeper's *Directory for Midwives* and William Sermon's *English Midwife*, but not Chamberlen. I think it is significant that Sharp chose Chamberlen, not the more widespread version of the text, implicitly rejecting some of the sexualized readings of the female body in the *Compleat Midwifes Practice*. I do not discuss Sharp extensively here because much of her text derived from texts I have discussed above, such as Culpeper's *Directory for Midwives*.
[6] *Aristoteles Master-piece, or, The secrets of generation displayed in all the parts thereof* (London: Printed for J. How, and are to be sold next door to the Anchor Tavern in Sweethings Rents in Cornhil, 1684), Wing2 A3697fA.
[7] See above, pp. 187–88 for the medieval period see Cadden, *The Meanings of Sex Difference*, esp. 105–34.   [8] *Compleat Midwife* (1663), 86–7.

female. Male seed is both hotter and thicker than female, powerful claims to superiority in an Aristotelian framework. Having put female seed in its place, the text then acknowledges that 'it is not to be denied, but that the seed of the Woman gives a mutual assistance to the seed of the Man, in the work of generation'. Then even this somewhat grudging acknowledgement is overturned. Female seed, the text asserts, is menstrual blood.[9] The *Compleat Midwife* almost creates a kind of hybrid between the one-seed and the two-seed models. In the one-seed model, the female contribution to conception is menstrual blood, which is not seed. Making menstrual blood into seed is a kind of half-step away from the hierarchical one-seed model. This half-step draws upon the connotations of blood as merely matter and upon negative connotations of menstrual blood in particular to re-create a male/female hierarchy.

It is as if the *Compleat Midwife* gives with one hand and takes away with the other. Yes, there is female seed—but it is none other than menstrual blood, usually understood not as seed but as the raw material upon which (male) seed works. The rhetorical structure of the discussion adds to this sense that female seed is a problematic category, no sooner invoked than repressed. Again and again in this passage, the *Compleat Midwife* dares its readers to disagree: 'we deny not', 'it is not to be denied', 'but it being unquestionable'.[10] It is as if the peculiar status of female seed needs to be hedged in with especially firm assertion.

Dr. Chamberlain's Midwifes Practice and *A Discourse Touching Generation* grant female seed much more power than did the *Compleat Midwife*. Both of these texts argue for the full two-seed model, saying that men and women produce seed and that the fetus is nourished with menstrual blood. Peter Chamberlen asserts the equality of the contributions of male and female seed to the shaping of the fetus, 'of both seeds mingled together are framed and pro-created equally together at one and the same time all the parts of the body'.[11] He highlights the similarity of the seeds, 'there being in both sexes ordained organs and instruments for the preparing and leading thereof, and the same causes of delight and pleasure in the spending or evacuation of the same in

---

[9] *Compleat Midwife* (1663), 87. Rueff puts the difference more generously than does the compiler of the *Compleat Midwife*. As Rueff summarizes, 'the seeds doe mutually grow, and increase together, by the vertue of both of them'; *Expert Midwife*, 9, 10. See also his more positive valuation of menstruation. He also notes that female seed is menstrual blood, but again conveys this fact in a positive light, noting that the Germans call the menses flowers, because without them there will be no fruit. The English also call the menses 'flowers' but, pointedly, the *Compleat Midwife* omits this sentence from its borrowing of Rueff. Rueff, *Expert Midwife*, 11.   [10] *Compleat Midwife* (1663), 87.
[11] Chamberlen, *Midwifes Practice* (1665), 31. He goes on to clarify what he means by the body in this instance. He means something like the plan of the body or the foundation of it. The actual tissues or specific organs (what he calls the proper parenchymata) are formed at different times, as virtually every text on the subject agrees.

both'.[12] The material cause of generation is the mother's blood, the principle upon which the seeds work. Here, menstrual blood is recast as maternal blood. Chamberlen allows that maternal blood 'is of the same nature of that which is purged every month by the Womb', but he emphasizes that it is originally ordained 'for the generation and nourishment of the Infant'.[13] He closes his extensive discussion of maternal blood by reminding the reader that after the birth, the blood moves 'by known and accustomed wayes' up to the breasts to be converted into milk for the baby.[14]

Similarly, Lemnius's *Discourse Touching Generation* asserts that women make seed and that female seed is not the same as menstrual blood. He argues that women make seed by pointing out that Nature does nothing in vain—and so the seminary vessels in women must be there for a purpose.[15] More telling, however, is his extended discussion of the perils attendant upon frustrated seed. If a woman does not expend her seed in sexual intercourse, the seed becomes corrupt, and 'grows to be of a venemous quality'. Young women in love are described as of a swarthy weaselish colour, with shortness of breath, tremblings, and racing heartbeats—all because their seed is corrupting within them. Once they marry and have sex, 'you shall presently see them look fresh as a Rose, and be very amiable and pleasant and not so crabbid and testy'.[16] Of course, if a husband does not satisfy his wife, 'you shall see the House turn'd upside down'.[17] In effect, Lemnius takes a late medieval stereotype about women—that they are the lustier sex—and explains its origins in his version of female physiology. One of the reasons that women so desire sex is that they experience greater pleasure than men, because they both receive male seed and emit their own.[18] Where Chamberlen's text emphasizes a kind of equality between male and female seed, Lemnius makes female seed very powerful. That female power, as we shall see, is often double-edged. Women make seed—but they can also be poisoned by their own seed if it turns venomous.

Discussions of male and female seed are part of larger concerns about the relative contributions of each parent to his or her child. One of the most powerful ways that popular medical books debated the relative contributions of each parent was to use agricultural metaphors to describe reproduction. In all three texts of the 1660s analysed here, discussions of seed are framed in agricultural terms. Human reproduction is compared to growing grain and cultivating fruit trees. These agricultural metaphors, especially the fruit-tree ones, afforded many opportunities to discuss how and why certain characteristics are passed from one generation to the next. As we shall see, sometimes the same

[12] Chamberlen, *Midwifes Practice* (1665), 66.   [13] Ibid. 67.   [14] Ibid. 71.
[15] Lemnius, *Discourse*, 72–3.   [16] Ibid. 74.   [17] Ibid. 75.   [18] Ibid. 76.

images could be used by one writer to emphasize the importance of mothers, and by another to highlight the role of fathers.

As described in the previous chapter, the 1656 first edition of the *Compleat Midwifes Practice* highlighted the role of fathers in making babies. In its discussions of the primacy of male seed and its emphasis on male sexual pleasure, this book makes fathers the authors of their children. In the section added in 1659, a series of agricultural metaphors adds another dimension to this emphasis on fathers. Making babies is like growing grain, since man 'doth naturally draw his Original and Beginning, from the sperm and seed of Man, projected and cast forth into the Womb of Woman, as into a Field'.[19] The metaphor is expanded to describe why some women have trouble conceiving:

the qualities which render a woman fruitful, are cold and moisture, the Womb holding the same proportion with mans seed, that the earth doth with Corn or any other Grain; and we see, that if the earth want cold and moisture, the seed will not prosper . . .[20]

Women are naturally colder and moister than men in the humoral system of medicine that was dominant in Europe throughout the early modern period. As this quote suggests, however, women's wombs had to be cold and wet in the right degree—too much was as bad as too little. Men were naturally warmer and drier than women, and a womb that was too 'male'—too hot and dry—shrivelled seeds and prevented conception.

Peter Chamberlen's version of the *Compleat Midwife*, like many other subsequent texts, expands this agricultural metaphor. If the womb is like a field, the penis is like a plow: 'The Yard is an officiall member, the Cultor or Tiller of the Field of Mans generation.'[21] In this image, men's and women's reproductive bodies become microcosms of the social and gender order of early modern England. Men plowed and tilled the land, and plowing was one of the most stereotypically male forms of labour.[22] Women weeded, harvested, and gleaned in fields of grain, but they did not plow. In these images, men's roles in making babies become very important and active while women's are more passive. As the suggestions about fields/wombs that are too cold or too wet to be fertile suggest, women's passivity did not mean that their role was completely inert. Rather, men were the action figures, the doers, and women the acted-upon.

---

[19] *Compleat Midwife* (1663), 243–4.   [20] Ibid. 252.
[21] Chamberlen, *Midwifes Practice* (1665), 12; see also 23. Jane Sharp adopts this metaphor from Chamberlen.
[22] See e.g. the ballad in which the inversion of gender roles is characterized by a woman plowing and a man collecting eggs from the henhouse, *The Woman to the Plow and the Man to the Hen-roost* ([London]: Printed for J. Wright, J. Clarke, W. Thackeray, and T. Passinger, [1681–4]), Bodleian Don. b.13(106), Wing (CD-ROM) P448B. This ballad was first published by Francis Grove, probably *c.*1630.

For Lemnius and Chamberlen, however, agricultural images of reproduction emphasize the roles of mothers as well as fathers. As described above, these books argue that male and female seeds mix in the womb, and then the ensuing embryo is nourished by maternal blood that would otherwise be evacuated as menses. Because babies get two contributions from their mothers (seed and blood) and only one from their fathers (seed), they tend to resemble their mothers. As Chamberlen summarizes, the reason that offspring resemble their mothers is because 'the Female affordeth more matter to the generation than the Male'. Lemnius makes the same argument by inverting the male-work implications of the agricultural metaphors about conception: 'For as Plants receive more from fruitful ground, than they do from the Industry of the Husbandman; so the Infant receives all things more plentifully from the Mother.' He continues by suggesting that a child loves his or her mother more than the father because, in effect, more of the child's substance derives from the mother than from the father.[23] The same image—of a husbandman planting his fields—could thus be used to opposite ends, emphasizing the maternal or the paternal contribution to reproduction.

This process of making women's bodies into landscapes has a rich and long history. In England throughout the early modern period, the ownership of land was crucial to male identity in the upper classes. As the phrase 'landed gentry' suggests, men of gentle or noble status owned land. The women to whom they were married did not own land because as married women they did not have their own legal status—theirs was subsumed into that of their husbands, a practice known as *feme covert*. As Amy Erickson has shown, the realities of female property-owning were more complex than the stark legal picture might suggest. However, women were much more likely to own movable goods—beds, clothes, plates, books—than land.[24] So when popular medical books made women's reproductive bodies into agrarian fields, they were playing on at least two social facts. First, labouring men plowed those fields, making women the passive ground upon which men acted. Second, men of somewhat higher status owned that land, making women's reproductive bodies equivalent to property owned by men.

While popular medical books strive to make their comparisons of reproduction to grain-growing seem 'natural', the connections to male work suggest that these images were also profoundly social. It is striking how few analogies these books make to female work. For example, dairying has long been used for such

---

[23] Chamberlen, *Midwifes Practice* (1665), 96; Lemnius, *Discourse*, 76–7.

[24] Amy Louise Erickson, *Women and Property in Early Modern England* (London: Routledge, 1993). For an anthropological perspective on the gendering of alienable and inalienable property (i.e. moveables and land), see Annette Weiner, *Inalienable Possessions: The Paradox of Keeping-While-Giving* (Berkeley: University of California Press, 1992).

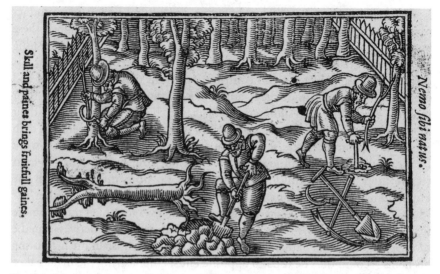

Fig. 7.1. Men's work growing fruit trees. William Lawson, *A New Orchard & Garden* (1676). Courtesy of the Folger Shakespeare Library

comparative purposes. Both Aristotle and the Bible, in the book of Job, compare the formation of the fetus to the process of making cheese.[25] As Job asks, 'Hast thou not poured me out as milk, and curdled me as cheese?' (10: 10). Medical books occasionally use language that echoes this vision of conception as cheese-making, but they never develop these echoes into a figurative system. Thus the *Compleat Midwife* describes the mixture of seeds in the womb as 'coagulated and curdled together' and Chamberlen's text refers to this moment as 'being like milk coagulated together, covered with a cream or film'.[26] Neither text expands on this comparison by situating the work of the seeds and the womb in women's work in the dairy.

While some of these grain-growing metaphors highlight the role of fathers in reproduction, another set of agricultural images could pull the other way. In all three of the 1660s texts I consider here, conception and generation are compared with the growing of fruit. At first glance, these metaphors also emphasize active male work upon a passive female body. Making fruit trees grow was a labour-intensive process in early modern England. As Fig. 7.1 suggests, almost

[25] On dairying as women's work see Valenze, '"The Art of Women, the Business of Men"'. See also Sandra Ott, 'Aristotle Among the Basques: "The Cheese Analogy" of Conception', *Man*, n.s. 14 (1979), 699–711 for this analogy as it has been developed in a Basque community.

[26] *Compleat Midwife* (1663), 89; Chamberlen, *Midwifes Practice* (1665), 73.

every aspect of the process involved hard work, usually performed by male labourers. The image is from William Lawson's *A New Orchard & Garden*, one of the many popular manuals on orchard-keeping sold in this period. One man is planting a sapling, another removes a sucker from a tree, and a third is digging a hole. The orchard is clearly the product of much human labour, and is carefully surrounded by a palisade or fence.[27]

In the *Compleat Midwife*, the male work involved in growing fruit trees results in a model of orderly inheritance:

Nature ingendereth things like unto itself; for every thing doth naturally covet and desire the form and likeness of that from which it is bred: hence it comes to pass, that Apples grow not from Pears, nor Pears from any other kind of fruit, unless it be so brought about, by means of Grafting or Planting.[28]

This idea, that like begets like, was a commonplace, especially described in terms of trees and fruit. Among the proverbs that John Ray collected in the later seventeenth century is 'such as the tree is, such as the fruit'. Other contemporary proverbs include 'an evil tree brings forth ill fruit'; 'he that sows thistles shall reap prickles'; and 'such seed such harvest'. The first female author of an English midwifery text, Jane Sharp, used a variant of the proverb collected by John Ray to persuade her readers of the truth of her remarks in 1671. In a discussion on the care of infants and the selection of a wet-nurse, she says: 'If a Nurse be well-complexioned her milk cannot be ill; for a Fig-Tree bears not Thistles: a good Tree will bring forth good Fruit.'[29] Comparisons between fruit trees and human reproduction could, therefore, emphasize the orderly transmission of characteristics from parent to child.

However, both Chamberlen and Lemnius use fruit-tree images for the opposite purpose. They invoke fruit trees as models of untidy reproduction. When Chamberlen uses the fruit-tree analogy, he says

It is found likewise in plants, that the graffe bears the fruit of that Tree it was taken from; but in the seed of that fruit remains the form of the stock it was graffed upon: As

[27] William Lawson, *A New Orchard and Garden* (London: Printed for George Sawbridge, at the Sign of the Bible on Ludgate-Hill, 1676), Wing (CD-ROM) L736. This book was first published in 1618 and went through least a dozen 17th-c. editions.
[28] *Compleat Midwife* (1663), 247. This is in the section first included in 1659.
[29] John Ray, *A Collection of English Proverbs* (Cambridge: printed by John Hayes for W. Morden, 1670), 163; Tilley, *Dictionary*, s.v. 'seed'; G. L. Apperson, *English Proverbs and Proverbial Phrases: A Historical Dictionary* (London: J. M. Dent, 1929), 591, 592; Ray, *Collection*, 210; Sharp, *Midwives Book*, 362–3. On the use of proverbs by historians, see Natalie Zemon Davis, *Society and Culture in Early Modern France* (Stanford: Stanford University Press, 1975), 227–67; James Obelkevich, 'Proverbs and Social History', in Peter Burke and Roy Porter (eds.), *The Social History of Language* (Cambridge: Cambridge University Press, 1987), 43–72. On proverbs more generally see Wolfgang Mieder, *Proverbs Are Never Out of Season* (Oxford: Oxford University Press, 1993). Thanks to Suzanne Yang for this last reference.

if you graffe an Apricock upon a Pear-stock, he will bring fair Apricocks, but set a stone of one of those Apricocks, and he will produce a Pear-tree.[30]

Unlike the *Compleat Midwife*, Chamberlen emphasizes that here resemblance and paternity (or maternity) did not go together. The stone of an innocent-looking apricot would produce a pear tree.

This understanding of heredity differs from our own. We would not expect that apricot stone to produce a pear tree. However, in early modern England, heredity was a more flexible concept than our own. Grafting was one of a number of well-known techniques for manipulating inheritance in fruit trees. Mid-seventeenth-century gardening books, such as Ralph Austen's *Treatise of Fruit-Trees*, Leonard Meager's *English Gardener*, and William Lawson's *New Orchard and Garden*, all devote considerable space to such methods and techniques.[31] *The Expert Gardener* explains how to use grafting to alter the nature of fruit. Grafting using a preparation of ox dung will produce fruit without stones. Dipping the sprout or scion into pike's blood will make the fruit turn red, as will grafting onto an alder stump. Boring a hole in the tree trunk and filling it with honey will make fruits sweet on a tree that formerly bore sour fruit. As this text summarizes, it is better to graft like to like, but if the reader 'try divers kindes, he may see and make many wonders'. Similarly, John White's book of secrets describes how to make grapes grow without seeds, how to alter the colour and taste of fruit by boring a hole in the tree trunk and inserting dyes or spices, and how to grow a yellow rose by grafting a white rose onto a (yellow) broom or furze bush.[32]

Texts such as these suggest that many readers knew that grafting was not a simple or straightforward process but rather one in which patterns of inheritance might be altered in surprising ways. The wishes, desires, and fancies of a gardener could take literal shape through the practices of grafting, becoming

[30] Chamberlen, *Midwifes Practice* (1665), 98. This is another image that Sharp borrows from Chamberlen.

[31] R. A. Austen, *A Treatise of Fruit-Trees* (Oxford: printed for Tho: Robinson, 1653), Wing2 A4238, Thomason E.701[5], 46–59; Lawson, *New Orchard and Garden*, 33–40; Leonard Meager, *The English Gardener* (London: Printed for Parker at the first shop on the right hand in Popes-Head-Alley going out of Cornhil, 1670), Wing (CD-ROM) M1568, 9–20.

[32] [Thomas Barker], *The Country-mans Recreation, or the Art of Planting, Graffing, and Gardening, in Three Books* (London: printed by T. Mabb, for William Shears, and are to be sold at the signe of the Bible in St. Pauls Church-yard, near the little north door, 1654), Wing2 B784, Thomason E.806[16], 6, 17, 19. This section was also published separately as *The Expert Gardener* (first published 1640, STC2 11562), although this too derives from an older text, *A Short Instruction Verie Profitable and Necessarie for All Those That Delight in Gardening* (first published in English in 1591). John White, *A Rich Cabinet, with Variety of Inventions in Several Arts and Sciences, The fifth edition, with many additions* (London: printed for William Whitwood at the sign of the Golden Bell in Duck-Lane near Smith-field, 1677), Wing2 W1792, 51–2 [1st edn. is 1651]. Austen pours scorn on just such methods; *Treatise*, 84–97.

embodied in a spicy peach or a yellow rose. When applied to human reproduction, however, desire was much more complex. When Chamberlen described that apricot grafted to a pear tree, he applied it to human reproduction in terms of the relationship between the forming faculty of the womb and the imagination. The womb followed the general rule that like produces like, and thus an infant resembled the parents from whom the seed derived. The imagination, however, disrupted this process just like a gardener who grafted one fruit tree onto another.

The maternal imagination was a rich and deep concept that explained many troubling aspects of reproduction—and produced others. Peter Chamberlen describes the three central stories about the maternal imagination common in seventeenth-century England. First, one of the most often mentioned examples of the maternal imagination is the biblical story of Jacob and his sheep. Laban agreed that his son-in-law Jacob would be paid for his stewardship of the flocks of sheep and cattle with all of the next generation of animals who were born spotted or streaked. Jacob took branches of hazel, poplar, and chestnut and peeled bits of the bark from them, so that the branches were spotted and streaked. He placed them over the watering troughs, so that when the ewes and cows drank, they saw spots and those spots were impressed upon their unborn offspring, resulting in much larger numbers of animals for Jacob than nature alone would have provided. In popular midwifery books, Jacob's strategy is presented as cunning but not wrong.[33] As Lemnius explains, such methods are still employed: 'So we make painted Birds, Dogs, and Horses dapled, and with divers spots.'[34]

The second often repeated story about the maternal imagination was the tale in which Galen counselled an Ethiopian couple who wished to have a white child. He told them to hang a painting of a white man in the marital bedchamber, so that at the moment of conception, the mother-to-be would see the image and it would be impressed upon her child.[35] This story was retold in many different ways in the early modern period, and we should not interpret it as narrowly racist. Just as often, the story is told of a white couple wishing to have a black baby. Another version has Hippocrates valiantly rescuing a

---

[33] For the original, see Genesis 30: 27–43. Chamberlen, *Midwifes Practice* (1665), 98; Lemnius, *Discourse*, 44–5. Interestingly, the midwifery books mostly refer to Jacob's use of this method with sheep and overlook the eugenic aspects of his work with cows. Jacob only put the spotted rods in view of the stronger cows, leaving weaker cows to reproduce naturally, thus ensuring that he got more of the stronger calves, leaving Laban with weaker ones.

[34] Lemnius, *Discourse*, 45.

[35] Chamberlen, *Midwifes Practice* (1665), 98. See e.g. John Baptista Porta, *Natural Magick* (London: Printed for John Wright next to the sign of the Globe in Little-Britain, 1669), Wing2 P2982A, 51. On this theme, see Mary E. Fissell, 'Hairy Women and Naked Truths: Gender and the Politics of Knowledge in *Aristotle's Masterpiece*', *William and Mary Quarterly*, 60 (2003), 43–74.

princess accused of adultery because her child is of another colour. Hippocrates explains the workings of the maternal imagination and the princess is saved from execution.[36]

As this last example suggests, when the maternal imagination was not governed or directed by men, the results were often negative. The third major tale about the maternal imagination, in addition to Jacob's sheep and the black parents/white baby (or vice versa), was the story of the hairy virgin. A mother prayed before an image of St John the Baptist in the desert while she was pregnant. She 'brought forth a female Child full of hair, like the hair of a Camell', because in the picture, St John was clothed in a camel skin.[37] As Marie-Hélène Huet has suggested, this story emphasizes the frailness of women's understanding—the mother's poor comprehension transformed an ascetic saint dressed in skins into a hairy, animalesque person, and transformed a long-haired male saint into a female monster.[38] In Protestant England, of course, this woman's fault was worse than mere frailty. Gazing at images of saints was a papist practice, frowned on by the Anglican church. This story was so well known that it featured as the frontispiece to *Aristotle's Masterpiece*, the popular midwifery guide derived from both Lemnius and the *Compleat Midwife*, first published in 1684 (see Fig. 7.2).

The problem of the maternal imagination was more troubling than just female weakness. It was a kind of desire that was seen as profoundly dangerous yet necessary. In popular medical books and in other forms of cheap print, women's sexual feelings produced instability and trouble. Yet, as these same texts acknowledged, without female desire, the human race itself would disappear. One of the most telling examples of this double-edged quality to female desire is in Lemnius's story about the power of maternal love. He says that he himself saw a flock of lambs put on a ship to be transported. Their mothers, a flock of 300 sheep, 'were not frighted with the Seas violence, but with incredible desire followed, still the Sea flowing up, drowned them all'. Ostensibly, this spectacle was not meant to horrify the reader. Instead, Lemnius uses it to reproach those parents who love their children insufficiently, or insincerely, 'but from the lips outward' as he puts it.[39]

Without desire, the human race would cease altogether. As Lemnius says, God put in men and women 'a greedy desire of procreating their like . . . he added allurements and a desire of mutual Embracing, that when they did use procreation, they should be sweetly affected'. For unless men and women

[36] Pierre Boaistuau, *Certaine Secrete wonders of Nature* (Imprinted at London, by Henry Bynneman dwelling in Knightrider streat, at the signe of the Mermaid Anno 1569), STC 10787, fo. 13ᵛ.
[37] Chamberlen, *Midwifes Practice* (1665), 95.   [38] Huet, *Monstrous Imagination*, 21.
[39] Lemnius, *Discourse*, 39.

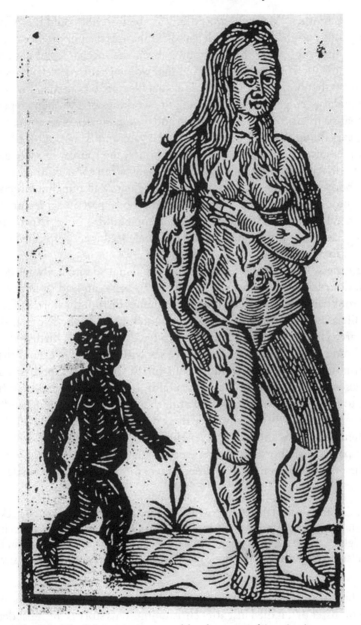

Fig. 7.2. The hairy woman, created by the maternal imagination gone awry. Frontispiece to *Aristoteles Master-piece* (1684). Courtesy of the National Library of Medicine

desired each other, 'Mankind would quickly be lost, nor could the Affairs of Mortals long endure'.[40] Chamberlen also emphasizes the importance of female sexual desire, suggesting that without it, even the mechanics of conception would not work. It was widely believed that women emitted their seed only at orgasm, so that both male and female sexual pleasure was needed for conception. Chamberlen goes further, making the workings of a woman's reproductive organs a microcosm of imagination and desire. He describes the clitoris in detail, explaining that it is analogous to the yard and is the source of female sexual pleasure. In women, however, the stones, the sources of seed, are not near the clitoris, the source of pleasure. So imagination connects these two disparate body parts. The 'imagination is wrought to call out that which lieth deeply hidden in the body'.[41] It is as if one body part imagines or desires another, calling the seed to itself. Just as humankind is only perpetuated by means of desire, so too the production of female seed is accomplished only by means of imagination.

As in the story of the 300 sheep, however, female desire is always double-edged, destructive as well as creative. Women's lusts can lead to imperfect or monstrous babies while pregnant women's desires disrupt the norms of human social life as well. Lemnius describes how Dutch women who live near the sea and marry sailors are particularly prone to have problematic births. Mariners come home after a long voyage and have sex with their wives even if they are menstruating, which leads to monstrous births. Initially, it appears that the fault lies with the husbands' lack of restraint, but Lemnius quickly shifts the blame to their wives, who 'voluntarily put themselves on their Husbands, and suck the seed from them, as hungry dogs do a bone, or Cerberus his bait'.[42] Here female desire is animalistic, even deadly.

In a particularly horrible story, Lemnius relates how one sailor's wife gave birth first to a misshapen lump of flesh, then to a monster described in demonic terms:

A Monster came forth of the Woman with a crooked back, and a long round neck, with brandishing eyes, and a pointed tail, and it was very nimble footed. As soon as it came to the light, it made a fearfull noyse in the room, and ran here and there to find some secret place to bury it self: at last the Women with Cushions fell upon it, and strangled it.[43]

Last, a little baby boy was born whose flesh had been so consumed in the womb by the monster that it died just after christening. This story is the most detailed

[40] Lemnius, *Discourse*, 33. See also Chamberlen, *Midwifes Practice* (1665), 52.
[41] Chamberlen, *Midwifes Practice* (1665), 51–2.   [42] Lemnius, *Discourse*, 92.
[43] Ibid. 100.

and gruesome discussion of a monster birth that I have read in any popular medical book. The pairing of the monster who runs around the birthing room with the innocent baby whose flesh has been consumed by its monster sibling is reminiscent of the paradoxical nature of female desire. Without desire, there would be no babies—but here the destructive potential of desire (the monster) seems to overwhelm or consume its more benign twin.

Female desire was disruptive of human society in yet another way in these texts. As we have seen, it might mark an unborn child with an item the mother longed for, or might create monsters. It might also disrupt paternity and the orderly functioning of the family. If female desire were working properly, during sexual intercourse a woman would be focused on her partner, her lawful husband. Therefore an image of her husband would be in her imagination and this image would be imprinted on any conception. The mixing of male and female seeds, the contribution of maternal blood, and the effects of the maternal imagination would all work together to produce a baby who looked like its father and mother. Social relations would be literally embodied in the child who resembled its parents. But as we have seen, such orderly transmission of characteristics from parents to children could be disrupted rather than guaranteed by female desire. More troubling still was the possibility of female deception linked to desire. A woman who was having an adulterous affair might imagine her husband although she was having sex with her lover—and then a baby would look like the husband, not the lover.[44] Lemnius quotes a long verse by Sir Thomas More to amplify this point, describing how a man with five sons rejected four of them as bastards because they did not look like him. The fifth, which did resemble him, was the only one not actually his—but this son was 'begot in fear' of discovery, and so looked like the man on the mother's mind at the moment of conception rather than her adulterous lover, the actual father.[45]

These concerns with the dangers of female desire, the potential for female deception, and the possible confusions of paternity are evident in other forms of cheap print besides medical texts. Broadside ballads resonate with these themes in the 1660s and 1670s. Changes in ballads' discussions of paternity and maternity can help us understand how and why medical books come to focus on these themes in the Restoration. Broadside ballads were the cheapest form of print available. Printed on a single side of a piece of paper, usually in black-letter, and illustrated with a woodcut, these songs sold for about a penny, the cost of a pot of ale. People heard them sung in streets and alehouses, and saw them pasted up as decoration in homes, taverns, and inns. Because these ballads were sung or spoken, even the illiterate were familiar with them. Ballads addressed many themes. Some were 'godly', describing virtues or telling a

---

[44] Lemnius, *Discourse*, 46.   [45] Ibid. 47.

moral tale. Others discussed and memorialized a recent event, such as a battle or the execution of a noted criminal or a great fire or storm. Throughout the seventeenth century, many ballads were devoted to relations between men and women, especially the process of courtship and marriage.[46]

Because ballads were the cheapest form of printed matter, they were also among the most quickly discarded. Most of the ballads extant today were amassed by seventeenth-century collectors, such as John Selden or Samuel Pepys. Since many ballads survived because they caught the fancy of a collector, we cannot make elaborate quantitative arguments about the shape of the ballad market based on ballads extant today. The exact date of a ballad's origin is also often difficult to determine, both because publishers rarely dated an individual ballad and because we are often unsure whether a ballad is new or a reprint of an older one that no longer survives. Despite these caveats, we can see certain patterns in the portrayal of gender relations in seventeenth-century ballads that seem to resonate with concerns expressed in popular medical books.[47] While Restoration medical books ponder the problems of paternity— how is it that a child looks like the parents? What do fathers contribute to their offspring? How does the maternal imagination erase paternity?—ballads take up similar themes, often in more comic ways.

Both ballads and popular medical books enquire into the age-old problem of paternity: how can a father know that a child is truly his? A number of ballads published after 1660 explore this very problem. Some ballads show fathers tricked by their wives into accepting a baby that is not theirs. *The Lass of Lynn's*

---

[46] On ballads, see Hyder Edward Rollins, 'The Black-Letter Broadside Ballad', *PMLA* 34 (1919), 258–339; Joy Wiltenburg, *Disorderly Women and Female Power in the Street Literature of Early Modern England and Germany* (Charlottesville, Va.: University of Virginia Press, 1992); Fox, *Oral and Literate Culture*, esp. 299–334; Helen Weinstein, 'Hammer and Anvil: Metaphors of Sex in the Seventeenth-Century English Ballad', paper presented at the Ninth Berkshire Conference on the History of Women, Vassar College, June 1993, as well as the more specialized works on the publishers and printers of ballads cited below.

[47] My analysis is based on reading the four major collections of 17th-c. ballads: the Pepys collection at Magdalene College, Cambridge; the holdings of the Bodleian Library, Oxford, such as the Douce and Wood collections; the Bagsworth Ballads in the British Library; and the Roxburghe Ballads, also in the British Library. These four collections combined yield thousands of ballads on all topics. I have identified approximately 140 ballads that deal with cuckoldry or uncertain paternity. Because of the difficulties in dating ballads accurately, I have relied on the crudest division in my analysis: those printed before the Restoration and those printed afterwards, up to about 1690. In 1649, a law instituted stiff penalties for printing or singing ballads, a part of a larger crackdown on popular recreations. In relation to the decades before and after, the 1640s and 1650s seem to have produced fewer ballads. I give approximate dates in square brackets; these are based on the invaluable scholarship of the compilers and editors of these collections, as well as the germinal works by Cyprian Blagden and Roger Thomson: Cyprian Blagden, 'Notes on the Ballad Market in the Second Half of the Seventeenth Century', *Studies in Bibliography*, 6 (1954), 162–81; Roger S. Thomson, 'The Development of the Broadside Ballad Trade and its Influences upon the Transmission of English Folksongs' (D.Phil. thesis, Cambridge University, 1974). Thanks to Helen Weinstein for much help with ballads.

New Joy is typical. This ballad was the third appearance of the Lass of Lynn—publishers often built on the success of one ballad by continuing the story in another ballad or offering another character's 'answer' to the original ballad. In the first ballad, the Lass of Lynn consents to have sex with a man even though he is clear that he will not marry her. In the second, she bemoans her fate: her belly is almost up to her chin, yet 'I'm neither Widow, Wife, nor Maid'.[48] Her problems are solved in the third ballad, when she marries George, a tapster at the Bull tavern. Five months later, she gives birth to a boy. George counts up five months, and doubts that the child could be his. The midwife revises his counting, saying that it is five months of days and five months of nights that make up ten months of pregnancy. Then she turns to the question of resemblance, telling George 'Had it been spit out of your Mouth, more like you it could not be.' George is persuaded, taps a barrel of ale for the gossips, and all is well.[49]

George is not the only ballad father to find himself in such circumstances. The 'Buxom Lass of Bread-street' describes the twelve different men with whom she has had sexual relations, and declares that if none of them will father her child, she'll go back to her rural village and marry her old sweetheart, making him a father in five months.[50] The 'Somerset Damsel' presents her husband with not one but two babies after five months. Her baker husband is told by the midwife that the wife is just very fruitful, hence the early arrival of the twins.[51] The five-months interval in these ballads may be mere coincidence, but it also fits well with early modern women's experiences. Pregnancy was only assured at quickening, which usually occurred around four months. A speedy

[48] *The Thankfull Country Lass, or The Jolly Batchelor Kindly Entertained* ([London]: Printed for J. Bissel, at the Bible and Harp near the Hospital-Gate in West-Smithfield), *Pepys*, v. 398. (All ballads are presumed to have been printed in London unless otherwise noted. Although they rarely specify 'London', the addresses for the printers and booksellers make this clear.) ESTC dates this as *c*.1701 but Wing suggests dates of 1687–96 for Bissell. The Pepys version is in white letter, which only came into use for ballads around 1700, so this may be a later version of an earlier ballad, since the third Lass of Lynn ballad is in black letter *c*.1685–90. *Answer to I Marry and Thank ye Too; or The Lass of Lyn's Sorrowfull Lamentation for the Loss of her Maiden-head* ([London]: Printed for Brooksby at the Golden ball in Pye-Corner, J. Deacon at the Angel in Gilt-spur Street, J. Blare at the Looking-Glass in London Bridge, near the church, J. Back at the Black Boy on London Bridge, near the Draw-bridge [*c*.1690]), Wing (CD-ROM) A3359A, *Pepys*, v. 245.

[49] *The Lass of Lynn's New Joy for finding a father for her Child* ([London]: Printed and sold by J. Millet, next door to the Flower-de-Luce in Little-Brittain, [1685–1690]), Wing (CD-ROM) L462E, *Pepys*, iii. 300.

[50] *The Buxom Lass of Bread-street, or, Lamentation for the Loss of her Maiden-head* ([London]: Printed for Brooksby, J. Deacon, J. Blare, J. Back, [1682–96]), Wing (CD-ROM) B6341C, *Pepys*, iii. 295. The 'lamentation' formula in the title seems to be very popular and does not necessarily indicate expressions of genuine regret.

[51] *The Sommerset-shire Damsel beguil'd; or, The Bonny Baker chous'd in his bargain* ([London]: Printed for J. Blare, at the sign of the Looking-Glass on London Bridge, [1685–8; dated from the licensor]), Wing (CD-ROM) S4653, *Pepys*, iv. 22.

bride who went to term would then indeed give birth five months after the wedding.

Other men met fatherhood even sooner after the wedding. Tom the tailor's wife gave birth a mere seven weeks after the wedding. The so-called 'Buxom Virgin' produced her baby at around the same time, less than two months after the nuptials. The prize, however, goes to the man in the ballad titled *The Blind Eats many a Flye*, for he became a father three days after the ceremony. Like the baker's wife, his bride was a country girl who came to London to solve her problem. As this ballad explains, 'it now appeareth plain, if a Girl be undone, She is quickly made whole again, if she goes up to London'.[52] This father consoles himself with an old proverb: 'marriage goes by destiny', he says, omitting the gloomier and more usual version, 'marriage and hanging go by destiny'.[53] The ballad suggests that he deserved his fate, for he married a woman other than his true love.

This theme, in which an unwitting man parents a child who is not biologically his, was not brand new in the Restoration. A well-known ballad called *Rock the Cradle John* was printed around 1631, if not earlier. In this song, a man marries a wealthy woman who presents him with twins a month after the wedding. This basic outline resembles the later ballads on the same theme, but once we look at the details, we can see important differences. John is a figure of fun. The midwife laughs at him when he decides that he's become a father so soon because his wife is very fruitful. In later ballads, the midwife and the gossips conspire with the wife to make an early birth explicable, but here the midwife refuses to be a party to any coverup or to John's *naïveté*. John's neighbours also make fun of him. The pictures accompanying the ballad make it clear that he is understood to be a cuckold, a man whose wife has sexually betrayed him, by portraying him with horns.[54]

---

[52] *The Ansvver to the Buxome Virgin, or the Farmer well-fitted* ([London]: Printed for J. Deacon, at the Angel in Guiltspur-street. [1685–99; I date this from the specific address although Deacon was in business for a much longer period, 1671–1704]), Bodleian Library, Douce 1(4b), Wing (CD-ROM) A3393. See another edition, *Pepys*, iii. 189. *Roger the Millers Present sent by the Farmers Daughter to his cousin Tom the Taylor in London* ([London]: Printed for J. Blare, at the Looking-Glass on London Bridge, [1685–8, dated from licensor]), Wing (CD-ROM) R1792A, *Pepys*, iii. 211. *The Blind Eats many a Flye, or The Broken Damsel Made Whole* ([London]: Printed for Brooksby at the Golden-Ball, in Pye-Corner, [1672–1700]), Wing (CD-ROM) B3191, *Roxburghe*, viii. 684. A ballad of this title was entered in the Stationers Company in 1627 by John Wright. A number of these ballads portray the pregnant woman leaving the place of seduction, seeking a husband elsewhere. It is more likely that a rural woman would have moved to a city to work as a servant, and, finding herself pregnant, gone back to the country than the reverse, but these patterns of migration are another way in which ballads echo social realities.   [53] Ray, *Collection*, 44.

[54] *Rock the Cradle, John: or, Children after the rate of Twenty-four in a yeere* (Printed at London for E.B. [probably Edward Blackmore, who entered this title at Stationers Hall in 1631]), STC 20320, *Roxburghe*, vii. 162; see also the edition in *Pepys*, i. 404.

This image points to one of the fundamental characteristics of the cuckold in the first half of the seventeenth century: his submission to his wife. Historians have discussed how a man's sexual command of his wife was equated with his ability to run his household. A man's ability to govern other men was assessed in his government of his wife and household. For example, Cynthia Herrup has shown how the scandal surrounding the Earl of Castlehaven in the 1620s was especially shocking, not because of accusations of sodomy, but because the Earl so clearly failed to govern his family and household.[55] In less elite households, men were also expected to govern. Community rituals, such as skimmingtons and charivaris, functioned to police appropriate domestic relations by publicly making fun of the hapless man who did not exercise sufficient domestic authority. As Laura Gowing, Elizabeth Foyster, and others have shown, men who permitted their wives too much power could expect community ridicule as well as shaming rituals.[56]

In their characterizations of cuckoldry and good government, however, these historians have overlooked a crucial shift in definitions of manhood.[57] Before the 1640s, masculinity, as they say, was crucially linked to the sexual reputation of a man's wife. A husband whose wife cheated on him had only himself to blame; cuckoldry was not so much a product of a woman's lust as a man's ineptitude. Indeed, a special word was used to describe such a man: he was a 'wittol', a weak man who let his wife do what she pleased. In the ballad *Rock the Cradle John*, the reader is given many details that show us that John is just such a man. Before they are married, the woman specifies the many unmanly tasks that she will expect John to perform. He will make up the fire first thing in the morning, fix his wife's breakfast, brush her gown, polish her shoes, make the bed, serve at table, and much more. The title of the ballad refers to just such gender inversion: it is the wife who should be rocking any cradle, not John. John, however, consents to all of this because, as he puts it, 'My heart doth fry in Cupid's fire'.[58] A better man can be found in the contemporary ballad that plays off this one, called *Rocke the Babie Joane*, in which a

<hr>

[55] Cynthia Herrup, *A House in Gross Disorder: Sex, Law, and the Second Earl of Castlehaven* (Oxford: Oxford University Press, 1999).

[56] Gowing, *Domestic Dangers*, esp. 94–9; Elizabeth Foyster, *Manhood in Early Modern England. Honour, Sex and Marriage* (London: Longman, 1999), esp. 103–46.

[57] Gowing's study, based on defamation suits in church courts, ends in 1640 with the demise of those courts. Foyster also grounds a good portion of her analysis in church court records but draws on ballads and plays, and is less attentive to the possibility that definitions of masculinity are not static. A number of studies of gender end in 1640, or characterize the entire early modern period or the entire 17th c., thus inadvertently emphasizing continuity over change.

[58] *Rock the Cradle, John*, [1631].

man makes his wife nurse a bastard he had fathered after its mother dies.[59] While this song does not valorize extramarital sexual activity, it does emphasize that a wife should be submissive to her husband even in this difficult circumstance. Here the wife acknowledges both the authority of her husband and the needs of the baby, who will die without care.

Ballads about cuckolds dating from the 1620s and 1630s often place the blame for extramarital sexual activity on the man's shoulders even when it is the wife who errs. For example, there is the foolish older man who marries a much younger wife, who cuckolds him.[60] Or there is the man who marries too quickly, and repents at leisure. The original 'Essex Man', for example, comes to London and marries too quickly to discover that his wife is a whore.[61] These men are guilty of folly, but they are also portrayed as weak, unable to control their wives as they should. In ballads from the first half of the century, becoming a cuckold is almost incidental to becoming henpecked. As one such man complains in *Cuckolds Haven*, 'Whatever I doe say, Shee will have her owne way; She scorneth to obey.'[62] Ostensibly, this man is warning other men not to marry such a dominant wife—but he is also providing a pattern of inadequate masculinity that other men should seek to avoid.

In other pre-1640 ballads, a woman's extramarital sexual relations are not assigned to any specific failing of either spouse. It is as if a kind of force of nature acts on all the participants, creating a situation beyond their control. In the single most popular seventeenth-century ballad involving cuckoldry, a woman's fall from honour is presented as a kind of inevitable result of another man's pursuit of her. Versions of *A Lamentable Ditty of Little Mousgrove and Lady Barnet* were published at least seven times over the century. It is a tragic tale, cast in the language and emotions of the chivalric romance so popular in chapbook form.[63] Mousgrove first sees Lady Barnet in church on a 'high holy

---

[59] *Rocke the Babie Joane: or Iohn his Petition to his louing Wife Ioane* (Printed at London: for H.G. [1630s? H.G. is presumably Henry Gosson, who worked between 1601 and 1640, but the tune to this ballad, 'Over and Under', was first registered in 1631, according to Ebsworth. 'Over and Under' is also the tune to *Rock the Cradle, John*.]), STC 21138.5, *Pepys*, i. 396.

[60] *No Fool to the Old Fool: or, A Cuckold in Querpo* (London: printed for F. G. [dated by the Bodleian from the ballad on the verso to c.1650; Francis Grove published from 1623 to 1661]), Bodleian Wood 401(40ᵛ, 39ʳ). Not in Wing.

[61] *The Essex Man Cozened by a VVhore* (Printed at London for H. Gosson, [1601–40?]), STC 5420.5, *Pepys*, i. 290; see also *Joy and Sorrow Mixt Together* (London: printed for Iohn Wright the younger dvvelling in the Old Bayley, [1634–40]), STC 5424, *Roxburghe*, i. 509.

[62] *Cuckolds Haven, or, The Marry'd Mans Miserie* (Printed at London: by M. P. for Francis Grove, neere the Sarzens Head without Newgate [dated by STC to 1638]), STC 6101, *Roxburghe*, i. 148. See also *The Discontented Married Man* (London: printed for Richard Harper in Smithfield [1635–42]), STC 17232, *Roxburghe*, i. 295, in which the sexual misdeeds of the wife are secondary to her identity as a scold.

[63] On this language, see Spufford, *Small Books and Pleasant Histories*, esp. 224–37.

day' and vows to have her. She consents, and a page betrays them to Lord Barnet. The lord catches the adulterous couple in bed, and orders Mousgrove to get up and get dressed, for he will not slay a naked man. Lord Barnet kills Mousgrove in a duel, and then slays Lady Barnet and himself. As one version of the ballad concludes, 'This sad mischief by lust was wrought, then let us call for grace, That we may shun the wicked vice, and fly from sin apace.' Only God's grace, it seems, can help humans withstand the onslaught of lust, characterized here almost as a natural force, like a storm, rather than an individual human desire.[64]

In another 1630s ballad, an adulterous wife is portrayed as blameless, or at least her culpability is utterly ignored. On her deathbed, this woman tells her husband that only one of their four sons is actually his. She will not reveal which one it is, saying 'They are my children, every one'. After the father's death, judges decide on a bizarre test of paternity to settle the estate. They hang the father's corpse from a tree, and invite the four sons to shoot at it, claiming that the one whose arrow lands nearest to the heart will be revealed as the genuine son of the father. The first three arrows pile in on top of each other into the corpse's heart. The fourth son refuses to treat his father's body so uncivilly. In a judgement reminiscent of the biblical Solomon, the judges say that 'the other three, They were unnaturall' and award the estate to the fourth son. The tale ends happily with the son sharing his new wealth with his brothers.[65] Like *Little Mousgrove*, this ballad seems to take place somewhere far away, in this case in Thrace. Again, the adulterous woman is presented as without fault. Harmony and good household are restored when her fourth son treats her other three sons equitably, making family ties derive from social as well as bio-logical fact.

After the Civil War, women become sexual suspects in ballads, although the results of their misdeeds are usually comic rather than the tragic ones of *Little Mousgrove*. While many older themes are repeated, such as the henpecked husband and the man who marries in haste only to repent at leisure, a new set of themes makes cuckolds blameless and their wives responsible.[66] The older

---

[64] *The Lamentable Ditty of Little Mousgrove, and the Lady Barnet* (London: Printed for H. Gosson [c.1630]), STC 18316.3, *Pepys*, i. 364. The edition in the Wood collection at the Bodleian has a manuscript note that the protagonists in the story were alive in 1543. This ballad has a very remote feel to it compared with other ballads, which are clearly meant to be about contemporary times.

[65] *A Pleasant History of a Gentleman in Thracia* (Printed at London: for H.G. [dated by STC to 1633]), STC 24047, *Roxburghe*, ii. 262.

[66] For older themes see e.g. *The Cuckold's Lamentation of a Bad Wife* ([London]: Printed for Brooksby at the Golden Ball in Pye-corner, [1672–1700]), Wing (CD-ROM) C7455, Bodleian Douce 1(41a); *The Hen-peckt Cuckold: or, the Cross-Grain'd Wife* ([London]: Printed and sold by J. Millet, next door to the Flower-de-Luce in Little Brittain [1682–92]), Wing (CD-ROM) H1453A, *Pepys*, iv. 129.

themes depict a wife's adultery as potentially tearing apart the social fabric. In *Little Mousgrove*, only the death of all concerned restores honour and peace. Social harmony is only restored in the tale about the four Thracian sons by the generosity of the son who inherits.

In the new post-war ballads, this threat to social harmony is offset by the many ballads that make cuckoldry merely an item of fun, the inevitable result of female sexuality. In ballads, men tell each other that there are cuckolds everywhere, and that there is no point in getting upset about it. In *The Catalogue of Contented Cuckolds*, a group of men meet in a tavern and resolve that 'the best of us all / Cannot be our Wives Keepers, they are subject to Fall'.[67] If men cannot be reconciled immediately to their cuckolded status, many ballads try to show them the way, sometimes via the money that their wives make from sexual encounters. *The Rich and Flourishing Cuckold* argues that jealousy causes men unnecessary grief. As the accompanying woodcut counsels, 'This it is to be contented Brother'! (see Fig. 7.3).[68] Or ballads advise men that there are so many cuckolds that there is no point in worrying about the issue. In *The London Cuckold*, a husband goes to see the troops mustered on Hounslow Heath by James II, intended to intimidate Londoners after the Duke of Monmouth's rebellion in 1685. While he is away, his wife dallies with another. In the answer to this ballad, the adulterous wife tells her husband not to cry over spilt milk, reassuring him that he is far from unique: 'we see how many daily flourish, that are of the horned crew'.[69] Although it is implied that the husband is elderly, he is not at fault for marrying a younger woman—cuckoldry can happen to anyone. No longer were cuckolds 'wittols'—weak men whose inability to govern produced domestic instability.[70]

Although the cuckold was no longer a wittol, he was a figure of great interest. Edward Ravenscroft borrowed the ballad title *The London Cuckold* for his

[67] *The Catologue* [sic] *of Contented Cuckolds: or, A Loving Society of Confessing Brethren of the Forked order* (London: printed for J. C. in Little Britain [1662–88]), Wing (CD-ROM) C1307A, *Pepys*, iv. 130. See also the similar themes in *The Bulls Feather; Being the Good-fellows Song* (Printed for F. Coles, T. Vere, J. Wright, and J. Clarke, [1674–9]), Wing (CD-ROM) B5437, *Pepys*, iv. 152.

[68] *The Rich and Flourishing Cuckold Well Satisfied* ([London]: Printed for F. Coles, T. Vere, J. Wright, and J. Clarke, [1674–9]), Wing (CD-ROM) R1366, Bodleian Wood E 25(123).

[69] *The London Cuckold: or, An Ancient Citizens Head Well Fitted with a Flourishing Pair of Fashionable Horns* ([London]: Printed for J. Back, at the Black-Boy on London-Bridge, near the Drawbridge, [1685–8]), Wing (CD-ROM) L2894, *Pepys*, iv. 122; *An Answer to the London Cuckold, Lately Fitted with a Large Pair of Horns of the New Fashion* ([London]: printed for J. Deacon, at the Angel in Guiltspur-street [1686–7, from internal evidence and licensing]), Wing (CD-ROM) A3417A, *Pepys*, iv. 123. The troops remained on the Heath until Aug. 1688.

[70] See *Father a Child that's None of My Own* for a specific disavowal of wittol status by a man reconciled to raising a baby he knew was not his. *Father a Child that's None of My Own* ([London]: Printed for Brooksby, near the Hospital-gate, in West-smithfield, [1672–96]), Wing (CD-ROM) F545aA, Bodleian Douce 1(77a).

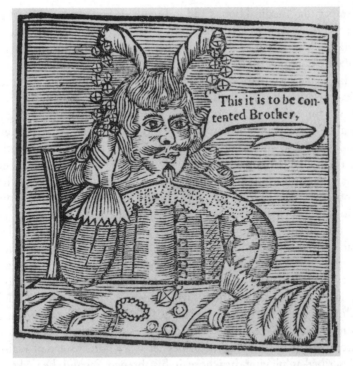

This it is to be con-
tented Brother,

Fig. 7.3. Cuckolds be contented! A ballad suggests that any man might
become a cuckold through little or no fault of his own, and make some
money in the bargain. *The Rich and Flourishing Cuckold Well Satisfied*
(1674–9). Courtesy of the Bodleian Library

play *The London Cuckolds*. Other plays presented on London stages in this
period include Nahum Tate's *Cuckold's Haven* (also the title of a ballad and a
landmark on the banks of the Thames); Joseph Harris's *The City Bride: or, The
Merry Cuckold* (a reworking of John Webster's *A Cure for a Cuckold*); John
Dryden's *The Husband his own Cuckold*; Reuben Bourne's *The Contented
Cuckold* (also deriving from a ballad title); Thomas Southerne's *The Wives
Excuse: or, Cuckolds Make Themselves*; and Richard Brome's *The Debauchee: or,
The Credulous Cuckold*.[71]

This cultural fascination with cuckolds was not wholly new, but its intensi-
fication in the Restoration is part of the larger crisis in paternity that I have

---

[71] See also the pamphlets that expand on ballad themes, such as *Bull-Feather Hall: Or, the Antiquity
and Dignity of Horns Amply Shown* (London: Printed for the Society of Bull-Feathers Hall, 1664),
Wing B5420; *Hey for Horn Fair: The General Market of England. Or Room for Cuckolds* (London:
printed for F. Coles, T. Vere, and J. Wright, 1674), Wing H1658A.

traced in popular medical books and in broadside ballads. In its most general terms, this crisis problematizes paternity, giving new weight to the old insight that a father can never truly know which children are his. Thus popular medical books argue about why and how children resemble their parents, destroying any easy equation between resemblance and what we would call a biological relationship. Ballads and midwifery books emphasize women's propensity for sexual duplicity—even honest women might imagine the wrong man or be frightened by a hare and mark their fetuses accordingly. Others, less honest, could conjure up the image of their husband at the very moment of sexual congress with a lover. Where pre-Civil War culture emphasized that a man's honour and credit depended on his control of his wife's sexuality, post-war masculinity shifted the blame for sexual irregularity onto the wife. Husbands shrugged, saying that all women were sexual suspects.

The roots of the redefinition of male and female sexuality are tangled. The political context of Restoration England provided powerful incentives to rework notions of masculinity, femininity, and inheritance. In the ballad *Father a Child that's None of My Own*, a sailor recounts how he went to sea for seven years, and returned to find his wife nursing a baby who could not be his. The sailor struggles with his fate, and in the ballad we see him trying out a range of positions and defences of his masculinity. First, he labels his wife a whore. The extended title of the ballad describes her as 'a whore instead of a saint', and she is described as 'playing the whore' in his absence. Second, he makes it clear that he is not responsible for his wife's misdeeds. She may be a whore, but he is not a wittol. He suggests that he was 'made a Cuckold by chance' and says that 'a Wittal is ten times worse' than the kind of ignorant cuckold that he has become. Nor will he grieve about his situation, because many a man is overthrown by woman.[72]

In one of the most suggestive parts of the ballad, however, the sailor defines appropriate masculinity as appropriate paternity. He does not want to 'father a child that's none of my own'—a line that echoes one in *Rock the Cradle John*. He states: 'Neither did I spring out of that race / to call that my Seed which another hath sown.' This sailor reasserts a kind of biological paternity that is superior to the social reality that a child born to a married woman was presumptively and legally her husband's. In the next line, the sailor situates himself very precisely in historical time. He says, 'Then ne'er let me look King Charles in the face / if I father a child that's none of my own.' At first glance, the sailor's comment about his king makes little sense. King Charles II was known, not for

---

[72] *Father a Child.* The tune to this ballad was first used sometime after 1659. The tune seems to migrate from political ballads in the 1660s to ballads about gender relations in the 1670s, being used for two other such. The reference to King Charles places the end date for the ballad to 1685.

fathering children none of his own, but for fathering bastards aplenty. He had great affection for his illegitimate children, making them peers and often keeping them at court. However, the inversion hinted at by the sailor's remark makes sense when we begin to understand the tremendous anxieties that surrounded the topic of royal succession. Charles married Catherine of Braganza in 1663, but the marriage proved childless. The heir presumptive to the throne was Charles's brother James. While Charles enjoyed a fair measure of popular approval, the same cannot be said of James, who was widely understood to be Catholic, and whose authoritarian tendencies were disliked.

The possibility of a papist on the throne was inflammatory to most of the English in the later seventeenth century. From our perspective, the threat of Catholicism does not seem very great. Although accurate numbers will never be possible, only a tiny fraction of English people worshiped as Catholics.[73] The threat of invasion by Louis XIV of France or by a Spanish force (the two Catholic superpowers of the Continent) seems remote. However illogical the threat of papistry might seem to us, it was very real to English men and women in the seventeenth century, who rehearsed a whole roster of papist dangers.[74] Guy Fawkes had tried to blow up the houses of Parliament back in 1605 as a part of a Catholic conspiracy. Catholics were widely believed to have set the fire in 1666 that became the Great Fire of London. They were at the heart of the so-called Popish Plot, a tangled fabrication of 1678–81 that led to the execution of a number of Catholic priests and an endless stream of political propaganda, innuendo, accusation, and counter-accusation. Londoners staged all kinds of protests and demonstrations against the supposed threat, the best-known of which were the annual pope-burning processions performed on 5 November, the anniversary of the discovery of the Gunpowder Plot.[75] Even those who did not live in London could become vicarious audiences for such processions by means of cheap print. Figure 7.4 is a broadside depicting the pope-burning procession of 1680. It serves both to make the viewer a kind of virtual participant and, by means of the careful captions to the various figures, to create a

---

[73] On English Catholicism, see John Bossy, *The English Catholic Community, 1570–1850* (Oxford: Oxford University Press, 1976). Recent scholarship has emphasized works printed abroad for English Catholics, providing us with a richer picture of English Catholic life. See e.g. Walsham, '"Domme Preachers?"'.

[74] On anti-popery, see Peter Lake, 'Anti-Popery: The Structure of a Prejudice', in Richard Cust and Ann Hughes (eds.), *Conflict in Early Stuart England: Studies in Religion and Politics, 1603–1642* (London: Longmans, 1989); Alexandra Walsham, '"The Fatall Vesper": Providentialism and Anti-Popery in Late Jacobean London', *Past & Present*, 144 (1994), 36–87; Robin Clifton, 'The Fear of Popery', in Conrad Russell (ed.), *The Origins of the English Civil War* (New York: Barnes and Noble, 1973), 144–67.

[75] Tim Harris, *London Crowds in the Reign of Charles II: Propaganda and Politics from the Restoration until the Exclusion Crisis* (Cambridge: Cambridge University Press, 1987); Odai Johnson, 'Pope-Burning Pageants: Performing the Exclusion Crisis', *Theatre Survey*, 37 (1996), 34–57.

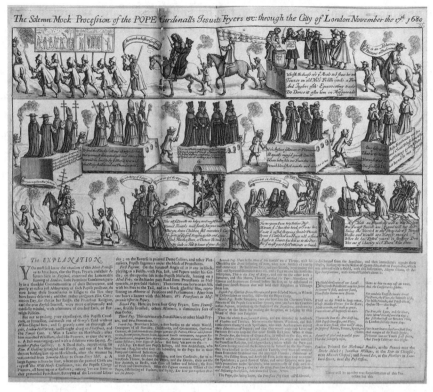

Fig. 7.4. A pope-burning procession, London, 1680. *The Solemn Mock Procession of the Pope Cardinalls Jesuits Fryers & c* (1680). Courtesy of the British Library, shelf mark C.20.f.6.(26)

litany of papist villains and victims. In villages and in towns, political contests often centred on religious differences in this period, connecting high politics with particular local issues.[76]

The Catholic threat was imagined as both near and far. On the one hand were the male Catholic monarchs on the Continent. But equally if not more threatening were the Catholics at the English court. Charles's mother and his wife were both openly Catholic, one French, the other Spanish. His mistresses were all too often Catholic, such as the much-reviled Louise de Kerouaille.

---

[76] See e.g. Newton E. Key and Joseph Ward, '"Divided into Parties": Exclusion Crisis Origins in Monmouth', *English Historical Review*, 115 (2000), 1159–83. On the growth of social stability in smaller towns, see Steve Hindle, 'The Growth of Social Stability in Restoration England', *European Legacy*, 5 (2000), 563–76. Lines of division were not just between Catholic and Protestant. Persecutions of dissenters created and promoted many further fracture lines.

Ballads contrasted the King's home-grown mistress Nell Gwynn with Louise de Kerouaille, always to the latter's disadvantage.[77] And who knew what kinds of temptations towards Catholicism Charles himself might have experienced during his long years of exile in France? As Frances Dolan has recently suggested, the threat of Catholicism was often feminized, thereby becoming more complex and scary.[78] So much of English national identity became gendered in such a context: upright masculine Protestant Englishmen were encouraged to define themselves in opposition to duplicitous feminized foreign Catholics.

Thus the remark by the sailor in the ballad about Charles II takes on deeper meaning when we understand the fraught political context of Charles's role as father. Tracing this context of criticism and contention is not straightforward. The plethora and diversity of cheap print that flourished in the 1640s without censorship did not thrive in the Restoration. The government licensed publications, and so we cannot fully trace the kinds of opposition and contestation in cheap print of the later period that is so abundant in the earlier one, although by the 1680s censorship weakened. Often, political dissent was as much oral or manuscript as print in these decades. For instance, it is exactly in this moment that the coffee house became a London institution. Not only could one read the licensed newspapers there for the cost of a cup of coffee, one could also read the occasional unlicensed newspaper and hear scabrous poems critical of the court or read them in manuscript. The government was well aware of the seditious potential of coffee houses and tried to crack down on them more than once. A cup of coffee was cheap—perhaps tuppence—and the government was not being overly paranoid to see coffee houses as potential nurseries of sedition.[79] In some measure, public opinion had been created in England in the unfettered press of the 1640s and 1650s, and that genie could not be put back into the bottle.

Many of these poems critical of the court have survived in manuscript while others were published only after 1688, when James II was replaced by William and Mary in the bloodless coup known as the Glorious Revolution. Some of

[77] *A Pleasant Dialogue Betwixt Two VVanton Ladies of Pleasure; Or, the Dutchess of Porsmouths Woful Farwel to Her Former Felicity* ([London]: Printed for J. Deacon in Guiltspur-street, [1685]), Wing (CD-ROM), P2543B, *Bagford,* ii. 599–602; *Portsmouths Lamentation, Or, a Dialogue Between Two Amorous Ladies, E. G. and D.* ([London]: Printed for C. Dennisson, at the Stationers-Arms, within Aldgate, [1685]), Wing (CD-ROM), P3008, *Bagford,* ii. 606–8.

[78] Frances Dolan, *Whores of Babylon: Catholicism, Gender, and Seventeenth-Century Print Culture* (Ithaca: Cornell University Press, 1999).

[79] On popular politics, see Harris, *London Crowds.* On coffee houses, see Steve Pincus, ' "Coffee Politicians Does Create": Coffeehouses and Restoration Political Culture', *Journal of Modern History,* 67 (1995), 807–34; Lawrence E. Klein, 'Coffeehouse Civility, 1660–1714: An Aspect of Post-courtly Culture in England', *Huntington Library Quarterly,* 59 (1997), 30–51; Brian Cowan, 'What Was Masculine about the Public Sphere? Gender and the Coffeehouse Milieu in Post-Restoration England', *History Workshop Journal,* 51 (2001), 127–57.

these poems resonate with the themes I have described as a crisis in paternity. It is as if the concerns in ballads and popular medical books have been transposed into a different key in critiques of the King and his court. First, as Harold Weber has shown, many of these poems emasculate the King. Charles's fondness for his mistresses is presented as a kind of effeminacy, a fatal weakness that makes him more like a woman than a man, the weakness that the ballad sailor so wanted to avoid. Charles's propensity for fathering bastards was well known. The perhaps apocryphal story has Charles himself responding to the title 'father of his country' with the quip 'I believe that I am, of a good number of them'.[80] But in the hands of satirical writers, what might seem a kind of hypermasculine over-sexuality is transmuted into effeminacy. A real man/monarch would spend less time in bed and more time on the battlefield.

Just as in ballads and medical books, the fault is said to lie not only with Charles himself, although his weakness is regrettable. As Weber has shown, the real evil can be traced to his scheming mistresses. It is they who seduce him away from the cares of state.[81] In this context, the mistresses are dangerous exemplars of women's sexual natures. In many ballads, the same tendency is used to comic effect. A number of Restoration ballads portray a woman who has had sex with many men. She is a temptress perhaps, but a comical one. For example, there are the seven journeymen tailors of Yorkshire, who find themselves in court for child support. The woman in question has had sex with each of them and cannot say which is the father—so each man is assessed a penny a day 'to defray this extraordinary cost'.[82] Or there is the London lass who says without shame of the father of her unborn child: 'So many men I dealt withal that I could not begin to conjecture / Whether it were some Citizen or dejected hector.'[83] Her problem is solved when she goes to the soldiers' encampment (probably the one on Hounslow Heath again!) A soldier blushes when he sees her pregnant belly. His blush functions to reveal his paternity in a kind of comic betrayal, and the two are happily wed. These ballads, in which women have sex with large numbers of men without shame or even censure, point to

---

[80] Quoted in Harold Weber, *Paper Bullets: Print and Kingship under Charles II* (Lexington: The University Press of Kentucky, 1996), 90.   [81] Ibid. 88–127.

[82] *The Lamentation of Seven Journeymen-Taylors, Being Sent up in a Letter From York-shire* ([London]: Printed for I. Deacon, at the Angel in Guilt-spur-street, [1671–1704]), Wing L287, Bodleian Douce 1(113a). Here too, 'lamentation' is formulaic, as is the occupation of tailor. In ballads such as these, millers are the lusty seducers, and tailors the ones who take the blame or father the baby, as in *Roger the Millers Present to his Cousin Tom the Taylor* discussed above.

[83] *The Answer to the London Lasses Folly: Or, the New-Found Father Discovered at the Camp* ([London]: Printed for C. Dennisson, at the Stationers Arms within Aldgate, [1685, from internal evidence and the licensor]), Wing (CD-ROM) A3418, Bodleian Douce 1(18). Interestingly, in the ballad to which this one is the answer, she has sex with only one man, but it is at night and she had no idea who he is.

the larger cultural understanding of women as unable to resist their sexual impulses.

The same theme about a woman not being able to name the father of her child was rehearsed in a much more consequential way at the very centre of the court. Charles II's favourite illegitimate son was the handsome and personable Duke of Monmouth.[84] Rumours circulated constantly about the possibility that Charles might legitimize Monmouth, turning a bastard into a 'legitimate' heir to the throne. More telling are the rumours that were disseminated in cheap print and in coffee-house gossip about the parentage of Monmouth. Many stories circulated about the so-called 'black box' that supposedly held a marriage certificate showing that Charles had married Monmouth's mother Lucy Walter; in others Lucy was portrayed as a whore who had sex with so many men that Monmouth's paternity could never be truly known.

Although these two possibilities—that Monmouth was the legitimate son of the King, or that he was not the King's son at all—seem like diametric opposites, they were used together in satiric ballads and poems. Benjamin Harris was one of the few publishers in Restoration London to print works critical of the government. After publishing an opposition newspaper and a number of broadsides and pamphlets, he fled to New England to avoid prosecution— although not before he too was libelled as a cuckold.[85] Harris tried to suggest that Monmouth was Charles's son and a worthy successor to the throne by publishing a story about how Monmouth cured the King's Evil. If true, this would have been the most striking form of resemblance for a king's son to possess, far more persuasive than any facial or bodily similarities. Since the Middle Ages, English monarchs had had the power to heal what was known as the King's Evil, a swelling of glands of the neck known more prosaically as scrofula. Merely the touch of the king's hand on the sufferer was sufficient to

---

[84] For Monmouth's appeal, see the ballad *Young Jemmy. An Excellent New Ballad, to an Excellent New Tune* (London: printed for Alexander Banks, 1681), Wing Y102A, Bodleian Firth b.20(84), as well as Robin Clifton, *The Last Popular Rebellion: The Western Rising of 1685* (New York: St. Martin's Press, 1984), and some of the evidence cited in Melinda Zook, *Radical Whigs and Conspiratorial Politics in Late Stuart England* (University Park, Pa.: Penn State University Press, 1999), 126–8. On the Exclusion Crisis (the attempt to bar James II from succession), see Mark Knight, *Politics and Opinion in Crisis, 1678–81* (Cambridge: Cambridge University Press, 1994).

[85] *The Protestant Cuckold: a New Ballad. Being a Full and Perfect Relation How B.H. the Protestant-news-forger, Caught His Beloved Wife Ruth in Ill Circumstances* (London: printed for Francis Smith, 1681), Wing (CD-ROM), P3829, Bodleian Wood 417(58); *The Saint Turn'd Curtezan: Or, a New Plot Discover'd* ([London]: Printed for the use of the Protestant-Cobler in Pell-Mell, [1681]), Wing S359, Bodleian Wood 417(65). On Harris, see W. C. Ford, 'Benjamin Harris, Printer and Bookseller', *Proceedings of the Massachusetts Historical Society*, 57 (1923–4), 34–68. Harris also published early editions of *Aristotles Masterpiece*.

ensure a cure. When Charles II was restored to the throne, he began to conduct large public ceremonies at which he touched for the Evil.[86] These pageants were very public demonstrations of the divine aspects of kingship, and as such were a kind of wordless reproach to the Englishmen who had executed Charles's father, thinking to extinguish monarchy itself.

In 1681 Harris published a very circumstantial account of Monmouth's healing of Elizabeth Parcet, a 20-year-old woman of the parish of Crookhorn in Somerset, attested to by the minister of the parish and eight reliable witnesses. The meaning of this cure was made clear in the pamphlet: 'Heaven by this Miracle proclaim his legitimacy, and God Almighty declare for the *Black Box.*'[87] 'Legitimacy' here meant both that Monmouth was born to a married woman (the marriage certificate stored in the black box) and that he was the heir to the throne. The pamphlet continues by carefully demarcating the Protestant nature of such cures. Not only did the Duke of Monmouth cure the King's Evil, but his sister Mrs Fanshaw also healed a young man of the complaint. It is carefully specified that she was 'formerly a Roman Catholick' but had been brought round to 'the true sincere Protestant faith' by her husband.[88] When the pamphlet details the history of monarchical cures of the King's Evil, it describes Edward the Confessor, the first to so heal, as 'a Good King, though a *Popish Saint*'.[89] Having ruled centuries before Luther, Edward could scarcely have been anything other than 'popish', but the pamphlet's author considered it necessary to excuse or explain his religious allegiance nonetheless.

In addition to the monarch, there was another type of person who could heal the King's Evil: the seventh son of a seventh son. Londoners in particular had reason to know this fact because in 1666 Valentine Greatrakes had come to London from his home in Ireland in order to exercise his healing talents. He became known as 'Greatrakes the Stroker' for his skill in healing the King's Evil, supposedly due to his status as a seventh son.[90] Ballads and poems satirizing Monmouth's supposed cure of the King's Evil reminded readers of Greatrakes's

---

[86] See Weber, *Paper Bullets*, 50–87. On the more general problem of monarchical succession in this period, see Howard Nenner, *The Right to be King* (London: Macmillan, 1995).

[87] *A Collection of Wonderful Miracles, Ghosts and Visions* (London: Printed for Benjamin Harris, and sold by Langley Curtis in Goatham Court, 1681), Wing (CD-ROM) C3915, 1.

[88] Ibid.   [89] Ibid. 2.

[90] On Greatrakes, see Eamon Duffy, 'Valentine Greatrakes, the Irish Stroker: Miracle, Science, and Orthodoxy in Restoration England', in Keith Robbins (ed.), *Religion and Humanism: Papers Read at the 18th Summer Meeting and 19th Winter Meeting of the Ecclesiastical History Society* (Oxford: Blackwell, 1981), 251–73; Barbara Beigun Kaplan, 'Greatrakes the Stroker: The Interpretation of his Contemporaries', *Isis*, 73 (1982), 178–85; Nicholas Steneck, 'Greatrakes the Stroker: The Interpretation of Historians', *Isis*, 73 (1982), 161–77; Alan Marshall, 'The Westminster Magistrate and the Irish Stroker: Sir Edmund Godfrey and Valentine Greatrakes, Some Unpublished Correspondence', *Historical Journal*, 40 (1997), 499–505.

skill and the reason for his possession of it. Rather than being a seventh son, Monmouth might have had seven fathers:

> If *Seventh Sons* do Things so Rare
> In You *Seven-fathers* have a share
> Shew us some more of these fine Mocks
> Shew us your *Black Art*, shew your *Black Box.*[91]

Or as another poem that describes Monmouth as 'Base as thy Mothers Prostituted Womb' suggests, Monmouth had too many fathers: 'You shew us all your Fathers but the KING.'[92] Too many fathers, too few legitimate parents, black boxes containing marriage certificates, corporeal tests of legitimacy including healing the King's Evil—cheap print describing the Duke of Monmouth was full of problematic paternity which could never, it seemed, be fully known. Again, it is striking that the faults here are never those of the father; they are displaced repeatedly and creatively onto the sexually suspect mother and the potentially unfilial son.

Thus one source of the Restoration crisis of paternity lay in the problem of monarchical succession. Charles II was a paradoxical patriarch, father to all but the one so necessary for political stability. The crisis also took shape in relation to memories of the turmoil of civil war, what one historian has called 'the intertwining of present fears with public memory'.[93] The two, of course, were intimately related: the anxieties about Charles's successor were coloured by memories of civil war. The potential of a world turned upside down again made the plots of the 1670s and 1680s, such as the Rye House Plot and the Popish Plot, threatening to contemporaries even as they seem so improbable to us, while persecution of religious minorities reminded people of the proliferation of religious radicalism in the 1640s and 1650s. Women's political activism of the 1640s was satirized and remembered as female sexual licence, and so gender disorder came to represent all the other kinds of disorder experienced in the 1640s. As Patricia Crawford has suggested, images of unruly women came to function as cultural icons, emblems of the disruptions of the Civil War period.[94] It is as if the traumas of the 1640s were constantly reworked in cheap print twenty or thirty years later. Memories of the 1640s were condensed and consolidated around certain specific themes and images, so that a few tropes come to function as signifiers for all of the tumult of civil war. Often, the world

---

[91] *Collection of Wonderful Miracles*, 5. A few lines earlier, Greatrakes is dismissed as a fraud.
[92] *The Ghost of Tom Ross to his Pupil the D. of Monmouth* (n.p., n.d. [London, 1683]), Wing G640B. See also *The Waking Vision; or, Reality in a Fancy* (London: Printed by N.T., 1681), Wing W282, *Bagford*, ii. 788–93. Here the character of Monmouth declares 'What though my Mother was his Concubine? The fault was hers, I'm sure, it was not mine.'
[93] Scott, 'Restoration Process', 619. [94] Crawford, 'The Challenges to Patriarchalism'.

turned upside down came to be re-represented as women inadequately subordinated to men.

For example, the idea of a parliament of women, used to satirize women's political activities as sexual ones in the 1640s and 1650s, was revived in the Restoration. *An Account of the Proceedings of the New Parliament of Women* rehearsed many of the themes. The laws these women consider all have to do with sex. Maidens present a petition complaining that widows have had three or four husbands each while they languish without any. The names of the supposed members of parliament are a catalogue of sexual puns: Mary Make-horn, Alice Allcock, Rachell Rouzeall, as well as references to a more general misogyny: Rebeccah Ragmanners, Elinor Empty-braine, Dorothy Drinkwell.[95] The central image is one of women's boundless sexual desire, which makes them unable to consider anything as profound as matters of state. The married women in the parliament cheerfully admit that their husbands are not sufficient and that they 'violate the bonds of matrimony by wronging the Bridall bed'.[96] In this fantasy, men are punished for sexual inadequacy by being cuckolded or even gelded, and women are granted total sexual liberty. By comparison the 'real' Parliament seems tame, even emasculated.[97]

The Civil War was re-remembered as gender trouble in pictures as well as words. The same woodcuts that were used to slander women's political activism sexually in the 1640s (see Ch. 3) migrated back to their original uses as illustrations for ballads about gender relations. One example will suggest the ways in which an image used in the Restoration might have a complex web of associations. Figure 7.5 is a woodcut that illustrated a number of pre-Civil War ballads about henpecked and cuckolded husbands. The Pepys version of *Rock the Cradle John*, in which a wife presents her husband with twins two months after the wedding, featured this image.[98] The husband holds up a hornbook, a favourite visual pun in cuckold ballads, and wears horns, while the wife threat-

[95] *An Account of the Proceedings of the New Parliament of Women Sitting at Gossips-hall* ([London]: Printed for J. Coniers at the Black Raven in Duck Lane, [1683]), Wing A370.

[96] Ibid. sig. A3ᵛ.

[97] On this theme, see also *The Cuckholds Petition to the Parliament of Women* (London: printed for A. Chamberlain in St. John-Street [1684]), Wing (CD-ROM) C7455A; *The Gossips Meeting. Or, the Merry Market-women of Taunton* ([London]: Printed for F. Coles, T. Vere, J. Wright, and J. Clarke, [1674–9]), Wing G1317, Bodleian Wood E 25(120), a ballad sung to a tune called the 'Parliament of Women'; and *Great News from a Parliament of Women, Now Sitting in Rosemary-Lane* (London: Printed for A. Chamberlain in St. Johns-Street, 1684), Wing (CD-ROM) G1714. The idea of a parliament of women was even expanded into a novel-length work, which concludes with a doctor claiming to have found a method to make men pregnant. *The Parliament of Women* (London: Printed for John Holford, at the Crown in the Pall-Mall, 1684), Wing (CD-ROM) P506A.

[98] *Children after the Rate of 24 in a Yeare, Thats 2 Euery Month as Plaine Doth Appeare . . .* (London: printed for E.B., [c.1635]), STC 20320.5, *Pepys*, i. 404.

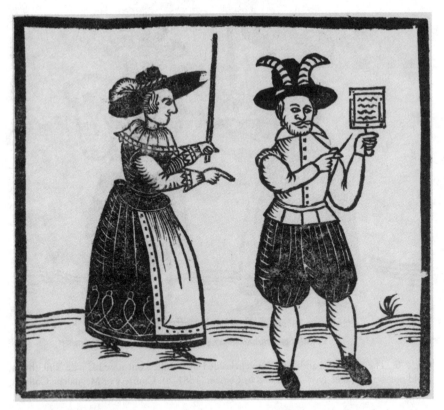

Fig. 7.5. The cuckold dominated by his scolding wife. *Children after the Rate of 24 in a Yeare.* Courtesy of Magdalene College, Cambridge

ens to beat him with a stick. He is doubly emasculated, both cuckolded and positioned as a child learning his letters. During the 1640s this same image was used to illustrate one of the mock-petitions of women to Parliament, implying that women wanted their husbands to go to war just so that they could cuckold them. Here the wife has lost her stick but instead the words 'Go to the wars' have been inserted (see Fig. 3.1 above).[99] After the Civil War, this image migrated back to gender-relation ballads, being used, for example, to illustrate *A Cuckold by Consent.* The husband has lost his hornbook but the wife still has her stick, and the husband's horns make the message clear (Fig. 7.6).[100] Images

[99] *The Resolution of the Women of London to the Parliament* ([London]: for William Watson, 1642), Thomason E.114[140]. Thomason's copy is dated 26 Aug. This appears to be a different woodblock than the above, but the image is the same.

[100] *A Cuckold by Consent: Or, the Frollick Miller That Intic'd a Maid* ([London]: Printed for J. Wright, J. Clarke, W. Thackeray, [1681–4]), Wing (CD-ROM) C7453AC, *Pepys*, iv. 124.

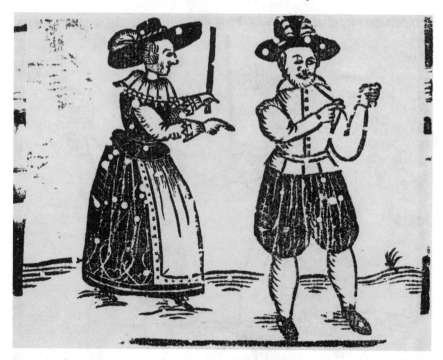

Fig. 7.6. The same husband, this time cuckolded by a miller, but now his wife is neither a scold nor a political activist. *A Cuckold by Consent* (1681–4). Courtesy of Magdalene College, Cambridge

such as these are another example of the ways in which gender relations and political discourse remained intertwined during the Restoration, so that invoking disorder in one implied disorder in the other.

Finally, it seemed that life imitated art, or at least life imitated cheap print. In 1688, James II's wife Mary of Modena gave birth to a baby boy, heir to the throne. Or did she? Rumours quickly circulated that the baby was not hers. Instead, it was suggested, a different baby had been smuggled into the birthing room, hidden in a warming pan. Here was a crisis in paternity and succession at the very centre of English life. After the previous two decades of plots, counter-plots, sham plots, and a rebellion led by an illegitimate son, the so-called Warming-Pan Baby Scandal quickly caught the public imagination, fuelled by a stream of propaganda generated by William of Orange.[101] When

[101] Lois Schwoerer, 'Propaganda in the Revolution of 1688–89', *American Historical Review*, 82 (1977), 843–74; Weil, *Political Passions*, 86–104; W. A. Speck, 'The Orangist Conspiracy Against James II', *Historical Journal*, 30 (1987), 453–62.

William invaded England and ultimately was offered the crown jointly with Mary, the birth of a supposititious heir to James II was prominent in his justifications.

The stories about the birth of James Francis Stuart, later known as 'The Old Pretender', were not uniform. Instead, like the stories about the Duke of Monmouth's parentage, various versions of the tale played on cultural stereotypes, mixing and matching elements already commonplace. At least three different stories circulated widely. The simplest one had another baby substituted for a stillborn prince, smuggled into the birthing room in a warming pan or through a door adjoining the royal bed. A different version had it that James was incapable of fathering a son, and that the father of the baby was the Queen's Jesuit confessor Father Petre or the papal nuncio. Another variant claimed that the whole pregnancy was a sham, and that the baby was really the child of a miller and his wife. As we shall see, elements of these three stories were intermixed in all kinds of ways that played on cultural commonplaces.

Many different forms and genres of cheap print offered readers stories about the birth of the Prince of Wales. Some ballads and poems straightforwardly celebrate the birth of an heir to the throne.[102] But many other pamphlets and broadsides recount various versions of the Prince's nativity. Many of the themes in these works were crystallized in a deck of playing cards published in 1689, after James II had fled and William of Orange had been offered the throne jointly with Mary.[103] Playing cards as political propaganda were relatively new: the first deck that we know of dates only from 1659. But this form seems to have been very attractive, since a number of decks were produced in the Restoration. The so-called Rye House Plot featured in a deck of cards, as did the Duke of Monmouth's Rebellion.

The 1689 deck was probably widely circulated in alehouses, taverns, and coffee houses—places where people gathered to play cards, gamble, and gossip about the news. As David Kunzle has observed, this deck is numbered chronologically, forming a kind of pictorial history that almost overrides the usual structure of the four suits.[104] The cards are almost all picture, with only brief

[102] *England's Happiness or, A Health to the young Prince of VVales. The tune: Now, now, the fight's done* (London: printed by R.M. for James Deane, in St. Jame's Market, 1688), Wing (CD-ROM) E2978A; *Englands triumph for the Prince of Wales, or, A short description of the fireworks, machines & c.* (London: Printed for L. P., 1688), Wing2 E3065A; *The Princely triumph: or, Englands joy in the birth of the young Prince of Wales: born on the 10th. of June, 1688. to the great content and satisfaction of all loyal subjects. To the tune of, Packington's Pound. This may be printed, R. P.* ([London]: Printed for Brooksby, at the Golden Ball in Pye Corner, near West-Smithfield, [1688]), Wing (CD-ROM), P3491B, *Pepys*, ii. 251.

[103] Francis Barlow [?], *The Revolution*. Playing cards, Department of Prints and Drawings, British Museum.

[104] David Kunzle, *The Early Comic Strip; Narrative Strips and Picture Stories in the European Broadsheet from c.1450 to 1825* (Berkeley: University of California Press, 1973), nos. 5–20.

captions. On the one hand, this meant that a person did not have to be able to read to understand the import of the cards. On the other, as we shall see, the pictures only make sense within a dense network of contemporary references. In order to understand the meanings of the images, a viewer of the cards would have needed either familiarity with cheap print or a kind of saturation in the rumours and gossip that circulated in coffee houses and other places of recreation.

The first card that makes reference to the rumours about the Prince of Wales is number 19, a lady making pilgrimage to St Winifred's Well. This card is in the midst of a series depicting papist practices taking place in public. Number 17 shows the processing of the Host through St James Park, and number 20 depicts a Jesuit preaching against the English Bible. Both pictures were highly inflammatory, given the virulently anti-Catholic mood of many Londoners. However, the lady going to worship at the well of a saint is more than just another papist practice renewed or newly pursued in public. Rumours circulated that Mary of Modena, desperate for a child, had gone to this well in the hope of regaining her reproductive health.[105]

Card number 21 is 'Madam W-ks at Confession'. Here too, only the knowledge that Judith Wilks is the Queen's midwife reveals the full import of this image. The picture almost seems to prefigure the supposed fraudulent birth, allegedly accomplished by means of a concealed door by the birthing bed. Here the little window between Wilks and her confessor hints at the little space through which the suppositious prince will be smuggled through a wall. The pose of Wilks echoes that of her mistress two cards earlier, and the viewer is reminded thereby that these weak women are in the hands of cunning papists.

The next image again situates the birth in a Catholic context. It shows praying to Our Lady of Loreto for the Queen. Mary of Modena did pray to Our Lady for a successful pregnancy; her mother made a pilgrimage to Loreto itself, and many sources also note that a large offering was made to the statue. Another deck of cards depicts Mary gazing up at the statue, with her offering in her hands (see Fig. 7.7).[106]

---

[105] *An Account of the Reasons of the Nobility and Gentry's Invitation of His Highness the Prince of Orange into England. Being a Memorial from the English Protestants Concerning their Grievances. With a Large Account of the Birth of the Prince of Wales. Presented to their Highnesses the Prince and Princess of Orange* (London: printed for Nathanael Ranew, and Jonathan Robinson, in St. Paul's Church-yard, 1688), Wing (CD-ROM) A379, 23.

[106] *The Reign of James II.* Playing cards, Department of Prints and Drawings, British Museum. It was Mary's mother, the Duchess of Modena, who made the actual pilgrimage to Loreto for her daughter.

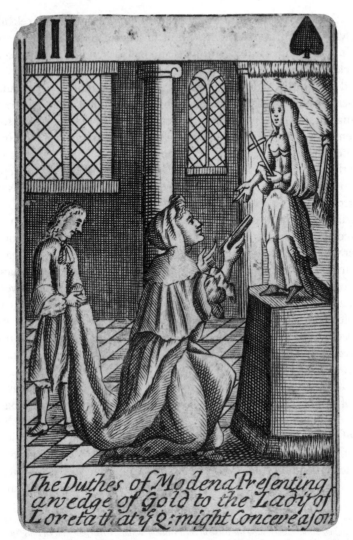

The Duthes of Modena Presenting
a wedge of Gold to the Lady of
Loreta that if Q: might Conceve a son

Fig. 7.7. The Duchess making offerings to a statue of Our Lady of Loreto
in hopes of restoring the Queen's fertility. Francis Barlow, *Reign of James II*.
Courtesy Department of Prints and Drawings, British Museum

Each of these two versions refers to one of the most contested aspects of the birth: the date of conception. Cheap-print sources endlessly conjectured about the timing of the pregnancy. Mary of Modena originally believed that she had become pregnant just after her offering to the Lady of Loreto. Were this dating

correct, the Prince would have been born at eight months. A few weeks after the
birth, Mary evidently changed her mind, and decided that the pregnancy had
dated from a month earlier. Pamphlets and ballads revelled in the uncertainty.
Some claimed that she should have known exactly when she conceived, since
she had lain with the King only twice: on 6 September at Bath and on 6
October at Windsor.[107] Another pamphlet made fun of Mary of Modena by
pointing out that most wives lie with their husbands every night, and so can be
forgiven a little confusion about dates—but since she slept with the King twice
only, she should have been certain.[108] Most of the Williamite propaganda suggested that Mary of Modena deliberately lied about the date of conception in
order to confuse people about when she would deliver the child, thus making
the introduction of a sham prince easier.[109]

Praying to an image of Our Lady of Loreto was the kind of popish practice
so feared and disliked by the English. In this context, it calls up the story of the
mother who looked so long at the image of John the Baptist that she gave birth
to a hairy baby—in the English context, worshiping at images was a dangerous
thing for women to do. At the same time, as we have seen, the power of the
maternal imagination was understood to be very great. English disgust at Mary
of Modena's worship seems coloured by little-articulated fears that perhaps her
prayers might be answered—that perhaps the maternal imagination might be
triggered by looking intensely at the greatest mother of them all, the Virgin
Mary.

The next card in the deck makes these fears more articulate and plays on the
kinds of problematic paternity we have seen in popular medical books and in
ballads. The picture is of the papal nuncio and an attendant priest bringing
Mary of Modena a smock that had formerly been worn by a statue of the Virgin
Mary in Rome (see Fig. 7.8). The papal nuncio, who had the misfortune to
bear the surname D'Adda, was often credited as being the real father of the
Prince.[110] As one pamphlet cheerfully detailed, King James II was unable to

[107] *The Several Declarations, Together with the Several Depositions Made in Council, on Monday the 22d of October, 1688, Concerning the Birth of the Prince of Wales. N.B. Those mark'd thus * were Roman Catholicks* (London: printed and sold by the booksellers of London and Westminster, 1688), Wing S2760, 34–5. This was the testimony of the King's physician, and is the clearest statement of the confusions about the date of conception.

[108] *A Full Answer to the Depositions; and to All Other the Pretences and Arguments Whatsoever, Concerning the Birth of the Prince of Wales* (London: printed for Simon Burgis, 1689), Wing (CD-ROM) F2342, 10.

[109] Ibid. 13. Many pamphlets commented on the fact that Princess Anne was inconveniently at Bath when the Queen lay in, so that one of the most desirable witnesses to the birth was absent. As Rachel Weil has pointed out, the Princess's absence was certainly convenient for Williamites spreading rumours about a suppositious birth. Weil, *Political Passions*, 90.

[110] See e.g. the broadside *The Audience* ([London: s.n., 1688]), Wing A4193; *The Sham Prince Expos'd in a Dialogue Between the Popes Nuncio and Bricklayers Wife, Nurse to the Supposed Prince of Wales* ([London: s.n.], 1688), Wing S2961.

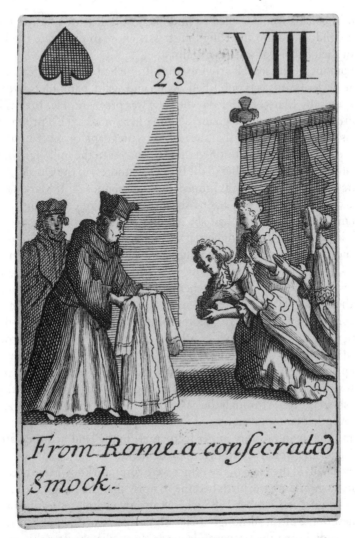

Fig. 7.8. Card 23. Jesuits bring Mary of Modena a smock worn by a statue of the Virgin. Francis Barlow?, *The Revolution*. Courtesy Department of Prints and Drawings, British Museum

conceive due to 'infirmity of Male agent', implying venereal disease. Even if the King's mistresses claimed to have had his children, this pamphlet argues, everyone knew that these women must have slept with many others and that women 'always lay the child to those best can keep it'.[111] Just like the unwed young

---

[111] *Full Answer*, 4.

women in ballads who searched to find likely, if dull-witted fathers for their unborn children, so too the King's mistresses chose to designate the King as father of their babies for reasons of gain.

The picture of the smock arriving from Rome had another referent by the time the deck of cards was published. Again and again, pamphlets refer to the smocks worn by Mary of Modena while she was pregnant. Her breasts leaked milk often while she was pregnant, staining her smocks. This production of milk was either seen as proof that she really was pregnant, or as yet another part of the fraud. Many women testified that they had seen the milk, ranging from grand ladies of the bedchamber to the humble laundress to the Queen.[112] These women's earnest testimony was immediately lampooned.[113] If Mary had really had milk in her breasts, why hadn't she shown it to Princess Anne, a reliable Protestant witness? Or why had she allowed the Prince of Wales to be dry-nursed, instead of feeding him herself with that abundant milk?[114]

The next card refers to the highly staged birth of the Prince on 10 June 1688 (Fig. 7.9). It depicts the Lord Chancellor at the foot of the bed. He is here shown as incompetent, standing where he cannot see the crucial moment of the birth that he ought to witness. A satire suggested that he too was a cuckold, too incompetent or foolish to accomplish his task.[115] It also noted that the birthing room was so stuffed with Catholics that there was hardly any room for the Lord Chancellor.[116] This image, like the previous ones, refers to many items of gossip and rumour, such as the idea that there was a secret door next to the bed through which the sham prince was smuggled. One pamphlet even gave a map to show the route through the palace by which the sham prince was intro-duced. Another lampoon suggested that the bed itself had some unusual fea-tures, and that by now every joiner [carpenter] in the land had the pattern of the bedstead and would replicate it upon demand.[117]

Many details of the birth of the Prince were common knowledge because the rumours surrounding the birth became so noisy that the King called a special panel of enquiry in October 1688 where forty-two witnesses testified to what they knew of the birth. Although their testimony was swiftly published, James II was already losing the propaganda battle. Immediately after the testimony appeared in print, a satirical poem went through the same material, making

---

[112] *Several Declarations;* see 7, 8, 9, 13, 14, 15, 17, 22, 23.

[113] See e.g. *The Deponents* ([London: s.n., 1688?]), Wing D1077. There are multiple editions of this two-page satire but Wing does not currently distinguish amongst them.

[114] *Full Answer,* 5–6. One pamphlet suggested that the imposture was poor, and that the Jesuits should have made a better job of it. After all, as this pamphlet reminds us, the Catholic Church had relics of the Virgin Mary's milk in churches all over Europe, so making milk appear in Mary of Modena's breasts should have been better managed (*An Account,* 19).

[115] *Deponents,* 2.   [116] Ibid.   [117] *Full Answer,* [22]; *Sham Prince.*

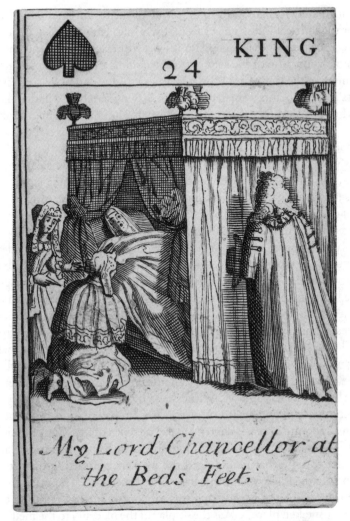

Fig. 7.9. Card 24. The birth of the Prince of Wales, witnessed (inadequately) by the Lord Chancellor. Francis Barlow?, *The Revolution.* Courtesy Department of Prints and Drawings, British Museum

fun of point after point brought forward by the witnesses. One of the publications of the testimony even undermined itself by putting an asterisk next to the name of every Catholic who testified,[118] which implicitly denied the truth value of their statements in many English people's eyes.

[118] *Several Declarations.*

Unfortunately for James, the publication of the testimonies provided more grist for the satirical mills. The Queen, it was said, chose to lie in on a Sunday morning specifically because good Protestant witnesses would be at church and thus the introduction of the sham prince would be easier.[119] Many pamphlets made much of the lack of appropriate witnesses. One pamphlet suggested that Princess Anne's doctors were in on the plot, having sent her to Bath to keep her out of the way.[120] Another faulted the Queen for not having a man-midwife in attendance, a very unusual practice at that time.[121] Another claimed that the King had forwarded the so-called Seven Bishops Case just so that leading bishops were imprisoned in the Tower and were therefore unavailable as witnesses to the birth.[122] The figure of the Lord Chancellor, then, stands in for a whole series of inadequate or compromised witnesses whose stories filled the pages of cheap print.

The next card in the deck shows the infant prince being dressed by the fire (Fig. 7.10). Here too, a reader or gossiper would have brought many details to this picture. The testimonies gathered by the King were full of details about the newborn baby, details that were quickly satirized. A number of witnesses noted that the baby looked black and seemed stunned. Indeed, the baby did not cry right after it was born, and the Queen cried out, fearing it was dead. The male witnesses to the birth were careful to note the progress of the baby from the bed to the fireside in the next room. At the same time, some of these men were acutely uncomfortable in the birthing room. The Lord Chancellor, for example, described the baby as 'black and reeking'. The Earl of Middleton said that the baby was 'very foul'.[123] Witnesses said that the baby looked weak, and as a strengthening remedy, it was given three drops of blood from the navel-string in a spoonful of black-cherry water. The scorn of the King's physician for such 'women's medicine' comes through the printed page centuries later. He was careful to note that he indulged the women, permitting them to give a medicine that he knew was both harmless and useless.[124] The detail that there was fresh blood in the navel-string was, of course, further evidence that the birth had just taken place, as was the display of the placenta to the medical men present. Once again, though, the blood from the navel-string quickly entered the realm of satire, being used to make the witnesses seem credulous.[125]

---

[119] *An Account*, 21. On this theme, see also *Several Declarations*, 9.

[120] *The Great Bastard, Protector of the Little One Done out of French; and for Which a Proclamation, with a Reward of 5000 Lewedores, to Discover the Author, Was Published* (Reprinted at Cologne: [s.n.], 1691), Wing2 G1663A, 21. This pamphlet went through many editions. It is highly unlikely that it was printed in Cologne.   [121] *Full Answer*, 7.

[122] *A Melius Inquirendum into the Birth of the Prince of Wales: or an Account of Several New Depositions and Arguments Pro and Con* (London: printed for J. Wilks in St. James's Street, 1689), Wing (CD-ROM) M1646, 2; see also *Deponents*, 1.

[123] *Several Declarations*, 24, 30.   [124] Ibid. 34.   [125] *Deponents*, 2.

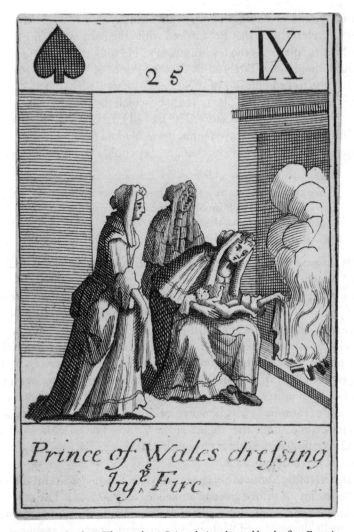

Fig. 7.10. Card 25. The newborn Prince being dressed by the fire. Francis Barlow?, *The Revolution*. Courtesy Department of Prints and Drawings, British Museum

A number of the witnesses referred to marks by which they knew that this was the Prince of Wales. The baby's nurse, Mrs Delabadie, testified about the newborn that 'she was glad to see the same Marks upon his Eye, as the Queen's former Children had'.[126] The idea of 'marks' or signs that this was indeed the

---

[126] *Several Declarations*, 20.

Prince of Wales seems to have been in the minds of other witnesses also. The Earl of Craven testified that he watched while the baby was being cleaned in front of the fireplace. As the testimony says, 'He took that particular Mark of this Child, that he may safely averr, that the Prince of Wales is that very child that then was so brought out of the Queen's Great Bedchamber.'[127] The idea that there was some special sign or mark by which the prince might be known quickly entered the realm of satire. The Earl of Craven's testimony was transmuted into the idea that Craven himself was marked for a fool.[128] The *Lullaby* ballad made fun of everyone who thought they could know a prince by a special mark:

> They knew the sweet babe from a thousand they cry'd
> 'Twas born with the Print of a Tile on his Side
> This shews he came of the Royal Race,
> And therefore ought indeed to take place [i.e. take the throne].[129]

What is missing from all these accounts is any discussion of paternal resemblance. No one here echoes the ballads in which the midwife assures the anxious father that the baby is just like him. Instead, the satires create a plenitude of possible fathers, structurally always leaving open the possibility for yet another story about the origins of the Prince of Wales. There are a number of reasons for this openness. For the pieces published while James was still on the throne, of course, a certain caution was indicated. From the perspective of publishers of cheap print and of Williamite conspirators, the more stories the better. For Williamites, one story that might be disproved was not as effective as a climate of rumour in which many stories circulated, entertaining as well as confusing people about the origins of the Prince. For publishers, of course, tales that combined the threat of popish plots with salacious details of royal bedrooms were moneymakers.

Yet another story about the origins of the Prince is suggested in card number 27. Here the infant Prince gives an audience (see Fig. 7.11). The crucial detail in this image is the toy in the baby's hands. It is a windmill. This device was used frequently by the makers of Williamite propaganda, and refers to the story that the Prince was actually the son of a miller.[130] As like bred like, so the infant returned to the playthings of his true father. This image was used in a number of prints made by Dutch and English printmakers.[131] It also migrated to a more

---

[127] *Several Declarations*, 26–7.   [128] *Deponents*, 2.
[129] *Father Peter's Policy Discovered: Or, the Prince of Wales Prov'd a Popish Perkin* (London: [s.n.], printed in the year 1689), Wing (CD-ROM) F549.   [130] See e.g. *Melius Inquirendum*, 8.
[131] Frederic George Stephens, *Catalogue of Political and Personal Satires Preserved in the Department of Prints and Drawings in the British Museum* (London: British Museum Publications Ltd., 1954), i. items 1164, 1166, 1167, 1174.

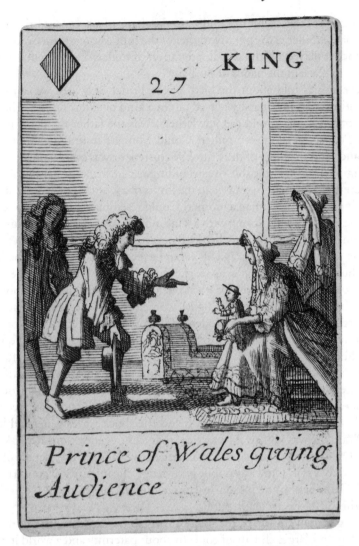

Fig. 7.11. Card 27. The infant Prince, playing with a windmill, a sign of
his supposed father, a miller. Francis Barlow?, *The Revolution*. Courtesy
Department of Prints and Drawings, British Museum

expensive form of representation, the commemorative medal.[132] Millers were
renowned in ballads for foisting their babies off on other men. The 'Buxom
Virgin', for example, was made pregnant by one of three millers, but fathered
the child onto a farmer.[133] Or there is Roger the Miller who sent a 'present' to

---

[132] Stephens, *Catalogue*, items 1159, 1163, 1187.   [133] *The Answer to the Buxome Virgin*.

his cousin Tom the Taylor in London in the shape of a pregnant bride.[134] The choice of the miller as the putative father of the supposititious prince was a clever one, since it played off the sexual reputation of millers and provided a handy emblem to place in the hands of the baby.

In the stories told about the birth of the Prince of Wales, we can see the Restoration crisis in paternity played out in a kind of comic reprise. This baby had at once too many and too few fathers. Was the father the papal nuncio? Father Peters? An unknown miller? Could women's testimony about Mary's pregnancy and the birth of the Prince be trusted, or was every woman a sexual (or religious) suspect, capable of cuckolding her husband or her faith? Could the maternal imagination transcend the limits of a woman's own body, making a seemingly infertile woman a mother? Could resemblance be a key to related-ness (the infant Prince playing with a windmill) or were all such signs unstable?

When I embarked on this book, I never expected to end up in a royal birthing room. My interests as a historian have always been in the experiences and beliefs of ordinary people, not social elites, let alone kings and queens. The stories told about this particular royal birth, however, tell us much about his-torical changes that reshaped all English women's experiences of pregnancy and childbirth. Nothing Mary of Modena did would have seemed extraordinary to an Englishwoman of the 1530s. She gave offerings to a statue of the Virgin Mary. She wore a smock sanctified by its association with such a statue, and went to a well associated with a healing saint. She employed a midwife who shared her faith, and had her son baptized in her faith. Unfortunately for Mary of Modena, English beliefs and practices about reproduction had been pro-foundly changed by the Reformation and the shock waves generated by the Civil War. She was vilified for practices that earlier generations had taken for granted, and which were common in her native land. While details of royal births are always in some way public knowledge, the intensity of concern about James's Catholicism, and his son-in-law's manipulations from the Netherlands, made this birth spectacularly public.

More generally, however, the many efforts to portray this birth as dubious depended on a larger climate of concern about paternity and a world in which women's bodies could stand in for a range of social relations. It is as if my story has come full circle. By the Restoration, cheap print had exploded the range of possibilities for talking about women's bodies. No longer did male writers apologize for discussing the processes of conception, pregnancy, and delivery. No longer did they grant primary authority to speak about women's reproduc-tive bodies to women, allocating themselves only a minor role as occasional trespassers. Instead, men wrote eagerly and openly about women's bodies. For

---

[134] *Roger the Millers Present.*

reasons of space, this chapter has discussed only a few of the most significant male-authored vernacular midwifery manuals published in the Restoration—there were at least another six I have not analysed here, including a book by one of King Charles's physicians.[135] Readers were offered a cacophony of views about women's bodies, and women's bodies had become a language of politics.

[135] *The English Midwife Enlarged, Containing Directions to Midwives; Wherein Is Laid down Whatever Is Most Requisite for the Safe Practising Her Art* (London: printed for Rowland Reynolds, next door to the Golden bottle in the Strand, at the middle Exchange door, 1682), Wing (CD-ROM) E3104; *Every Woman Her Own Midwife, Or, a Compleat Cabinet Opened for Child-bearing Women* (London: Printed for Simon Neale, 1675), Wing E3553; François Mauriceau, *The Accomplisht Midwife, Treating of the Diseases of Women with Child* (London: printed by John Darby; and are to be sold by Benjamin Billingsley, at the Printing-Press in Cornhil near the Royal-Exchange, 1673), Wing (CD-ROM) M1371A; William Sermon, *The Ladies Companion, Or, the English Midwife* (London: Printed for Edward Thomas, 1671), Wing2 S2628; James Wolveridge, *Speculum Matricis Hybernicum, Or, the Irish Midwives Handmaid* (London: Printed by E. Okes, and are to be sold by Rowland Reynolds, 1670), Wing2 W3319; Nicholas Sudell, *Mulierum Amicus: Or, the Womans Friend; Plainly Discovering All Those Diseases That Are Incident to That Sex* ([London]: Printed for the author, and is to be sold by J. Hancock in Popes-head-Alley in the year, 1666), Wing2 S6143.

Conclusions

While I was writing this book, two hoardings appeared in my neighbourhood. The first showed a tiny pink dot, about to be inundated by white sperm-shaped objects. The caption read 'Don't like the odds? Don't have sex!' The second depicted the Mona Lisa, her enigmatic smile explained by the caption 'Who's the Daddy?' She advertised a DNA paternity-testing service. While the medium is modern, the messages resonate with many of the concerns in this book. Images of women's reproductive bodies—whether depicted as a blank field and a pink dot, or by the delicate smile of the Mona Lisa, inherited from a tradition of portraying the Madonna—carry powerful and often conflicting messages. Indeed, the two hoardings, just yards from each other, can be read in oppositional terms. That small helpless pink dot (why is an ovum pink?) suggests a passive woman at the mercy of invading men/sperm. The Mona Lisa, on the other hand, smiles as if to say that only she knows for sure who the father of her child might be. Men are powerless to decode that smile. Only modern science can help them decipher her mystery.

This book is about how we moved from the Mona Lisa to that picture of the egg and invading sperm. In the hoarding Mona Lisa, the female reproductive body is mysterious and powerful. Without the most advanced tools of modern science, the Mona Lisa's body remains secret, known only to her. The diagram of egg and sperm is just the opposite. Here, the innermost recesses of a woman's body are laid open, stripped of wonder or mystery.

This book traces these changes, arguing that women's bodies came to bear social meanings as well as babies. Before the Reformation, women's bodies were women's work. The imagery associated with pregnancy and childbirth drew upon commonplaces of female labour. The fetus and the infant, for example, were imagined as guests, whom women fed and welcomed. The fetus was cared for and nourished within the female body like a guest within the home. Once born, the baby was offered hospitality in the form of luxury foods like butter, sugar, and wine, like an honoured visitor. Labour and delivery were female work of a more gruelling sort, undertaken in the company of other women who both cheered the birthing woman and urged her to labour appropriately. This female world excited both wonder and fear in men. Somehow, women's bodies transformed a little bit of semen into a new being, a wondrous act indeed. Miraculously, the womb expanded from a tiny organ the size of a walnut to encompass a full-term infant. Just underneath these connotations of wonder, however, lay fear and uncertainty. What were those gossips in the birthing room talking about, if not male inadequacies? What would happen if irreverent men read the birthing manuals written for women and joked about these wondrous things?

England's slow transition from a Catholic to a Protestant nation gradually changed many of these ideas about female bodies and childbirth. First, those practices which explicitly linked the wonder of each pregnancy to that of the Virgin Mary were changed. No longer would women in childbirth call upon the Virgin Mary to ease their pains, no longer were they to understand their suffering as cognate with hers, and no longer would they make thank-offerings to her statue in the local church. Much more slowly, those connotations of wonder that made each pregnancy a pale echo of the conception of Christ were extinguished. While the womb retained some associations of wonder and mystery, its powers were now understood as potentially dangerous. A disordered womb might kill a woman rather than make a baby.

In other words, as England gradually moved towards a Protestant faith, women's bodies were reimagined or reformulated. Just as the interiors of churches were whitewashed, and rich wall paintings replaced by sentences of Scripture and the royal coat of arms, older beliefs about the wondrous properties of women's bodies were replaced by newer ones that emphasized the dangers inherent in female bodies. However, just as in many a parish church, it was only after many decades that the old wall paintings and old beliefs were finally obscured and gone from memory. By the time that Mary of Modena wore a smock of the Virgin Mary to aid in her pregnancy, few if any Protestant Englishwomen would realize or remember that their great-grandmothers had routinely worn girdles of the Virgin to aid them in childbirth. Instead, the smock was further evidence of Mary's superstitious foreign beliefs.

Although some of the Warming-Pan Baby Scandal can be understood in relation to England's transformation into a Protestant nation, other aspects of the affair point us towards the other crisis that reshaped women's bodies. The Civil War that erupted in the 1640s was often represented as 'the world turned upside down'. Every form of authority was called into question: that of the king over his people, of bishops over the church, of priests over their parishioners, of landlords over their tenants, and of men over women. In this crisis, women took on new roles as political petitioners and as preachers. Men, however, were horrified by the spectacle of women speaking in public, be it about politics or religion. As in many other revolutions, radical reform often stopped short of gender roles.

In the Interregnum, ideas about women's bodies changed, but just as important, ways of writing about women's bodies changed. Nicholas Culpeper was a radical in many regards, shaped by themes associated with the Leveller movement and adamant about the inequities preserved and perpetrated by learned physicians. His books offered medical learning to anyone who could read basic English. When it came to women's bodies, however, Culpeper's work re-embedded gender hierarchies inside the body itself. He introduced men's bodies into midwifery books, implicitly and explicitly making women's bodies inferior versions of men's bodies. On a deeper level, he transformed the meanings that could be ascribed to the female body. He writes about midwifery without any of the reservations or anxieties displayed by earlier male writers. Instead of worrying about his role as a man writing about women's bodies, he jokes about it, and makes it clear that he has knowledge that is superior to that of midwives and other women. Culpeper thus pulls off a double feat: he makes a male writer (presumably never present at a birth) more authoritative than a female midwife who had attended many births, and he makes women's bodies testify to social facts beyond themselves. In his writing, women's bodies reveal a social hierarchy grounded in bodily facts, being made to show how they are inferior to men's bodies. They speak, not just about themselves, but about men and the relations between men and women as well. It is as if a new space for imagining gender relations has been opened up. That space is narrated and described by a male writer although it is inside the female body.

Henry Jessey, writing about Sarah Wight's body, constantly repositions himself as the authoritative reader of that body. Her body produces meanings as she fasts, but those meanings are only made clear through his transcriptions and interpretations. On the one hand, we can understand Wight as one of the many women who claimed new forms of religious authority in the 1640s. While others preached in public spaces, Wight made her bedside into a pulpit. On the other, we can see Jessey, like Culpeper, claiming interpretative authority over a female body, reinscribing familiar gender hierarchies in new and unsettling circumstances. Because much of Wight's testimony is in her own words, Jessey's book reveals much more interpretative struggle than does Culpeper's, which relies instead on a language of anatomy in which the subject, a dead female body, never speaks. Both works, however, reveal the ways in which men came to claim that they had authoritative knowledge of women's bodies, and both suggest the ways in which women's bodies came to signify social order.

One of the linchpins of that social order was the institution of the family. Contemporaries called the family a little commonwealth, underlining the way that governing the household was much like governing the nation. In the 1640s and 1650s the family was assailed from two different poles. The State attempted to remake certain moments when the institution of the family was publicly enacted. The government closed church courts, which regulated sexual misdemeanors, substituting a draconian but underenforced Adultery Act. Parliament sought to change the religious ceremonies that produced families, altering baptism, abolishing churching, and making marriage a civil ceremony. If the State was one focus of the attack on the family, radical religion was the other. In descriptions of groups like the Adamites and the Ranters, readers were presented with the terrifying yet seductive possibility of a world in which sexual relations between men and women were governed solely by desire. Just as Culpeper's text sought the sources of gender hierarchy deep within the body at the very moment when those sources seemed to be scarce in society, so too did texts of the 1650s attempt to re-create the family within the body itself. Pregnancy was reimagined as a relationship amongst father, mother, and infant. In earlier works, fathers were ignored, and mothers' roles completely dominated consideration of the fetus. Now, however, the sexual act (and thus men) assumed new importance in the creation of the fetus, and babies themselves were understood to initiate the birth process. The maternal body had to share the stage with those of the father and the baby.

Introducing fathers into the narratives of pregnancy and birth was not simple. It was one thing to point out, as Culpeper did, that male anatomy was superior to female. But careful consideration of the roles of fathers in pregnancy quickly led to considerable anxiety about paternity in general. As Englishmen and women worried about monarchical succession, they also worried about what we would call heredity. How are characteristics transferred from parents to children? Are children more like mothers than fathers? How can a father ever be certain which children are his? Where books from the 1650s seem to reach some sort of closure, recreating a gender hierarchy within the body, those of the 1660s and 1670s do not achieve the same kind of simple conclusion. Women's reproductive bodies seem to represent some of the confusions and uncertainties of the moment. They have come to signify much more than themselves.

While the crisis of paternity that shaped the tellings of the warming-pan baby stories was resolved by William's accession to the throne, female bodies did not suddenly revert to a set of simpler meanings. Female bodies continued to serve as interpretative spaces within which larger social issues might be worked through or reimagined. For example, as England became a premier commercial nation, whose economy was structured by mercantilist imperatives, Englishwomen's bodies were reformulated accordingly. By the 1690s pregnancy was compared to a merchant voyage. The women's body was like a ship, enclosing valuable cargo. Labour and delivery were just that—the delivery of goods, usually imagined as the ship coming to dock in a rock-strewn and dangerous harbour. No longer was pregnancy women's work. On the contrary, women were just the containers, loaded and unloaded by men.

The story I have outlined is one in which female bodies become freighted with many kinds of significances. In one way, bodies are always overloaded with meanings. Our bodies are a part of the social world in which we live, and we come to know those bodies through the lenses our culture offers us. What I have traced here are changes both in what female bodies meant and in how those meanings were produced and reproduced.

In other ways, however, my story is more specific to time and place. One of the central arguments of this book is that bodies are local. While the Reformation marked every European country, its impact varied from place to place. While I expect that gender relations and women's bodies were part and parcel of religious changes in other European countries, I suspect that different contexts made for considerable variation in the ways in which the meanings ascribed to female bodies changed. The upheavals in gender relations caused by the English Civil War were not immediately echoed on the Continent, and so the relationship between images of the female body and tensions in gender relations were probably different in England than in other European countries. Some of the connections between the female body and society drawn in England in the 1650s might be paralleled in France in the troubled times of the Revolution of the 1790s.

My emphasis on the local nature of understandings of the body is intended to add a layer of interpretation to the rich pan-European arguments of other scholars. Founding fathers of the history of the body such as Norbert Elias and Michel Foucault emphasized developments that took place all across Europe. They showed, for example, how the rise in centralized state power was echoed in new conceptions of the body. Thomas Laqueur also paints on a large canvas, drawing on a learned literature read by scholars in many countries and delineating a large-scale set of changes in models of the body. Because I focus on cheap print, the body stories I analyse are more particular and more contested.

The consequences of the Reformation and the Civil War for women were complex and unforseen. Eventually, transferring the right to speak about women's reproductive bodies from women to men led to improved care for labouring women. But what the nineteenth-century physician William Farr called 'a deep, dark and continuous stream' of maternal mortality was fundamentally altered only in the 1930s with the advent of sulfa drugs to treat post-partum fevers. Over the intervening centuries, Culpeper's sneers about midwifery's ignorance of anatomy took institutional form as man-midwives and then obstetricians claimed that birthing babies was their prerogative. A sphere of female expertise was slowly eclipsed. I do not wish to wax overly nostalgic about early modern midwifery or engage in ultimately unresolvable arguments about who had superior outcomes. Rather, I wish to highlight two related results of the shift from female to male authority. First, as suggested, an important arena of female work was slowly taken over by men. However, this book is about the second result: the ways in which women's reproductive bodies came to assume a whole range of meanings. Once women's bodies entered cheap print, and men assumed the right to speak about them, those bodies and the practices associated with them changed.

The two hoardings that open these Conclusions testify to this process. On the one hand, there is the image of the Mona Lisa, whose enigmatic smile here suggests that only she knows the father of her child. Unlike all the suspicious ballad fathers discussed in the previous chapters, however, today's man can wipe that smile off her face by employing DNA testing to resolve paternity. The secrets of the female body can be made known, can be open to male scrutiny as never before. The other hoarding, which imagines conception as a diagram resembling a football play, is an example of how women's reproductive bodies have assumed a range of meanings. Here, all the complexities of male and female sexual interactions are reduced to an onslaught of spermatozoa intimidating a little pink ovum. Something that happens deep inside a woman's body is opened up and made to represent a version of social reality. In this version, men are sexual aggressors, and women's role is to cower and say no. Compare this image of conception with one common in the sixteenth century, in which the womb decides whether or not it is in the mood, and if yes, opens itself to (non-threatening) semen. The womb then embraces the semen and forms a new being from it. The womb is a like woman—it desires or rejects, it embraces, it nourishes. It is not that this image of the body lacks social meanings, but those meanings are about women. Subsequent images of women's reproductive bodies make those bodies into arenas for all kinds of contests about gender relations, social structures, economic changes, and more. They open the womb to the world.

Bibliography

Primary Sources, Anonymous

An Account of the Proceedings of the New Parliament of Women Sitting at Gossips-hall ([London]: Printed for J. Coniers at the Black Raven in Duck Lane, [1683]), Wing A370.

An Account of the Reasons of the Nobility and Gentry's Invitation of His Highness the Prince of Orange into England. Being a Memorial from the English Protestants Concerning their Grievances. With a Large Account of the Birth of the Prince of Wales. Presented to their Highnesses the Prince and Princess of Orange (London: printed for Nathanael Ranew, and Jonathan Robinson, in St. Paul's Church-yard, 1688), Wing (CD-ROM) A379.

Acts and Ordinances of the Interregnum, ed. C. H. Firth and R. S. Rait (London: H.M. Stationers Office, 1911).

The Anabaptists Catechisme ([London]: Printed for R.A., 1645), Thomason E.1185[8].

Answer to I Marry and Thank ye Too; or The Lass of Lyn's Sorrowfull Lamentation for the Loss of her Maiden-head ([London]: Printed for P. Brooksby at the Golden ball in Pye-Corner, J. Deacon at the Angel in Gilt-spur Street, J. Blare at the Looking-Glass in London Bridge, near the church, J. Back at the Black Boy on London Bridge, near the Draw-bridge [c.1690]), Wing (CD-ROM) A3359A, *Pepys*, v. 245.

The Ansvver to the Buxome Virgin, or the Farmer well-fitted ([London]: Printed for J. Deacon, at the Angel in Guiltspur-street. [1685–99]), Wing (CD-ROM) A3393, Bodleian Douce 1(4b).

An Answer to the London Cuckold, Lately Fitted with a Large Pair of Horns of the New Fashion ([London]: printed for J. Deacon, at the Angel in Guilt-spur-street [1686–7]), Wing (CD-ROM) A3417A, *Pepys*, iv. 123.

The Answer to the London Lasses Folly: Or, the New-Found Father Discovered at the Camp ([London]: Printed for C. Dennisson, at the Stationers Arms within Aldgate, [1685]), Wing (CD-ROM) A3418, Bodleian Douce 1(18).

The Apprehension and Confession of Three Notorious Witches. Arreigned and by iustice condemned and executed at Chelmes-forde, in the Countye of Essex, the 5. day of Iulye, last past. 1589 ([London: E. Allde, 1589]), STC2 5114.

Aristoteles Master-piece, or, The secrets of generation displayed in all the parts thereof . . . (London: Printed for J. How, and are to be sold next door to the Anchor Tavern in Sweethings Rents in Cornhil, 1684), Wing2 A3697fA.

The Audience ([London: s.n., 1688]), Wing A4193.

The Blind Eats many a Flye, or The Broken Damsel Made Whole ([London]: Printed for P. Brooksby at the Golden-Ball, in Pye-Corner, [1672–1700]), Wing (CD-ROM) B3191, *Roxburghe*, viii. 684.

Bloody Newes from Dover ([London]: Printed in the Year of Discovery, Feb. 13. 1647), Thomason E.375[20].

Bull-Feather Hall: Or, the Antiquity and Dignity of Horns Amply Shown (London: Printed for the Society of Bull-Feathers Hall, 1664), Wing B5420.

The Bulls Feather; Being the Good-fellows Song ([London]: Printed for F. Coles, T. Vere, J. Wright, and J. Clarke, [1674–9]), Wing (CD-ROM) B5437, *Pepys*, iv. 152.

The Buxom Lass of Bread-street, or, Lamentation for the Loss of her Maiden-head ([London]: Printed for P. Brooksby, J. Deacon, J. Blare, J. Back, [1682–96]), Wing (CD-ROM) B6341C, *Pepys*, iii. 295.

The Byrth of Mankynde ([London]: Imprynted at London by T.R., 1540), STC2 21153.

The Catologue [sic] *of Contented Cuckolds: or, A Loving Society of Confessing Brethren of the Forked order* (London: printed for J. C. in Little Britain [1662–88]), Wing (CD-ROM) C1307A, *Pepys*, iv. 130.

Children after the Rate of 24 in a Yeare, Thats 2 Euery Month as Plaine Doth Appeare ([London]: printed for E.B., [*c.*1635]), STC 20320.5, *Pepys*, i. 404.

A Closet for Ladies and Gentlewomen Or, the Art of Preserving, Conserving, and Candying. . . . Also Divers Soveraigne Medicines and Salves for Sundry Diseases (London: printed by Richard Hodgkinson, 1641). Not in Thomason.

A Collection of Wonderful Miracles, Ghosts and Visions (London: Printed for Benjamin Harris, and sold by Langley Curtis in Goatham Court, 1681), Wing (CD-ROM) C3915.

The Compleat Midwifes Practice, in the most weighty and high Concernments of the Birth of Man (London: Printed for Nathaniel Brooke at the Angell in Cornhill, 1656), Wing2 C1817C; Thomason E.1588[3].

The Compleat Midvvife's Practice Enlarged . . . With a Full Supply of Those Rare Secrets Which Mr. Culpeper in His Brief Treatise of Midwifry, and Other English Writers, Have Kept Close to Themselves, Concealed, or Wholly Omitted ([London]: Printed for Nath. Brooke at the Angel in Cornhill, 1659), Wing2 C1817D; Thomason E.1723[1].

The Compleat Midvvife's Practice Enlarged . . . the Third Edition Enlarged, with the Addition of Sir Theodore Mayern's Rare Secrets in Midwifry (London: Printed for Nath. Brooke at the Angel in Corn-hill, 1663), Wing2 C1817E.

Continued Heads or Perfect Passages in Parliament ([London]: Printed at London for Andrew Coe, and are to be sold without Cripplegate, and in the Old-Bayley, 1649).

The Cony-catching Bride (Printed at London by T. F., 1643), not in Thomason.

The Cuckholds Petition to the Parliament of Women (London: printed for A. Chamberlain in St. John-Street [1684]), Wing (CD-ROM) C7455A.

The Cucking of a Scould. To the Tune Of, the Merchant of Em[d]en (Printed at London: by G.P., [*c.*1630]), STC2 6100.

A Cuckold by Consent: Or, the Frollick Miller That Intic'd a Maid ([London]: Printed for J. Wright, J. Clarke, W. Thackeray, [1681–4]), Wing (CD-ROM) C7453AC, *Pepys*, iv. 124.

Cuckolds Haven, or, The Marry'd Mans Miserie (Printed at London: by M. P. for Francis Grove, neere the Sarzens Head without Newgate [dated by STC to 1638]), STC 6101, *Roxburghe*, i. 148.

The Cuckold's Lamentation of a Bad Wife ([London]: Printed for P. Brooksby at the Golden Ball in Pye-corner, [1672–1700]), Wing (CD-ROM) C7455, Bodleian Douce 1(41a).

A Declaration of a Strange and Wonderful Monster (London: printed by Jane Coe, 1646), Thomason E.325[20].

The Deponents ([London: s.n., 1688?]), Wing D1077.

A Description of the Sect called the Familie of Love (London: printed 1641), Thomason E.168[2].

A Detection of Damnable Driftes, practized by three witches arraigned at Chelmissford in Essex (Imprinted at London for Edward White, at the little North-dore of Paules, [1579]), STC2 5115.

A Dialogue between the Crosse in Cheap, and Charing Crosse, by Ryhen Pameach [Henry Peacham] ([London]: printed Anno 1641), Thomason E.238[9].

A Dialogue between Mistris Maquerella, a Suburban Bawd, Ms Scolopendra, a noted Curtezan, and mr Pimpinello and Usher &c. (London: Printed for Edward Couch, 1650), Thomason E.607[13].

A Diary, or an Exact Journall ([London]: Printed for Matthew Walbancke, at Grayes-Inne Gate, 1644–6).

A Directory for the Publique Worship of God, Throughout the Three Kingdoms of England, Scotland, and Ireland (London: Printed for Evan Tyler, Alexander Fifield, Ralph Smith, and John Field; and are to be sold at the Signe of the Bible in Cornhill, neer the Royal-Exchange, 1644), Thomason E.273[17].

The Discontented Married Man (London: printed for Richard Harper in Smithfield [1635–42]), STC 17232, *Roxburghe*, i. 295.

A Discovery of Six Women-Preachers ([London?]: Printed, 1641), Thomason E.166[1].

Documents of the English Reformation, ed. Gerald Bray (Cambridge: J. Clarke, 1994).

The Dolefull Lamentation of Cheap-side Crosse (London, printed for F.C. and T.B., 1641), Thomason E.134[9].

England's Happiness or, A Health to the young Prince of VVales. The tune: Now, now, the fight's done (London: printed by R.M. for James Deane, in St. Jame's Market, 1688), Wing (CD-ROM) E2978A.

Englands triumph for the Prince of Wales, or, A short description of the fireworks, machines &c. (London: Printed for P.L., 1688), Wing2 E3065A.

The English Midwife Enlarged, Containing Directions to Midwives; Wherein Is Laid down Whatever Is Most Requisite for the Safe Practising Her Art (London: printed for Rowland Reynolds, next door to the Golden bottle in the Strand, at the middle Exchange door, 1682), Wing (CD-ROM) E3104.

The Essex Man Cozened by a VVhore (Printed at London for H. Gosson, [1601–40?]), STC 5420.5, *Pepys*, i. 290.

Every Woman Her Own Midwife, Or, a Compleat Cabinet Opened for Child-bearing Women (London: Printed for Simon Neale, 1675), Wing E3553.

The Examination and Confession of Certaine Wytches at Chensforde in the countie of Essex: before the Quenes Maiesties judges, the xxvi daye of July, anno 1566 (Imprynted at London: By Willyam Powell for Wyllyam Pickeringe dwelling at Sainte Magnus corner and are there for to be soulde, anno 1566.the.23.August), STC2 19869.5.

Father a Child that's None of My Own, Being the Seamans Complaint ([London]: Printed for P. Brooksby, near the Hospital-gate, in West-Smithfield, [1672–85]), Wing (CD-ROM) F545aA, Bodleian Douce 1(77a).

Father Peter's Policy Discovered: Or, the Prince of Wales Prov'd a Popish Perkin (London: [s.n.], printed in the year 1689), Wing (CD-ROM) F549.

A Full Answer to the Depositions; and to All Other the Pretences and Arguments Whatsoever, Concerning the Birth of the Prince of Wales (London: printed for Simon Burgis, 1689), Wing (CD-ROM) F2342.

The Ghost of Tom Ross to his Pupil the D. of Monmouth ([London, 1683]), Wing G640B.

Gods Handy-vvorke in VVonders. Miraculously Shewen Vpon Two Women Lately Deliuered of Two Monsters: with a Most Strange and Terrible Earth-quake, by Which, Fields and Other Grounds, Were Quite Remoued to Other Places (London: Printed [by George Purslowe] for I. W[right], 1615), STC2 11926.

The Gossips Meeting. Or, the Merry Market-women of Taunton ([London]: Printed for F. Coles, T. Vere, J. Wright, and J. Clarke, [1674–9]), Wing G1317, Bodleian Wood E 25(120).

The Great Bastard, Protector of the Little One Done out of French; and for Which a Proclamation, with a Reward of 5000 Lewedores, to Discover the Author, Was Published (Re-printed at Cologne: [s.n.], 1691), Wing2 G1663A.

Great News from a Parliament of Women, Now Sitting in Rosemary-Lane (London: Printed for A. Chamberlain in St. Johns-Street, 1684), Wing (CD-ROM) G1714.

The Hen-peckt Cuckold: or, the Cross-Grain'd Wife ([London]: Printed and sold by J. Millet, next door to the Flower-de-Luce in Little Brittain [1682–92]), Wing (CD-ROM) H1453A, *Pepys*, iv. 129.

Here after foloweth the Prymer in Englysshe sette out alonge, after the vse of Sarum ([Newly imprynted at Rown: by Nycholas le Roux, for F. Regnault, 1538]), STC 16004.

(Het Hoe, for a Husband,) or, The Parliament of Maides ([London]: Printed in the Yeare 1647), Thomason E.408[19].

Hey for Horn Fair: The General Market of England. Or Room for Cuckolds (London: printed for F. Coles, T. Vere, and J. Wright, 1674), Wing H1658A.

The Humble Petition of Many Thousands of Wives and Matrons (Printed at London for John Cookson, 1643), Thomason E.88[13].

Joy and Sorrow Mixt Together (London: printed for Iohn Wright the younger dvvelling in the Old Bayley, [1634–40]), STC 5424, *Roxburghe*, i. 509.

The Knowing of Women's Kind in Childing: A Middle English Version of Material Derived from Trotula and Other Sources, ed. Alexandra Barratt (Turnhout: Brepols, 2001).

The Ladies, A Second Time Assembled in Parliament ([London]: Printed in the Yeare 1647), Thomason E.406[23].

The Lamentable Complaints of Nick Froth the Tapster and Rulerost the Cooke ([London]: Printed in the year 1641), Thomason E.156[4].

The Lamentable Ditty of Little Mousgrove, and the Lady Barnet (London: Printed for H. Gosson [*c.*1630]), STC 18316.3, *Pepys*, i. 364.

The Lamentation of Seven Journeymen-Taylors, Being Sent up in a Letter From York-shire ([London]: Printed for I. Deacon, at the Angel in Guilt-spur-street, [1671–1704]), Wing L287, Bodleian Douce 1(113a).

The Lass of Lynn's New Joy for finding a father for her Child ([London]: Printed and sold by J. Millet, next door to the Flower-de-Luce in Little-Brittain, [1685–90]), Wing (CD-ROM) L462E, *Pepys*, iii. 300.

Letters and Papers, Foreign and Domestic, of the Reign of Henry VIII, ed. James Gairdner (London: Printed for Her Majesty's Printing Office by Eyre and Spottiswoode, 1887).

The London Cuckold: or, An Ancient Citizens Head Well Fitted with a Flourishing Pair of Fashionable Horns ([London]: Printed for J. Back, at the Black-Boy on London-Bridge, near the Drawbridge, [1685–8]), Wing (CD-ROM) L2894, *Roxburghe*, viii. 601.

Ludus Coventriae; or, the Plaie called Corpus Christi, ed. K. S. Block, EETS, e.s. 120 (Oxford: Oxford University Press, 1922).

The Man in the Moon Discovering a World of Knavery under the Sunne ([London]: Printed at the full of the moon, and are to be sold at the signe of Scorpio, for the good of the state, 1649).

The Mary Play from the N-Town Manuscript, ed. Peter Meredith (Exeter: University of Exeter Press, 1997).

Match me these Two: or the Convicton [sic] *and Arraignment of Britannicus and Lilburne. With An answer to a Pamphlet, entitled, The Parliament of Ladies* ([London]: Printed in the Yeere 1647), Thomason E.400[9].

A Melius Inquirendum into the Birth of the Prince of Wales: or an Account of Several New Depositions and Arguments Pro and Con (London: printed for J. Wilks in St. James's Street, 1689), Wing (CD-ROM) M1646.

Mercurius Brittanicus. Communicating Intelligence from All Parts, and Touching and Handling the Humors and Conceits of Mercurius Pragmaticus ([London: s.n., 1649]).

Mercurius Democritus ([London: printed by J. Crowch, and T[homas]. W[ilson]], 1652–4).

Mercurius Elenticus (For King Charles the II) ([London: s.n., 1650]).

Mercurius Pragmaticus ([London: s.n., 1649–50]).

The Middle English Stanzaic Versions of the Life of Saint Anne, ed. Roscoe Parker, EETS o.s. 174 (London: Milford, for Oxford University Press,1928).

The Mid-Wives Just Petition (Printed at London, 1643), Thomason E.86[14].

Mistris Parliament Brought to Bed of a Monstrous Childe of Reformation ([London]: Printed in the yeer of the Saints fear, 1648), Thomason E.437[24].

Mistris Parliament her Gossipping ([London]: printed in the yeer of the downfall of the sectaries, 1648), Thomason E.443[28].

Mrs. Parliament, her invitation of mrs. London, to a Thanksgiving dinner ([London]: Printed in the year. 1648), Thomason E.446[7].

Mistris Parliament presented in her bed ([London]: Printed in the yeer of the saints fear, 1648), Thomason E.441[21].

Moderare [sic] *Intelligencer. Comprising the Summe of All Occurrences in England, Scotland, and Ireland* (London: printed by Robert Wood, [1653]), Thomason E.711[17].

The Most Strange and Admirable Discouerie of the Three Witches of Warboys, Arraigned, Conuicted, and Executed at the Last Assises at Huntington, for the Bewitching of the Fiue Daughters of Robert Throckmorton Esquire (London: Printed by the Widdowe Orwin, for Thomas Man, and Iohn Winington, and are to be solde in Paternoster Rowe, at the signe of the Talbot, 1593), STC2 25019.

A Nest of Serpents Discovered. Or, a knot of old Heretiques revived, called the Adamites ([London]: Printed in the yeare 1641), Thomason E.168[12].

A Newe Boke, Conteyninge an Exhortacio[n] to the Sycke. The Sycke Mans Prayer. A Prayer With Thankes, at the Purification of Women. A Consolacion at Buryall ([London: T. Raynold?], M. D. XLVIII [1548]), STC2 3363.

Newes from Perin in Cornwall (London: Printed by E.A[llde] and are to be solde at Christ-Church gate, 1618), STC2 19614.

No Fool to the Old Fool: or, A Cuckold in Querpo (London: printed for F. G. [c.1650]), not in Wing, Bodleian Wood 401(40ᵛ, 39ʳ).

Original Letters Relative to the English Reformation, trans. and ed. Hastings Robinson, for the Parker Society (Cambridge: Cambridge University Press, 1846).

A Parliament of Ladies ([London]: Printed in the yeer 1647), Thomason E.388[4].

The Parliament of Women (London: Printed for John Holford, at the Crown in the Pall-Mall, 1684), Wing (CD-ROM) P506A.

A Perfect Diurnall of Some Passages in Parliament, and from Other Parts of this Kingdom ([London]: Printed for Francis Coles and Laurence Blaikelock: and are to be sold at their shops in the Old-Baily, and at Temple-Bar, [1643–9]).

Perfect Occurrences of Every Dayes Iournall in Parliament, and Other Moderate Intelligence (London: Printed for I[ane] Coe, and A[ndrew]. Coe, and are to be sold at Cripplegate, and in the Old-Baily, [1647–9]).

The Petition of the Weamen of Middlesex (London: Printed for William Bowden, 1641), Thomason E.180[17].

Pierce the Plowman's Crede, ed. Walter W. Skeat, EETS o.s. 30 (London: N. Trubner, 1873).

Pigges Corantoe, or Nevves from the North (London: Printed for L.C. and M.W., 1642), Thomason E.153[7].

A Pittilesse Mother. That Most Vnnaturally at One Time, Murthered Two of Her Owne Children at Acton Within Six Miles from London Vppon Holy Thursday Last 1616. ([London]: Printed [by G. Eld] for J. Trundle, and sold by J. Wright, [1616]), STC2 24757.

A Pleasant Dialogue Betwixt Two VVanton Ladies of Pleasure; Or, the Dutchess of Porsmouths Woful Farwel to Her Former Felicity ([London]: Printed for J. Deacon in Guiltspur-street, [1685]), Wing (CD-ROM) P2543B, *Bagford*, ii. 599–62.

A Pleasant History of a Gentleman in Thracia (Printed at London: for H.G. [dated by STC to 1633]), STC 24047, *Roxburghe*, ii. 262.

Portsmouths Lamentation, Or, a Dialogue Between Two Amorous Ladies, E.G. and D.P. ([London]: Printed for C. Dennisson, at the Stationers-Arms, within Aldgate, [1685]), Wing (CD-ROM) P3008, *Bagford*, ii. 606–8.

Thys primer of Salysbury use (Newly imprynted at London: By W. Rastell, the xxx day of Apryll in ye xxiiii yere of the reyn of kyng Henry the viii and in ye yere of our lorde MCCCCCxxxii.), STC 15976.

This Primer of Salysbury vse is a set out a long Latin (Parys: venudatur a F. Regnault, 1531), STC 15971.

This prymer of Salysbury use ([Parys: F. Regnault, 1535]), STC 15986.7.

The Princely triumph: or, Englands joy in the birth of the young Prince of Wales: born on the 10th. of June, 1688 ([London]: Printed for P. Brooksby, at the Golden Ball in Pye Corner, near West-Smithfield, [1688]), Wing (CD-ROM) P3491B, *Pepys*, ii. 251.

The Proctor and Parator their Mourning: Or, the lamentation of the Doctors Commons for their downfall ([London]: Printed in the year 1641), Thomason E.156[13].

The Protestant Cuckold: a New Ballad. Being a Full and Perfect Relation How B.H. the Protestant-news-forger, Caught His Beloved Wife Ruth in Ill Circumstances (London: printed for Francis Smith, 1681), Wing (CD-ROM) P3829, Bodleian Wood 417(58).

The Queens Closet Opened. Incomparable Secrets in Physick, Chirurgery, Preserving, Candying, and Cookery; as They Were Presented to the Qveen by the Most Experienced Persons of Our Times ([London]: Printed for Nathaniel Brook at the Angel in Cornhill, 1655), Thomason E.1519[1].

The Ranters Declaration (Imprinted at London, by J.C. MDCL), Thomason E.620[2].

The Ranters Monster: Being a True Relation of One Mary Adams, living at Tillingham in Essex (London: printed for George Horton, 1652), Thomason E.658[6].

The Ranters Ranting (London: Printed by B. Alsop, 1650), Thomason E.618[8].

The Ranters Religion. Or, A Faithfull and Infallible Narrative of Their Damnable and Diabolical Opinions (London: printed for R.H., 1650), Thomason E.619[8].

A Rehearsall Both Straung and True, of Hainous and Horrible Actes Committed by Elizabeth Stile, alias Rockingham, Mother Dutten, Mother Deuell, Mother Margaret, fower notorious witches, apprehended at Winsore in the countie of Barks (Imprinted at London: [By J. Kingston] for Edward White at the little north-doore of Paules, at the signe of the Gun, and are there to be sold, [1579]), STC2 23267.

The Reign of James II. Playing cards, Department of Prints and Drawings, British Museum.

Religious Lyrics of the XV Century, ed. Carleton Brown (Oxford: Clarendon Press, 1939).

The Resolution of the Women of London to the Parliament ([London]: for William Watson, 1642), Thomason E.114[140].

The Rich and Flourishing Cuckold Well Satisfied ([London]: Printed for F. Coles, T. Vere, J. Wright, and J. Clarke, [1674–9]), Wing (CD-ROM) R1366, Bodleian Wood E 25(123).

A Rich Closet of Physical Secrets (London: printed by Gartrude Dawson and are to be sold by William Nealand, at the Crown in Duck-Lane, 1652), Thomason E.670[1].

Rock the Cradle, John: or, Children after the rate of Twenty-four in a yeere (Printed at London for E.B.[1631?]), STC 20320, *Roxburghe*, vii. 162.

Rocke the Babie Ioane: or Iohn his Petition to his louing Wife Ioane (Printed at London: for H.G. [1630s]), STC 21138.5, *Pepys*, i. 396.

Roger the Millers Present sent by the Farmers Daughter to his cousin Tom the Taylor in London ([London]: Printed for J. Blare, at the Looking-Glass on London Bridge, [1685–8]), Wing (CD-ROM) R1792A, *Pepys*, iii. 211.

The Routing of the Ranters (n.p., n.d. [1650]), Thomason E.616[9].

The Saint Turn'd Curtezan: Or, a New Plot Discover'd ([London]: Printed for the use of the Protestant-Cobler in Pell-Mell, [1681]), Wing S359, Bodleian Wood 417(65).

The Sarum Missal in English (London: The Church Press, 1867).

The Seven Women Confessors (London: Printed for John Smith, [1641]), Thomason E.134[15].

*The Several Declarations, Together with the Several Depositions Made in Council, on Monday the 22d of October, 1688, Concerning the Birth of the Prince of Wales. N.B. Those mark'd thus * were Roman Catholicks* (London: printed and sold by the booksellers of London and Westminster, 1688), Wing S2760.

Several Proceedings of Parliament (London: printed by John Field, 1653).

The Sham Prince Expos'd in a Dialogue Between the Popes Nuncio and Bricklayers Wife, Nurse to the Supposed Prince of Wales ([London: s.n.], 1688), Wing S2961.

The Sisters of the Scabards Holiday: or, A dialogue between two reverent and very vertuous Matrons ([London]: Printed, 1641), Thomason E.168[8].

The Sommerset-shire Damsel beguil'd; or, The Bonny Baker chous'd in his bargain ([London]: Printed for J. Blare, at the sign of the Looking-Glass on London Bridge, [1685–8; dated from the licensor]), Wing (CD-ROM) S4653, *Pepys*, iv. 22.

A Spirit Moving in the VVomen-preachers (London: Printed for Henry Sheppard, at the Bible in Tower-Street, William Lay, at Pauls Chaine neere the Doctors Commons, 1646), Thomason E.324[10].

The Spirituall Courts Epitomized, in a dialogue beetwixt two Proctors ([London]: Printed 1641), Thomason E.157[15].

Strange Newes of a Prodigious Monster, Borne in the Towneship of Adlington in the parish of Standish in the Countie of Lancaster, the 17. day of Aprill last, 1613 ([London]: Printed by I. P[indley] for S. M[an] and are to be sold at his shop in Pauls Church-yard at the signe of the Ball, 1613), STC2 15428.

Strange Nevves out of Kent, of a Monstrous and Misshapen Child, Borne in Olde Sandwitch, Vpon the 10. Of Iulie, Last, the like (For Strangenes) Hath Neuer Beene Seene (Imprinted at London: By T. C[reede] for W. Barley, and are to be sold at his shop in Gratious-street, 1609), STC2 14934.

Sundrye strange and inhumaine murthers (Printed at London: By Thomas Scarlet, 1591), STC2 18286.5.

The Thankfull Country Lass, or The Jolly Batchelor Kindly Entertained ([London]: Printed for J. Bissel, at the Bible and Harp near the Hospital-Gate in West-Smithfield), not in Wing, *Pepys*, v. 398.

Three Chapters of Letters Relating to the Suppression of the Monasteries, edited from the originals in the British Museum, ed. Thomas Wright, Camden Society, 26 (1843).

To the Honourable House of Commons Assembled in Parliament. The humble petition of many thousand poore people, in and around the city of London (London: Printed for Will. Larner and T.B. This 31 of January 1642), Thomason 669.f.4[54].

To the Supream Authority of England The Commons Assembled in Parliament ([London: s.n., 1649]), Wing2 T1724A.

To the Supream authority of this nation (Imprinted at London, 1649), Thomason E.551[14].

The Trotula. A Medieval Compendium of Women's Medicine, ed. Monica H. Green (Philadelphia: University of Pennsylvania Press, 2001).

A True Copie of the Petition of the Gentlewomen, and Tradesmens-wives (London: Printed by R.O. and G.D. for John Bull, 1641), Thomason E.134[17].

The True Diurnall Occurances (London: printed for F.L. and Geo. Thompson, 1642).

Two Most Vnnaturall and Bloodie Murthers (Printed at London: By V. S[immes] for Nathanael Butter dwelling in Paules churchyard neere Saint Austens gate, 1605), STC2 18288.

The Virgins Complaint for the Losse of their Sweet-Hearts (London: printed for Henry Wilson, 1642), Thomason E.86[38].

Visitation Articles and Injunctions of the Period of the Reformation, ed. Walter Frere with the assistance of William Kennedy, Alcuin Club Collections, 15 (London: Longmans, Green, 1910).

The Waking Vision; or, Reality in a Fancy (London: Printed by N.T., 1681), Wing W282, *Bagford*, ii. 788.

The Widovves Lamentation (Printed at London for John Robinson, 1643), Thomason E.88[26].

The Woman to the Plow and the Man to the Hen-roost ([London]: Printed for J. Wright, J. Clarke, W. Thackeray, and T. Passinger, [1681–4]), Wing (CD-ROM) P448B, Bodleian Don. b.13(106).

A VVomans VVork Is Never Done (London: printed for John Andrews, at the White Lion in Pye-Corner, [1660?]), Wing (CD-ROM) W3326.

Young Jemmy. An Excellent New Ballad, to an Excellent New Tune (London: printed for Alexander Banks, 1681), Wing Y102A, Bodleian Firth b.20(84).

Primary Sources, Author Listed

AUSTEN, R. A., *A Treatise of Fruit=Trees* (Oxford: printed for Tho: Robinson, 1653), Wing2 A4238, Thomason E.701[5].

BARGRAVE, JOHN, *Pope Alexander the Seventh and the College of Cardinals, with a Catalog of Dr. Bargrave's Museum* (London: printed for the Camden Society, vol. 92, 1867).

BARKER, THOMAS, *The Country-mans Recreation, or the Art of Planting, Graffing, and Gardening, in Three Books* (London: printed by T. Mabb, for William Shears, and are to be sold at the signe of the Bible in St. Pauls Church-yard, near the little north door, 1654), Wing2 B784, Thomason E.806[16].

BARLOW, FRANCIS, [?], *The Revolution*. Playing cards, Department of Prints and Drawings, British Museum.

BECKE, EDMUND, *A Brefe Confutation of this Most Destestable, and Anabaptistical Opinion* (Imprinted at London by John Day dwellynge over Aldersgate, and William seres dwellynge in Peter College, 1550), STC2 1709.

BENTLEY, THOMAS, *The Monument of Matrones conteining seuen seuerall Lamps of Virginitie, or distinct treatises* ([London]: Printed by H. Denham, [1582]), STC 1892.

BERENGARIO DA CARPI, JACOPO, *Carpi Commentaria cum amplissimis additionibus super Anatomia Mundini una cum textu ejusdem in pristinum & verum nitorem redacto* (Bononiae, Impressum per Hieronymum de Benedictis, 1521).

BOAISTUAU, PIERRE, *Certaine Secrete wonders of Nature* (Imprinted at London, by Henry Bynneman dwelling in Knightrider streat, at the signe of the Mermaid Anno 1569), STC 10787.

BOKENHAM, OSBERN, *Legendys of Hooly Wummen*, ed. M. J. Serjeantson (London, EETS, by H. Milford, Oxford University Press, 1938).

CARY, MARY, *The Little Horns Doom & Downfall* (London: Printed for the Author, and are to be sold at the sign of the Black-spred Eagle, at the West end of Pauls, 1651), Thomason E.1274[1].

—— *A Word in Season to the Kingdom of England* (London: Printed by R.W. for Giles Calvert, and are to be sold at the Black-spred Eagle at the West end of Pauls, 1647), Thomason E.393[26].

CHAMBERLEN, PETER, *Dr. Chamberlain's Midwifes Practice: Or, a Guide for Women in That High Concern of Conception, Breeding, and Nursing Children* (London: printed for Thomas Rooks at the Lamb and Ink-Bottle, at the East-end of S. Pauls; who makes and sells the best ink for records, 1665), Wing (CD-ROM) C1817H.

CHIDLEY, KATHERINE, *The Justification of the Independent Churches of Christ* (London: Printed for William Larnar, and are to be sold at his Shop, at the Signe of the Golden Anchor, neere Pauls-Chaine, 1641), Thomason E.174[7].

—— *A New-Yeares-Gift, or a brief exhortation to Mr. Thomas Edwards* (s.l.: s.n., printed in the year, 1645), Thomason E.23[13].

COUCHMAN, OBADIAH, *The Adamites Sermon: Containing Their Manner of Preaching, Expounding, and Prophesying* ([London]: Printed for Francis Coules, in the Yeare, 1641), not in Thomason, Wing (CD-ROM) A475B.

CROOKE, HELKIAH, *Mikrokosmographia: A Description of the Body of Man* ([London]: Printed by William Iaggard dwelling in Barbican, and are there to be sold, 1615), STC2 6062.

CULPEPER, NICHOLAS, *Culpeper's School of Physick* (London: Printed for N. Brook at the Angel in Cornhill, 1659), Thomason E.1739[1].

—— *A Directory for Midvvives* (London: Printed by Peter Cole, at the sign of the Printing-Press in Cornhill, near the Royal Exchange, 1651), Thomason E.1340[1].

—— *An Ephemeris for the yeer 1651* ([London]: Printed by Peter Cole, and are to be sold at his shop at the sign of the Printing Press in Cornhil, near the Royal Exchange, 1651), Thomason E.1343[1].

—— *Pharmacopoeia Londinensis: or the London Dispensatory* (London: Printed for Peter Cole, at the sign of the Printing-Press in Cornhil neer the Royal Exchange, 1653), Wing (CD-ROM) C7525.

—— *A Physicall Directory or A Translation of the London Dispensatory* (London: Printed for Peter Cole and are to be sold at his Shop at the sign of the Printing-presse near to the Royall Exchange, 1649), Thomason E.576[1].

—— *A Physical Directory*, 2nd edn. (London: printed by Peter Cole, and are to be sold at his shop at the sign of the Printing-Press in Cornhil, near the Royal Exchange, 1650), Wing (CD-ROM) C7541.

DYMOND, DAVID, and PAINE, CLIVE (eds.), *The Spoil of Melford Church: The Reformation in a Suffolk Parish* ([Bury St. Edmunds]: Salient Press [Suffolk County Council], 1992).

EDWARDS, THOMAS, *Gangraena: Or a Catalog and Discovery of many of the Errours, heresies, blasphemies and pernicious practices of the sects* (London: Printed for Ralph Smith, at the Signe of the Bible in Corn hill near the Royall-Exchange, 1646), Thomason E.323[3].

—— *Reasons against the Independent Government of Particular Congregations* (London: printed by Richard Cotes for Jo. Bellamie, & Ralph Smith, dwelling at the signe of the three Golden Lions, in Corne-hill neere the Royall Exchange, 1641), Thomason E.167[16].

FONTANUS, NICHOLAS, *The Womans Doctour, Or, an Exact and Distinct Explanation of All Such Diseases as Are Peculiar to That Sex* (London: Printed for John Blague and Samuel Howes, and are to be sold at their shop in Popes Head-Alley, 1652), Thomason E.1284[2], Wing2 F1418A.

FORREST, PIETER VAN, *Observationum et Curationum Medicinalium Liber Vigesimusoctavus, De Mulierum Morbis. Una cum scholiis* ([Lugduni Batavorum] Ex Officina Plantiniana, apud Christophorum Raphelengium, 1599).

FOXE, JOHN, *The Acts and Monuments*, ed. George Townsend (New York: AMS Press, 1965).

GOODCOLE, HENRY, *Natures Cruell Step-dames: or, Matchlesse monsters of the female sex; Elizabeth Barnes, and Anne Willis* (Printed at London: [By E. Purslowe] for Francis Coules, dwelling in the Old-Baily, 1637), STC2 12012.

GOUGE, WILLIAM, *Of Domesticall Duties Eight Treatises* (London: Printed by John Haviland for William Bladen, and are to be sold at the signe of the Bible neere the great North doore of Pauls, 1622), STC 12119.

GREENE, ROBERT, *Penelopes VVeb: VVherein a Christall Myrror of Fæminine Perfection Represents to the Viewe of Euery One Those Vertues and Graces* (Imprinted at London: [by Thomas Orwin?] for T[homas] C[adman] and E[dward] A[ggas], [1587]), STC2 12293.

GREY, ELIZABETH, Countess of Kent, *A Choice Manual of Rare and Select Secrets in Physick and Chyrurgery; collected, and practised by the Right Honorable, the Countesse of Kent, late deceased* (London: printed by G.D. and are to be sold by William Shears, at the Sign of the Bible in S. Pauls Church-yard, 1653), Wing (CD-ROM) K310B.

GUILLEMEAU, JACQUES, *Child-birth Or, the Happy Deliuerie of VVomen. VVherein Is Set Downe the Gouernment of Women. In the Time of Their Breeding Childe* (London: Printed by A. Hatfield, 1612), STC2 12496.

H., L., *A Strange Wonder or Wonder in A Woman* (London: Printed for I.T., 1642), Thomason E.144[5].

HARRIS, EDWARD, *A True Relation of Brownists, Separatists, and Non-Conformists in Monmouthshire in Wales* ([London]: Printed in the yeare 1641), Thomason E.172[31].

HENRY, PHILIP, *The Diaries and Letters of Philip Henry, MA, of Broad Oak, Flintshire, 1631–1696*, ed. Matthew Henry Lee (London: Kegan Paul, Trench & Co., 1882).

HILLIARD, JOHN, *Fire from Heauen. Burning the body of one Iohn Hittchell* (Printed at London: [By E. Allde] for Iohn Trundle, and are to be sold at his shop in Barby can at the signe of Nobody, 1613), STC2 13507.3.

HOOPER, JOHN, *A Lesson of thee Incarnation of Christe* ([Imprinted at Londo[n]: In Paules Church yearde, at the signe of the Starre. By Thomas Raynalde, M. D. L.] [1550]), STC 13762.

HUTCHINSON, ROGER, *The Works of Roger Hutchinson*, ed. John Brice, for the Parker Society (Cambridge: Cambridge University Press, 1847).

JESSEY, HENRY, *The Exceeding Riches of Grace Advanced* (London: Printed by Matthew Simmons for Henry Overton, and Hannah Allen, and are to be sold at their shops in Popes-head Alley, 1647), Wing2 J687.

——*A Storehouse of Provision, to Further Resolution in Severall Cases of Conscience* (London: printed by Charles Sumptner for T[homas] Brewster and G[regory] Moule, and are to be sold at the three Bibles in Pauls-Church-yard neere the west-end, 1650), Wing (CD-ROM) J698.

JINNER, SARAH, *An Almanack and Prognostication for the Year of Our Lord 1659. Being the third after bissextile or leap year . . . By Sarah Jinner student in astrology* (London: printed by J.S. for the Company of Stationers, [1659]), Wing2 A1845.

JOCELINE, ELIZABETH, *The Mother's Legacie to her Vnborne Childe* (London: Printed by Iohn Hauiland, for William Barret, 1624), STC2 14624.

JORDEN, EDWARD, *A Briefe Discourse of a Disease Called the Suffocation of the Mother. Written Vppon Occasion Which Hath Beene of Late Taken Thereby, to Suspect Possession of an Euill Spirit, or Some Such like Supernaturall Power* (London: printed by Iohn Windet, dwelling at the signe of the Crosse Keyes at Powles Wharfe, 1603), STC2 14790.

LAKE, ARTHUR, 'A Sermon Preached at St. Cutberts in Welles When certaine persons did Penance for being at Conventicles where a Woman Preached', in *Sermons with Some Religious and Divine Meditations* (London: W. Stansby for Nathanial Butter, 1629), STC2 15134.

LATIMER, HUGH, *Sermons and Remains of Hugh Latimer*, ed. George Elwes Corrie, for the Parker Society (Cambridge: Cambridge University Press, 1845).

LAWSON, WILLIAM, *A New Orchard and Garden* (London: Printed for George Sawbridge, at the Sign of the Bible on Ludgate-Hill, 1676), Wing (CD-ROM) L736.

LEIGH, DOROTHY, *The Mothers Blessing. Or the Godly Counsaile of a Gentle-woman Not Long since Deceased* (Printed at London: For Iohn Budge, and are to be sold at the great South-dore of Paules, and at Brittaines Burse, 1616), STC2 15402.

LEMNIUS, LEVINUS, *A Discourse Touching Generation. Collected out of Lævinus Lemnius, a Most Learned Physitian. Fit for the Use of Physitians, Midwifes, and All Young Married People* (London: printed by John Streater, 1664), Wing (CD-ROM) L1043A.

——*A Discoruse* [sic] *Touching Generation*, 2nd edn. (London: By John Streater, 1667), Wing (CD-ROM) L1043B.

—— *The Secret Miracles of Nature* (London: printed by Jo. Streater, and are to be sold by Humphrey Moseley at the Prince's Arms in S. Paul's Church-Yard, John Sweeting at the Angel in Popes-Head-Alley, John Clark at Mercers-Chappel, and George Sawbridge at the Bible on Ludgate-Hill, 1658), Wing L1044.

LOCKE, JOHN, *A Strange and Lamentable Accident That Happened Lately at Mears Ashby* (Printed in London for Rich: Harper and Thomas Wine, and are to be sold at the Bible and Harpe in Smithfield, 1642), Thomason E.113[15].

LUPTON, THOMAS, *A Thousand Notable Things, of Sundry Sortes* (Imprinted at London: By Iohn Charlewood, for Hughe Spooner, dwelling in Lumbardstreete at the signe of the Cradle, [1579]), STC 16955.

Making the News: An Anthology of the Newsbooks of Revolutionary England, 1641–1660, ed. Joad Raymond (New York: St. Martin's Press, 1993).

MASSARIA, ALESSANDRO, *De Morbis Foemineis, the Womans Counsellour: Or, the Feminine Physitian* (London: printed for John Streater, and are to be sold by the booksellers in London, 1657), Wing2 M1028; Thomason E.1650[3].

MAURICEAU, FRANÇOIS, *The Accomplisht Midwife, Treating of the Diseases of Women with Child* (London: printed by John Darby; and are to be sold by Benjamin Billingsley, at the Printing-Press in Cornhil near the Royal-Exchange, 1673), Wing (CD-ROM) M1371A.

MEAGER, LEONARD, *The English Gardener* (London: Printed for P. Parker at the first shop on the right hand in Popes-Head-Alley going out of Cornhil, 1670), Wing (CD-ROM) M1568.

MIRK, JOHN, *Mirk's Festial: A Collection of Homilies, by Johannes Mirkus (John Mirk)*, ed. Theodore Erbe, part 1, EETS e.s. 97 (London: Kegan Paul Trench Trubner, 1905).

PARSONS, ROBERT, *The VVarn-vvord to Sir Francis Hastinges Wast-vvord* ([Antwerp: Printed by A. Conincx] Permissu superiorum, Anno 1602), STC2 19418.

PORTA, JOHN BAPTISTA, *Natural Magick* (London: Printed for John Wright next to the sign of the Globe in Little-Britain, 1669), Wing2 P2982A.

R., I., *A Most Straunge, and True Discourse, of the Wonderfull Iudgement of God. Of a Monstrous, Deformed Infant, Begotten by Incestuous Copulation, Betweene the Brothers Sonne and the Sisters Daughter, Being Both Vnmarried Persons* (Imprinted at London: [By E. Allde] for Richard Iones, 1600), STC2 20575.

RAY, JOHN, *A Collection of English Proverbs* (Cambridge: printed by John Hayes for W. Morden, 1670), Wing (CD-ROM) R386.

RAYNALDE, THOMAS, *The Byrth of Mankynde, otherwyse named the Womans booke* (London: Tho. Ray. [1545]), STC 21154.

RÖSSLIN, EUCHARIUS, *When Midwifery became the Male Physician's Province: The Sixteenth-Century Handbook, The Rose Garden for Pregnant Women and Mid-wives, Newly Englished,* trans. Wendy Arons (Jefferson, NC: McFarland & Co., 1994).

ROWLANDS, SAMUEL, *Tis Merrie VVhen Gossips Meete* (At London: Printed by W. W[hite] and are to be sold by George Loftus at the Golden Ball in Popeshead Alley, 1602), STC2 21409.

RUEFF, JACOB, *De Conceptu et Generatione Hominis, et iis quae circa hec potissimum* ([Zurich]: Christophorus Froschoverus excudebat Tiguri, anno M.D.LIIII. [1554]).

—— *The Expert Midwife, or An Excellent and Most Necessary Treatise of the Generation and Birth of Man* (London: Printed by E. G[riffin] for S. B[urton] and are to be sold by Thomas Alchorn at the signe of the Greene Dragon in Saint Pauls church-yard, 1637), STC2 21442.

SADLER, JOHN, *The Sicke-VVoman's Private Looking-Glasse* (London: Printed by Anne Griffin, for Philemon Stephens, and Christopher Merideth, at the Golden Lion in S. Pauls Church-yard, 1636), STC2 21544.

SERMON, WILLIAM, *The Ladies Companion, Or, the English Midwife* (London: Printed for Edward Thomas, 1671), Wing2 S2628.

SHARP, JANE, *The Midwives Book. Or the Whole Art of Midwifry Discovered. Directing Childbearing Women How to Behave Themselves in Their Conception, Breeding, Bearing, and Nursing of Children* (London: printed for Simon Miller, at the Star at the west end of St. Pauls, 1671), Wing2 S2969B. See the modern edition: Jane Sharp, *The Midwives Book*, ed. Elaine Hobby (Oxford: Oxford University Press, 1999).

SOWERBY, LEONARD, *The Ladies Dispensatory* (London: Printed for R. Ibbitson, to be sold by George Calvert at the Halfe-Moon in Watling street, 1652), Thomason E.1258[1].

SPIEGEL, ADRIAAN VAN DE, *De Formato Foetu Liber Singularis: Aeneis Figuris Exornatus* (Padua: Apud Jo. Bap. de Martinis, & Livium Pasquatum, expensis ejusdem Liberalis Cremae, [1626]).

STOWE, JOHN, *Three Fifteenth-Century Chronicles*, ed. James Gairdner, The Camden Society, 28 (London: 1880).

STRYPE, JOHN, *Annals of the Reformation*, in *Strype's Works* (Oxford: Clarendon Press, 1822).

—— *Ecclesiastical Memorials*, in *Strype's Works* (Oxford: Clarendon Press, 1822).

SUDELL, NICHOLAS, *Mulierum Amicus: Or, the Womans Friend; Plainly Discovering All Those Diseases That Are Incident to That Sex* ([London]: Printed for the author, and is to be sold by J. Hancock in Popes-head-Alley in the year, 1666), Wing2 S6143.

SWAN, JOHN, *A True and Breife Report, of Mary Glouers Vexation, and of Her Deliuerance by the Meanes of Fastinge and Prayer* ([London?: s.n.], Imprinted. 1603), STC2 23517.

T., D., *Certain Queries, or Considerations presented to the view of all that desire Reformation of Grievances* (London: printed for Giles Calvert, and are to be sold at the Sign of the Black spread-eagle at the West end of Pauls, 1651), Thomason E.647[10].

TAYLOR, JOHN, *The Needles Excellency* (London: Printed for James Boler and are to be sold at the Signe of the Marigold in Paules Churchyard, 1631), STC2 23775.5.

VORAGINE, JACOBUS DE, *The Golden Legend,* trans. William Granger Ryan (Princeton: Princeton University Press, 1993).

W., W., *A True and Iust Recorde, of the Information, Examination and Confession of All the Witches, Taken at S. Ofes in the Countie of Essex: Whereof Some Were Executed, and Other Some Entreated According to the Determination of Lawe* (Imprinted in London: At the three Cranes in the Vinetree by Thomas Dawson, 1582), STC2 24922.

WHITE, JOHN, *A Rich Cabinet, with Variety of Inventions in Several Arts and Sciences,* The fifth edition, with many additions (London: printed for William Whitwood at the sign of the Golden Bell in Duck-Lane near Smith-field, 1677), Wing2 W1792.

WIGHT, SARAH, *A Wonderful Pleasant and Profitable Letter Written by Mris Sarah Wight* (London: Printed by James Cottrel, for Ri. Moone, at the seven Stars in Pauls Churchyard, 1656), Thomason E.1681[1].

Witchcraft in England, 1558–1618, ed. Barbara Rosen (Amherst: University of Massachusetts Press, 1991).

WOLVERIDGE, JAMES, *Speculum Matricis Hybernicum, Or, the Irish Midwives Handmaid* (London: Printed by E. Okes, and are to be sold by Rowland Reynolds, 1670), Wing2 W3319.

YARB, SAMOTH [THOMAS BRAY], *A New Sect of Religion Descryed, called Adamites* ([London]: Printed anno. 1641), not in Thomason Wing (CD-ROM) B4281C.

Selected Secondary Sources

ACHINSTEIN, SHARON, 'Women on Top in the Pamphlet Literature of the English Revolution', *Women's Studies,* 24 (1994), 131–63.

AMUSSEN, SUSAN, *An Ordered Society: Gender and Class in Early Modern England* (Oxford: Oxford University Press, 1988).

APPERSON, G. L., *English Proverbs and Proverbial Phrases: A Historical Dictionary* (London: J. M. Dent, 1929).

ASTON, MARGARET, *England's Iconoclasts* (Oxford: Clarendon Press, 1988).

—— *Lollards and Reformers: Images and Literacy in Late Medieval Religion* (London: Hambledon, 1984).

ATKINSON, COLIN B. and JO B., 'The Identity and Life of Thomas Bentley, Compiler of *The Monument of Matrones*', *Sixteenth-Century Journal,* 31 (2001), 323–47.

—— and STONEMAN WILLIAM P. ' "These Griping Greefes and Pinching Pangs": Attitudes to Childbirth in Thomas Bentley's *The Monument of Matrones* (1582)', *Sixteenth-Century Journal,* 21 (1990), 193–205.

BARRY, JONATHAN, 'Introduction: Keith Thomas and the Problem of Witchcraft', in Jonathan Barry, Marianne Hester, and Gareth Roberts (eds.), *Witchcraft in Early Modern Europe* (Cambridge: Cambridge University Press, 1996), 1–45.

BECKWITH, SARAH, *Signifying God: Social Relations and Symbolic Act in the York Corpus Christi Plays* (Chicago: University of Chicago Press, 2001).

BEIER, LUCINDA MCCRAY, *Sufferers and Healers: The Experience of Illness in Seventeenth-Century England* (London: Routledge & Kegan Paul, 1987).

BENNETT, JUDITH M., 'Confronting Continuity', *Journal of Women's History,* 9 (1997), 73–94.

BERG, CHRISTINA, and BERRY, PHILLIPA, 'Spiritual Whoredom: An Essay on Female Prophets in the Seventeenth Century', in Francis Barker et al. (eds.), *1642: Literature and Power in the Seventeenth Century* (Proceedings of the Essex Conference on the Sociology of Literature, Colchester, 1981), 37–54.

BLAGDEN, CYPRIAN, 'Notes on the Ballad Market in the Second Half of the Seventeenth Century', *Studies in Bibliography,* 6 (1954), 162–81.

BOSSY, JOHN, *The English Catholic Community, 1570–1850* (Oxford: Oxford University Press, 1976).

BRAILSFORD, H. N., *The Levellers and the English Revolution* (London: Cresset Press, 1961).

BRAY, FRANCESCA, *Technology and Gender: Fabrics of Power in Late Imperial China* (Berkeley: University of California Press, 1997).

BRIGDEN, SUSAN, *London and the Reformation* (Oxford: Clarendon Press, 1989).

BRIGGS, ROBIN, *Witches and Neighbors: The Social and Cultural Context of European Witchcraft* (New York: Viking, 1996).

BROOKS, PETER, *Thomas Cranmer's Doctrine of the Eucharist,* 2nd edn. (London: Macmillan, 1992).

BURNS, WILLIAM E., 'The King's Two Monstrous Bodies: John Bulwer and the English Revolution', in Peter G. Platt (ed.), *Wonders, Marvels, and Monsters in Early Modern Culture* (Newark, Del.: University of Delaware Press, 1999), 187–202.

BUTLER, JUDITH, *Gender Trouble: Feminism and the Subversion of Identity* (London: Routledge, 1990).

BYNUM, CAROLYN WALKER, *Holy Feast and Holy Fast* (Berkeley: University of California Press, 1987).

—— *Jesus as Mother: Studies in the Spirituality of the High Middle Ages* (Berkeley: University of California Press, 1992).

CADDEN, JOAN, *The Meanings of Sex Difference in the Middle Ages: Medicine, Science, and Culture* (Cambridge: Cambridge University Press, 1993).

CAPP, BERNARD S., *Astrology and the Popular Press: English Almanacs 1500–1800* (London: Faber, 1979).

—— *The Fifth Monarchy Men: A Study in Seventeenth-Century English Millenarianism* (London: Faber and Faber, 1972).

CARLTON, CHARLES, *Going to the Wars: The Experience of the British Civil Wars, 1638–1651* (London: Routledge, 1992).

CHARTIER, ROGER, 'Culture as Appropriation: Popular Cultural Uses in Early Modern France', in Steven L. Kaplan (ed.), *Understanding Popular Culture: Europe from the Middle Ages to the Nineteenth Century* (Berlin: Mouton Publishers, 1984), 175–91.

CLARK, STUART, *Thinking with Demons: The Idea of Witchcraft in Early Modern Europe* (Oxford: Clarendon Press, 1997).

CLEMENT, C. J., *Religious Radicalism in England, 1535–1565* (Carlisle: Published for Rutherford House by Paternoster Press, 1997).

CLIFTON, ROBIN, 'The Fear of Popery', in Conrad Russell (ed.), *The Origins of the English Civil War* (New York: Barnes and Noble, 1973), 144–67.

—— *The Last Popular Rebellion: The Western Rising of 1685* (New York: St. Martin's Press, 1984).

CODY, LISA, ' "The Doctor's In Labour; or a New Whim Wham from Guilford" ', *Gender and History*, 4 (1992), 175–96.

COLLINSON, PATRICK, 'Night Schools, Conventicles and Churches: Continuities and Discontinuities in Early Protestant Ecclesiology', in Peter Marshall and Alec Ryrie (eds.), *The Beginnings of English Protestantism* (Cambridge: Cambridge University Press, 2002), 209–35.

COOK, HAROLD J., *The Decline of the Old Medical Regime in Stuart London* (Ithaca: Cornell University Press, 1986).

COSTER, WILL, 'Purity, Profanity, and Puritanism: The Churching of Women, 1500–1700', in W. J. Sheils and Diana Wood (eds.), *Women in the Church. Studies in Church History*, 27 (1990), 377–87.

COWAN, BRIAN, 'What Was Masculine about the Public Sphere? Gender and the Coffeehouse Milieu in Post-Restoration England', *History Workshop Journal*, 51 (2001), 127–57.

CRAWFORD, PATRICIA, 'Attitudes to Menstruation in Seventeenth-Century England', *Past & Present*, 91 (1981), 47–73.

—— 'The Challenges to Patriarchalism: How Did the Revolution Affect Women?', in John Morrill (ed.), *Revolution and Restoration: England in the 1650s* (London: Collins and Brown, 1992), 112–28.

—— 'Sexual Knowledge in England, 1500–1750', in Roy Porter and Mikulas Teich (eds.), *Sexual Knowledge, Sexual Science: The History of Attitudes to Sexuality* (Cambridge: Cambridge University Press, 1994), 82–106.

—— *Women and Religion in England, 1500–1720* (London: Routledge, 1993).

—— 'Women's Dreams in Early Modern England', *History Workshop Journal*, 49 (2000), 129–41.

—— and GOWING, LAURA (eds.), *Women's Worlds in Seventeenth-Century England* (London: Routledge, 2000).

CRESSY, DAVID, *Birth, Marriage and Death. Ritual, Religion, and the Life-Cycle in Tudor and Stuart England* (Oxford: Oxford University Press, 1997).

—— *Bonfires and Bells: National Memory and the Protestant Calendar in Elizabethan and Stuart England* (London: Weidenfeld and Nicolson, 1989).

—— 'Conflict, Consensus, and the Willingness to Wink: The Erosion of Community in Charles I's England', *Huntington Library Quarterly*, 61 (1998), 131–49.

—— *Literacy and the Social Order: Reading and Writing in Tudor and Stuart England* (Cambridge: Cambridge University Press, 1980).

—— 'The Protestation Protested, 1641 and 1642', *Historical Journal*, 45 (2002), 251–79.

—— 'Purifications, Thanksgiving and the Churching of Women in Post-Reformation England', *Past & Present*, 141 (1993), 106–46.

—— *Travesties and Transgressions in Tudor and Stuart England* (Oxford: Oxford University Press, 2000).

CROWTHER-HEYCK, KATHLEEN M., ' "Be Fruitful and Multiply": Genesis and Generation in Reformation Germany', *Renaissance Quarterly*, 55 (2002), 904–35.

CUST, RICHARD, 'News and Politics in Early-Seventeenth Century England', *Past & Present*, 112 (1986), 60–90.

DASTON, LORRAINE, and PARK, KATHARINE, *Wonders and the Order of Nature, 1150–1750* (New York: Zone Books, 1998).

DAVIS, J. C., *Fear, Myth and History. The Ranters and the Historians* (Cambridge: Cambridge University Press, 1986).

DAVIS, JOHN, 'Joan of Kent, Lollardy and the English Reformation', *Journal of Ecclesiastical History*, 33 (1982), 225–33.

DEWINDT, ANNE REIBER, 'Witchcraft and Conflicting Visions of the Ideal Village Community', *Journal of British Studies*, 34 (1995), 427–63.

DICKENS, A. G., *Lollards and Protestants in the Diocese of York, 1509–1558* (Oxford: Oxford University Press, 1959).

DOLAN, FRANCES E., *Dangerous Familiars: Representations of Domestic Crime in England, 1550–1700* (Ithaca: Cornell University Press, 1994).

—— *Whores of Babylon: Catholicism, Gender, and Seventeenth-Century Print Culture* (Ithaca: Cornell University Press, 1999).

DUFFY, EAMON, 'Holy Maydens, Holy Wyfes: The Cult of Women Saints in Fifteenth- and Sixteenth-Century England', in W. J. Sheils and Diana Wood (eds.), *Women in the Church: Studies in Church History*, 27 (1990), 175–96.

—— *The Stripping of the Altars: Traditional Religion in England 1400–1580* (New Haven: Yale University Press, 1992).

DUNN, M., 'Jacob Rueff (1550–1558) of Zurich and *The Expert Midwife*', *Archives of Disease in Childhood*, 85 (2001), 222–24.

DURSTON, CHRISTOPHER, *The Family in the English Revolution* (Oxford: Basil Blackwell, 1989).

EAMON, WILLIAM, *Science and the Secrets of Nature: Books of Secrets in Medieval and Early Modern Culture* (Princeton: Princeton University Press, 1994).

EARLE, PETER, 'The Female Labour Market in London in the Late Seventeenth and Early Eighteenth Centuries', *Economic History Review*, 2nd ser., 42 (1989), 328–53.

ELIAS, NORBERT, *The Civilizing Process*, trans. Edmund Jephcott (New York: Pantheon Books, 1982).

ERICKSON, AMY LOUISE, *Women and Property in Early Modern England* (London: Routledge, 1993).

EVENDEN, DOREEN, *The Midwives of Seventeenth-Century London* (Cambridge: Cambridge University Press, 1999).

EZELL, MARGARET, *The Patriarch's Wife: Literary Evidence and the History of the Family* (Chapel Hill, NC: University of North Carolina Press, 1987).

FISSELL, MARY E., 'Hairy Women and Naked Truths: Gender and the Politics of Knowledge in *Aristotle's Masterpiece*', *William and Mary Quarterly*, 60 (2003), 43–74.

—— and COOTER ROGER, 'Exploring Natural Knowledge: Science and the Popular in the Eighteenth Century', in *Cambridge History of Science*, iv: *Science in the Eighteenth Century*, ed. Roy Porter (Cambridge: Cambridge University Press, 2003), 145–79.

FLETCHER, ANTHONY, *Gender, Sex and Subordination in England, 1500–1800* (New Haven: Yale University Press, 1995).

—— *The Outbreak of the English Civil War* (New York: New York University Press, 1981).

FORD, W. C., 'Benjamin Harris, Printer and Bookseller', *Proceedings of the Massachusetts Historical Society*, 57 (1923–4), 34–68.

FOUCAULT, MICHEL, *Discipline and Punish: The Birth of the Prison*, trans. Alan Sheridan (New York: Pantheon Books, 1977).

FOX, ADAM, *Oral and Literate Culture in England, 1500–1700* (Oxford: Clarendon Press, 2000).

FOYSTER, ELIZABETH, *Manhood in Early Modern England: Honour, Sex and Marriage* (London: Longman, 1999).

FREIST, DAGMAR, *Governed by Opinion: Politics, Religion, and the Dynamics of Communication in Stuart London, 1637–1645* (London: Tauris Academic Studies, 1997).

FRIEDMAN, JEROME, *The Battle of the Frogs and Fairford's Flies* (New York: St. Martin's Press, 1993).

FURTH, CHARLOTTE, *A Flourishing Yin: Gender in China's Medical History, 960–1665* (Berkeley: University of California Press, 1999).

GENTLES, IAN, 'London Levellers in the English Revolution: The Chidleys and their Circle', *Journal of Ecclesiastical History*, 29 (1978), 281–309.

GIBSON, GAIL MCMURRY, 'Scene and Obscene: Seeing and Performing Late Medieval Childbirth', *Journal of Medieval and Early Modern Studies*, 29 (1999), 7–24.

—— *The Theater of Devotion: East Anglian Drama and Society in the Late Middle Ages* (Chicago: University of Chicago Press, 1989).

GIBSON, MARION, *Reading Witchcraft: Stories of Early English Witches* (London: Routledge, 1999).

GOWING, LAURA, *Common Bodies: Women, Touch and Power in Seventeenth-Century England* (New Haven: Yale University Press, 2003).

—— *Domestic Dangers: Women, Words, and Sex in Early Modern London* (Oxford: Clarendon Press, 1996).

—— 'Secret Births and Infanticide in Seventeenth-Century England', *Past & Present*, 156 (1997), 87–115.

GREEN, MONICA, 'From "Diseases of Women" to "Secrets of Women": The Gynecological Literature in the Later Middle Ages', *Journal of Medieval and Early Modern Studies*, 30 (2000), 5–39.

—— 'Obstetrical and Gynecological Texts in Middle English', *Studies in the Age of Chaucer*, 14 (1992), 53–88.

GREGORY, ANNABEL, 'Witchcraft, Politics and Good Neighborhood in Early Seventeenth Century Rye', *Past & Present*, 133 (1991), 31–66.

GRIFFITHS, PAUL, *Youth and Authority: Formative Experiences in England 1560–1640* (Oxford: Clarendon Press, 1996).

HACKETT, HELEN, *Virgin Mother, Maiden Queen: Elizabeth I and the Cult of the Virgin Mary* (Basingstoke: Macmillan, 1995).

HAIGH, CHRISTOPHER, *Reformation and Resistance in Tudor Lancashire* (Cambridge: Cambridge University Press, 1975).

HARRIS, TIM, *London Crowds in the Reign of Charles II: Propaganda and Politics from the Restoration until the Exclusion Crisis* (Cambridge: Cambridge University Press, 1987).

—— *Politics under the Later Stuarts: Party Conflict in a Divided Society, 1660–1715* (London: Longman, 1993).

—— 'What's New about the Restoration?', *Albion*, 29 (1997), 187–222.

—— SEAWARD, PAUL, and GOLDIE, MARK (eds.), *The Politics of Religion in Restoration England* (Oxford: Basil Blackwell, 1990).

HERRUP, CYNTHIA, *A House in Gross Disorder: Sex, Law, and the Second Earl of Castlehaven* (Oxford: Oxford University Press, 1999).

HILL, CHRISTOPHER, *The World Turned Upside Down: Radical Ideas during the English Revolution* (London: Maurice Temple Smith, 1972).

HINDLE, STEVE, 'The Growth of Social Stability in Restoration England', *European Legacy*, 5 (2000), 563–76.

HINDS, HILARY, *God's Englishwomen: Seventeenth-Century Radical Sectarian Writing and Feminist Criticism* (Manchester: Manchester University Press, 1996).

HOBBY, ELAINE, 'Discourses So Unsavoury: Women's Published Writings of the 1650s', in Isobel Grundy and Susan Wiseman (eds.), *Women, Writing, History 1640–1740* (Athens, Ga.: University of Georgia Press, 1992), 16–32.

HOFFER, PETER C., and HULL, N. E. H., *Murdering Mothers: Infanticide in England and New England, 1558–1803* (New York: New York University Press, 1981).

HOLMES, CLIVE, 'Women: Witnesses and Witches', *Past & Present*, 140 (1993), 45–78.

HOUSTON, ALAN, and PINCUS, STEVE (eds.), *A Nation Transformed: England after the Restoration* (Cambridge: Cambridge University Press, 2001).

HUDSON, ANNE, *The Premature Reformation: Wycliffite Texts and Lollard History* (Oxford: Clarendon Press), 1988.

HUET, MARIE-HÉLÈNE, *The Monstrous Imagination* (Cambridge, Mass.: Harvard University Press, 1993).

HUGHES, ANN, 'Gender and Politics in Leveller Literature', in Susan D. Amussen and Mark A. Kishlansky (eds.), *Political Culture and Cultural Politics in Early Modern England: Essays Presented to David Underdown* (Manchester: Manchester University Press, 1995), 162–88.

—— 'Women, Men and Politics in the English Civil War', Inaugural Lecture, 8 Oct. 1997 (Keele: University of Keele, 1997).

HULL, SUZANNE, *Chaste, Silent and Obedient: English Books for Women 1475–1640* (San Marino, Calif.: Huntington Library, 1982).

HUNT, E. W., *The Life and Times of John Hooper (c. 1500–1555), Bishop of Gloucester* (Lewiston, NY: Edward Mellen Press, 1992).

HUNT, WILLIAM, *The Puritan Moment* (Cambridge, Mass.: Harvard University Press, 1983).

HUTTON, RONALD, 'The English Reformation and the Evidence of Folklore', *Past & Present*, 148 (1995), 89–116.

—— *The Rise and Fall of Merry England: The Ritual Year 1400–1700* (Oxford: Oxford University Press, 1994).

INGRAM, MARTIN, *Church Courts, Sex, and Marriage in England, 1570–1640* (Cambridge: Cambridge University Press, 1987).

—— 'Puritans and the Church Courts, 1560–1640', in Jacqueline Eales and Christopher Durston (eds.), *The Culture of English Puritanism, 1560–1700* (New York: St. Martin's Press, 1996).

—— '"Scolding Women Cucked or Washed": A Crisis in Gender Relations in Early Modern England?', in Jennifer Kermode and Garthine Walker (eds.), *Women, Crime, and the Courts in Early Modern England* (Chapel Hill, NC: University of North Carolina Press, 1994), 48–80.

JACKSON, MARK (ed.), *Infanticide: Historical Perspectives on Child Murder and Concealment, 1550–2000* (Burlington, Vt.: Ashgate, 2002).

JOHNSON, ODAI, 'Pope-Burning Pageants: Performing the Exclusion Crisis', *Theatre Survey*, 37 (1996), 34–57.

KAPLAN, BARBARA BEIGUN, 'Greatrakes the Stroker: The Interpretation of his Contemporaries', *Isis*, 73 (1982), 178–85.

KEY, NEWTON E., and WARD, JOSEPH P., '"Divided into Parties": Exclusion Crisis Origins in Monmouth', *English Historical Review*, 115 (2000), 1159–83.

KING, HELEN, 'Once Upon a Text: The Hippocratic Origins of Hysteria', in Sander L. Gilman, Helen King, Roy Porter, G. S. Rousseau, and Elaine Showalter (eds.), *Hysteria beyond Freud* (Berkeley: University of California Press, 1993), 3–90.

—— 'The Power of Paternity: The Father of Medicine Meets the Prince of Physicians', in David Cantor (ed.), *Reinventing Hippocrates* (Aldershot: Ashgate, 2002), 21–36.

KLAPISCH-ZUBER, CHRISTIANE, 'Holy Dolls: Play and Piety in Florence in the Quattrocento', in her *Women, Family, and Ritual in Renaissance Italy*, trans. Lydia Cochrane (Chicago: University of Chicago Press, 1985), 310–29.

KLEIN, LAWRENCE E., 'Coffeehouse Civility, 1660–1714: An Aspect of Post-courtly Culture in England', *Huntington Library Quarterly*, 59 (1997), 30–51.

KNIGHT, MARK, *Politics and Opinion in Crisis, 1678–81* (Cambridge: Cambridge University Press, 1994).

KUNZLE, DAVID, *The Early Comic Strip: Narrative Strips and Picture Stories in the European Broadsheet from c.1450 to 1825* (Berkeley: University of California Press, 1973).

LAKE, PETER, 'Anti-Popery: The Structure of a Prejudice', in Richard Cust and Ann Hughes (eds.), *Conflict in Early Stuart England: Studies in Religion and Politics, 1603–1642* (London: Longmans, 1989).

—— 'Deeds against Nature: Cheap Print, Protestantism, and Murder in Early Modern England', in Peter Lake and Kevin Sharpe (eds.), *Culture and Politics in Early Modern England* (Stanford: Stanford University Press, 1994), 257–83.

—— 'Popular Form, Puritan Content? Two Puritan Appropriations of the Murder Pamphlet from Mid-Seventeenth-Century London', in Anthony Fletcher and Peter Roberts (eds.), *Religion, Culture and Society in Early Modern Britain: Essays in Honour of Patrick Collinson* (Cambridge: Cambridge University Press, 1994), 313–34.

—— with Michael Questier, *The Antichrist's Lewd Hat* (New Haven: Yale University Press, 2002).

LAQUEUR, THOMAS, *Making Sex: Body and Gender from the Greeks to Freud* (Cambridge, Mass.: Harvard University Press, 1990).

LAWRENCE, SUSAN, and BENDIXEN, KAI, 'His and Hers: Male and Female Anatomy in Anatomy Texts for U.S. Medical Students, 1890–1989', *Social Science and Medicine*, 35 (1992), 925–34.

LINDLEY, KEITH, *Popular Politics and Religion in Civil War London* (Aldershot: Scolar Press, 1997).

—— 'Riot Prevention and Control in Early Stuart London', *Transactions of the Royal Historical Society*, 5th ser., 33 (1983), 109–26.

LUDLOW, DOROTHY, '"Arise and Be Doing": English "Preaching" Women, 1640–1660' (Ph.D. diss., Indiana University, 1978).

MCARTHUR, ELLEN, 'Women Petitioners and the Long Parliament', *English Historical Review*, 24 (1909) 698–703.

MACCULLOCH, DIARMAID, *Thomas Cranmer: A Life* (New Haven: Yale University Press, 1996).

—— *Tudor Church Militant: Edward VI and the Protestant Reformation* (London: Allen Lane, 1999).

MACDONALD, MICHAEL, *Witchcraft and Hysteria in Elizabethan London: Edward Jorden and the Mary Glover Case* (London: Tavistock/Routledge, 1991).

MCGREGOR, J. F., 'The Baptists: Fount of All Heresy', in J. F. McGregor and Barry Reay (eds.), *Radical Religion in the English Revolution* (Oxford: Oxford University Press, 1984), 23–63.

MACK, PHYLLIS, 'The History of Women in Early Modern Britain: A Review Article', *Comparative Studies in Society and History*, 28 (1986), 715–22.

—— *Visionary Women: Ecstatic Prophecy in Seventeenth-Century England* (Berkeley: University of California Press, 1992).

McLaren, Angus, *Reproductive Rituals: The Perception of Fertility in England from the Sixteenth to the Nineteenth Century* (London: Methuen, 1984).

McLaren, Dorothy, 'Fertility, Infant Mortality, and Breast Feeding in the Seventeenth Century', *Medical History*, 22 (1978), 378–96.

—— 'Nature's Contraceptive: Wet-nursing and Prolonged Lactation, the Case of Chesham, Buckinghamshire, 1578–1601', *Medical History*, 23 (1979), 426–41.

McSheffrey, Shannon, *Gender and Heresy: Women and Men in Lollard Communities, 1420–1530* (Philadelphia: University of Pennsylvania Press, 1996).

Manning, Brian, *The English People and the English Revolution* (London: Heinemann, 1976).

Marland, Hilary (ed.), *The Art of Midwifery: Early Modern Midwives in Europe* (London: Routledge, 1993).

Marsh, Christopher W., *The Family of Love in English Society, 1550–1630* (Cambridge: Cambridge University Press, 1994).

Martenson, Robert, 'The Transformation of Eve', in Roy Porter and Mikulas Teich (eds.), *Sexual Knowledge, Sexual Science: The History of Attitudes to Sexuality* (Cambridge: Cambridge University Press, 1994), 107–33.

Martin, Emily, *The Woman in the Body* (Boston: Beacon Press, 1987).

Mazzio, Carla, 'The Sins of the Tongue', in David Hillman and Carla Mazzio (eds.), *The Body in Parts* (London: Routledge, 1997), 53–81.

Mendelson, Sara, and Crawford, Patricia, *Women in Early Modern England* (Oxford: Oxford University Press, 1998).

Mills, David, *Recycling the Cycle: The City of Chester and its Whitsun Plays* (Toronto: University of Toronto Press, 1998).

Morrill, John, 'The Impact of Puritanism', in his *The Impact of the English Civil War* (London: Collins and Brown, 1991), 50–66.

—— *The Revolt of the Provinces* (London: Unwin and Allen, 1976).

Morton, A. L., *The World of the Ranters: Religious Radicalism in the English Revolution* (London: Lawrence and Wishart, 1970).

Musacchio, Jacqueline Marie, *The Art and Ritual of Childbirth in Renaissance Italy* (New Haven: Yale University Press, 1999).

Neff, Amy, 'The Pain of *Compassio*: Mary's Labor at the Foot of the Cross', *Art Bulletin*, 80 (1998), 254–73.

Nenner, Howard, *The Right to be King* (London: Macmillan, 1995).

Newman, Karen, *Fetal Positions: Individualism, Science, Visuality* (Stanford: Stanford University Press, 1996).

Orlin, Lena Cowen, *Private Matters and Public Culture in Post-Reformation England* (Ithaca: Cornell University Press, 1994).

Ott, Sandra, 'Aristotle among the Basques: "The Cheese Analogy" of Conception', *Man*, n.s.14 (1979), 699–711.

Park, Katharine, 'The Life of the Corpse: Division and Dissection in Late Medieval Europe', *Journal of the History of Medicine and Allied Sciences*, 50 (1995), 111–32.

—— and DASTON, LORRAINE, 'Unnatural Conceptions: The Study of Monsters in Sixteenth- and Seventeenth-Century France and England', *Past & Present*, 92 (1981), 20–54.

PARKER, SIR WILLIAM, *The History of Long Melford* (London: Wyman & Sons, 1873).

PASTER, GAIL KERN, *The Body Embarrassed: Drama and the Disciplines of Shame in Early Modern England* (Ithaca: Cornell University Press, 1993).

PATEMAN, CAROLE, *The Sexual Contract* (Stanford: Stanford University Press, 1988).

PELLING, MARGARET, *Medical Conflicts in Early Modern London* (Oxford: Clarendon Press, 2003).

PINCUS, STEVE, ' "Coffee Politicians Does Create": Coffeehouses and Restoration Political Culture', *Journal of Modern History*, 67 (1995), 807–34.

POLLOCK, LINDA, *With Faith and Physic: The Life of a Tudor Gentlewoman, Lady Grace Mildmay, 1552–1620* (London: Collins & Brown, 1993).

POTTER, LOIS, 'The *Mistress Parliament* Dialogues', ed., with an introduction, *Analytical and Enumerative Bibliography*, 1 (1987), 101–70.

POYNTER, F. N. L., 'Nicholas Culpeper and his Books', *Journal of the History of Medicine and Allied Sciences*, 17 (1962), 152–67.

—— 'Nicholas Culpeper and the Paracelsians', in Allen Debus (ed.), *Science, Medicine and Society in the Renaissance: Essays to Honor Walter Pagel* (New York: Science History Publications, 1972), 201–20.

PURKISS, DIANE, 'Producing the Voice, Consuming the Body: Women Prophets of the Seventeenth Century', in Isobel Grundy and Susan Wiseman (eds.), *Women, Writing, History 1640–1740* (Athens, Ga.: University of Georgia Press, 1992), 139–58.

—— *The Witch in History* (London: Routledge, 1996).

—— 'Women's Stories of Witchcraft in Early Modern England: The House, the Body, the Child', *Gender and History*, 7 (1995), 408–32.

RAYMOND, JOAD (ed.), *News, Newspapers, and Society in Early Modern Britain* (London: F. Cass, 1999).

RIDDLE, JOHN M., *Contraception and Abortion from the Ancient World to the Renaissance* (Cambridge, Mass.: Harvard University Press, 1992).

—— *Eve's Herbs: A History of Contraception and Abortion in the West* (Cambridge, Mass.: Harvard University Press, 1997).

ROLLINS, HYDER EDWARD, 'The Black-Letter Broadside Ballad', *PMLA* 34 (1919), 258–339.

ROPER, LYNDAL, *The Holy Household: Women and Morals in Reformation Augsburg* (Oxford: Clarendon Press, 1989).

—— *Oedipus and the Devil* (London: Routledge, 1994).

ROSE, MARY BETH, 'Where Are the Mothers in Shakespeare? Options for Gender Representation in the English Renaissance', *Shakespeare Quarterly*, 42 (1991), 291–314.

SCARISBROOK, J. J., *The Reformation and the English People* (Oxford: Blackwell, 1984).

SCHOCHET, GORDON J., *Patriarchalism in Political Thought: The Authoritarian Family and Political Speculation and Attitudes especially in Seventeenth-Century England* (New York: Basic Books, 1975).

SCHWOERER, LOIS, 'Propaganda in the Revolution of 1688–89', *American Historical Review*, 82 (1977), 843–74.

SCOTT, JONATHAN, *Algernon Sidney and the Restoration Crisis, 1677–1683* (Cambridge: Cambridge University Press, 1991).

—— 'Restoration Process, Or, If this Isn't a Party, We're Not Having a Good Time', *Albion*, 25 (1993), 619–37.

SCRIBNER, ROBERT, 'The Impact of the Reformation on Daily Life', in *Mensch und Objekt im Mittelalter und in der frühen Neuzeit: Leben, Alltag, Kultur* (Vienna: Verlag der Österreichischen Akademie der Wissenschaften, 1990), 315–43.

SEAVER, PAUL, *Wallington's World: A Puritan Artisan in Seventeenth-Century London* (Stanford: Stanford University Press, 1985).

SERPELL, JAMES, 'Guardian Spirits or Demonic Pets: The Concept of the Witch's Familiar in Early Modern England, 1530–1712', in Angela Creager and William Chester Jordan (eds.), *The Animal/Human Boundary: Historical Perspectives* (Rochester: University of Rochester Press, 2002), 157–90.

SHAPIN, STEVEN, and SCHAFFER, SIMON, *Leviathan and the Air-Pump* (Princeton: Princeton University Press, 1985).

SHARPE, JAMES, *Instruments of Darkness: Witchcraft in Early Modern England* (Philadelphia: University of Pennsylvania Press, 1997).

—— 'Witchcraft and Women in Seventeenth-Century England: Some Northern Evidence', *Continuity and Change*, 6 (1991), 179–99.

SMITH, NIGEL, *Literature and Revolution* (New Haven: Yale University Press, 1994).

—— *Perfection Proclaimed: Language and Literature in English Radical Religion 1640–1660* (Oxford: Oxford University Press, 1989).

SPECK, WILLIAM A., 'The Orangist Conspiracy Against James II', *Historical Journal*, 30 (1987), 453–62.

SPUFFORD, MARGARET, 'First Steps in Literacy: The Reading and Writing Experiences of the Humblest Seventeenth-Century Spiritual Autobiographers', *Social History*, 4 (1979), 407–35.

—— *Small Books and Pleasant Histories: Popular Fiction and its Readership in Seventeenth-Century England* (Cambridge: Cambridge University Press, 1981).

STAVREVA, KIRILA, 'Fighting Words: Witch-Speak in Late Elizabethan Docu-Fiction', *Journal of Medieval and Early Modern Studies*, 30 (2000), 309–38.

STENECK, NICHOLAS, 'Greatrakes the Stroker: The Interpretation of Historians', *Isis*, 73 (1982), 161–77.

STEPHENS, FREDERIC GEORGE, *Catalogue of Political and Personal Satires Preserved in the Department of Prints and Drawings in the British Museum* (London: British Museum Publications Ltd., 1954).

STINE, JENNIFER K., 'Opening Closets: The Discovery of Household Medicine in Early Modern England' (Ph.D. diss., Stanford University, 1996).

STOERTZ, FIONA HARRIS, 'Suffering and Survival in Medieval English Childbirth', in Catherine Jorgenson Itnyre (ed.), *Medieval Family Roles: A Book of Essays* (New York: Garland, 1996), 101–20.

Symonds, Deborah, *Weep not for Me: Women, Ballads, and Infanticide in Early Modern Scotland* (University Park, Pa.: Penn State Press, 1997).

Thomas, Keith, 'The Puritans and the Adultery Act of 1650 Reconsidered', in Donald Penington and Keith Thomas (eds.), *Puritans and Revolutionaries: Essays in Seventeenth-Century History Presented to Christopher Hill* (Oxford: Clarendon Press, 1978), 257–82.

—— *Religion and the Decline of Magic* (New York: Charles Scribner's Sons, 1971).

Thompson, Roger S., 'The Development of the Broadside Ballad Trade and its Influences upon the Transmission of English Folksongs' (D.Phil. thesis, Cambridge University, 1974).

Tilley, Morris, *A Dictionary of the Proverbs in England in the Sixteenth and Seventeenth Centuries* (Ann Arbor: University of Michigan Press, 1950).

Tyacke, Nicholas (ed.), *England's Long Reformation 1500–1800* (London: University College Press, 1998).

Underdown, David, *A Freeborn People: Politics and the Nation in Seventeenth-Century England* (Oxford: Clarendon Press, 1996).

—— *Revel, Riot and Rebellion: Popular Politics and Culture in England, 1603–1660* (Oxford: Clarendon Press, 1985).

—— 'The Taming of the Scold: The Enforcement of Patriarchal Authority in Early Modern England', in Anthony Fletcher and John Stevenson (eds.), *Order and Disorder in Early Modern England* (Cambridge: Cambridge University Press, 1985), 116–36.

Valenze, Deborah, ' "The Art of Women, the Business of Men": Women's Work and the Dairy Industry c. 1740–1840', *Past & Present*, 130 (1991), 142–69.

Veith, Ilza, *Hysteria: The History of a Disease* (Chicago: University of Chicago Press, 1965).

Walsham, Alexandra, ' "Domme Preachers"? Post-Reformation English Catholicism and the Culture of Print', *Past & Present*, 168 (2000), 72–123.

—— ' "The Fatall Vesper": Providentialism and Anti-Popery in Late Jacobean London', *Past & Present*, 144 (1994), 36–87.

—— *Providence in Early Modern England* (Oxford: Oxford University Press, 1999).

Walter, John, 'Grain Riots and Popular Attitudes to the Law: Maldon and the Crisis of 1629', in John Brewer and John Styles (eds.), *An Ungovernable People: The English and their Law in the Seventeenth and Eighteenth Centuries* (New Brunswick, NJ: Rutgers University Press, 1980), 47–84.

Warner, Marina, *Alone of All Her Sex: The Myth and Cult of the Virgin Mary* (New York: Vintage Books, 1976).

Watt, Tessa, *Cheap Print and Popular Piety 1550–1640* (Cambridge: Cambridge University Press, 1991).

Weber, Harold, *Paper Bullets: Print and Kingship under Charles II* (Lexington: The University Press of Kentucky, 1996).

Webster, Charles, *The Great Instauration: Science, Medicine and Reform, 1626–1660* (London: Duckworth, 1975).

WEIL, RACHEL, *Political Passions: Gender, the Family, and Political Argument in England 1680–1714* (Manchester: Manchester University Press, 1999).

WEINSTEIN, HELEN, 'Hammer and Anvil: Metaphors of Sex in the Seventeenth-Century English Ballad', paper presented at the Ninth Berkshire Conference on the History of Women, Vassar College, June 1993.

WILLIAMS, ETHYN MORGAN, 'Women Preachers in the Civil War', *Journal of Modern History*, 1 (1929), 561–9.

WILLIAMS, GEORGE HUNSTON, *The Radical Reformation* (Philadelphia: The Westminster Press, 1962).

WILLIAMS, GORDON, *A Dictionary of Sexual Language and Imagery in Shakespearian and Stuart Literature* (London: Athlone Press, 1994).

WILLIAMS, TAMSYN, ' "Magnetic Figures": Polemical Prints of the English Revolution', in Lucy Gent and Nigel Llewellyn (eds.), *Renaissance Bodies: The Human Figure in English Culture c. 1540–1660* (London: Reaktion Books, 1990), 86–110.

WILLIS, DIANE, *Malevolent Nurture: Witch-Hunting and Maternal Power in Early Modern England* (Ithaca: Cornell University Press, 1995).

WILSON, ADRIAN, 'The Ceremony of Childbirth and its Interpretation', in Valerie Fildes (ed.), *Women as Mothers in Early Modern England: Essays in Memory of Dorothy McLaren* (London: Routledge, 1990), 68–107.

—— 'Childbirth in Seventeenth- and Early Eighteenth-Century England' (D.Phil. thesis, University of Sussex, 1982).

—— *The Making of Man-Midwifery: Childbirth in England, 1660–1770* (Cambridge, Mass.: Harvard University Press, 1995).

WILTENBURG, JOY, *Disorderly Women and Female Power in the Street Literature of Early Modern England and Germany* (Charlottesville, Va.: University of Virginia Press, 1992).

WISEMAN, SUSAN, ' "Adam, the Father of All Flesh": Porno-Political Rhetoric and Political Theory in and after the English Civil War', in James Holstun (ed.), *Pamphlet Wars: Prose in the English Revolution* (London: Frank Cass, 1992), 134–57.

—— 'Tis a Pity She's a Whore: Representing the Incestuous Body', in Lucy Gent and Nigel Llewellyn (eds.), *Renaissance Bodies: The Human Figure in English Culture, c. 1540–1660* (London: Reaktion Books, 1990), 180–97.

WRIGHTSON, KEITH, 'Infanticide in Earlier Seventeenth-Century England', *Local Population Studies*, 15 (1975), 10–22.

WRIGLEY, E. A., and SCHOFIELD, ROGER, *Population History of England and Wales 1541–1871: A Reconstruction* (Cambridge: Cambridge University Press, 1981).

ZARET, DAVID, *Origins of Democratic Culture: Printing, Petitions, and the Public Sphere in Early Modern England* (Princeton: Princeton University Press, 2000).

ZOOK, MELINDA, *Radical Whigs and Conspiratorial Politics in Late Stuart England* (University Park, Pa.: Penn State University Press, 1999).

ZWICKER, STEVEN, *Lines of Authority: Politics and English Literary Culture* (Ithaca: Cornell University Press, 1993).

Index